Advanced Health Assessment of Women

CLINICAL
SKILLS
AND
PROCEDURES

Second Edition

Helen A. Carcio, MS, MEd, ANP-BC, has been involved in women's health care, both educationally and clinically, for the past 20 years. She was an associate Clinical Professor at the University of Massachusetts at Amherst in the nurse practitioner program for 10 years, where she was awarded the distinguished teaching medal. During that time she wrote a column for the *Hampshire Gazette*, in Northampton, Massachusetts, titled "Women's Health Matters." The column addressed the health care needs of women in the community and offered a forum for women to address their concerns.

She has written four books on women's health for Lippincott, Williams & Wilkins, including the first edition of *Advanced Health Assessment of Women* (1999), and has published numerous articles. She recently received the national award "Nurse Practitioner Entrepreneur of the Year" by *Advance for Nurse Practitioners.*

Ms. Carcio practices independently and is the director and founder of the Health & Continence Institute of New England and offers workshops on Launching Continence Care Programs. She has established multiple bladder health centers nationally and continues to offer consultation services to others with the same focus. In addition, Ms. Carcio is a highly sought-after lecturer on women's health, bladder health issues, and incontinence. She is a frequent guest lecturer at Nurse Practitioner Associates of Continuing Education. She has written 11 feature articles in the nationally recognized publication *Advance for Nurse Practitioners*, where she is a member of the advisory board. Ms. Carcio was also the winner of the National Association for Continence (NAFC) "Continence Care Champion Award."

Mimi Clarke Secor, MS, MEd, FNP-BC, FAANP, is a Family Nurse Practitioner specializing in women's health at Newton Wellesley Obstetrics and Gynecology, Inc., in Newton, Massachusetts, and a Visiting Scholar at Boston College Graduate School of Nursing. She is a national speaker and consultant, and President Emerita and Senior Advisor for Nurse Practitioner Associates of Continuing Education (NPACE). Ms. Secor is a founding and current board member of the American College of Clinicians. Ms. Secor's 32 years of clinical experience as an NP have included emergency care, college health, private practice, prison nursing, and rural medicine. Before working for 7 years at Bethel Family Clinic, in Bethel, Alaska, she operated an independent Boston area NP practice for 12 years. Among other credits to her name, Ms. Secor is on the editorial board of *Clinician News,* was a former syndicated radio host of "Hot Topics in Women's Health," and has delivered numerous radio and TV presentations on Women's Health. She is a founder of the Massachusetts Coalition of Nurse Practitioners (MCNP), a member and fellow of the American Academy of Nurse Practitioners, and a member of the Association of Reproductive Health Professionals (ARHP), the National Association of Nurse Practitioners in Women's Health (NPWH), and the North American Menopause Society (NAMS).

Advanced
Health Assessment
of Women

CLINICAL
SKILLS
AND
PROCEDURES

Second Edition

HELEN A. CARCIO, MS, MEd, ANP-BC

MIMI CLARKE SECOR, MS, MEd, FNP-BC, FAANP

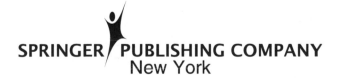

SPRINGER PUBLISHING COMPANY
New York

Special discounts on bulk quantities of our books are available to corporations, professional associations, pharmaceutical companies, health care organizations, and other qualified groups.
If you are interested in a custom book, including chapters from more than one of our titles, we can provide that service as well.

For details, please contact:
Special Sales Department, Springer Publishing Company, LLC
11 West 42nd Street, 15th Floor, New York, NY 10036-8002
Phone: 877-687-7476 or 212-431-4370; Fax: 212-941-7842
Email: sales@springerpub.com

Springer Publishing Company, LLC
11 West 42nd Street
New York, NY 10036
www.springerpub.com

Acquisitions Editor: Margaret Zuccarini
Production Editor: Pamela Lankas
Cover design: Mimi Flow
Cover art: Bernhard Springer
Composition: International Graphic Services
Ebook ISBN: 978-0-8261-2427-2

10 11 12 13/ 5 4 3 2

The author and the publisher of this Work have made every effort to use sources believed to be reliable to provide information that is accurate and compatible with the standards generally accepted at the time of publication. Because medical science is continually advancing, our knowledge base continues to expand. Therefore, as new information becomes available, changes in procedures become necessary. We recommend that the reader always consult current research and specific institutional policies before performing any clinical procedure. The author and publisher shall not be liable for any special, consequential, or exemplary damages resulting, in whole or in part, from the readers' use of, or reliance on, the information contained in this book. The publisher has no responsibility for the persistence or accuracy of URLs for external or third-party Internet Web sites referred to in this publication and does not guarantee that any content on such Web sites is, or will remain, accurate or appropriate.

Library of Congress Cataloging-in-Publication Data

Carcio, Helen Nelson.
  Advanced health assessment of women : clinical skills and procedures / Helen A. Carcio, Mimi Clarke Secor.—2nd ed.
    p. ; cm.
  Includes bibliographical references and index.
  ISBN 978-0-8261-2426-5 (alk. paper)
  1. Women—Medical examinations. I. Secor, Mimi Clarke. II. Title. [DNLM: 1. Diagnostic Techniques, Obstetrical and Gynecological. 2. Women's Health. WP 141 C265a 2010]
  RG110.C37 2010
  618'.0475—dc22
                          2009050239

Printed in the United States of America by Hamilton Printing

Contents

INVESTIGATIVE PROCEDURES

CONTRACEPTIVE DEVICES

ASSESSMENT OF WOMEN AT RISK

UNIT 6

EVALUATION OF THE MENOPAUSAL WOMAN

UNIT 7

EVALUATION OF THE PELVIC FLOOR

UNIT 8

ASSESSMENT OF THE INFERTILE WOMAN

UNIT 9

ADVANCED SKILLS

Contributors

Paula Brooks, MS, RN, CS, FNP
Long Pond Medical Center
Harwich, MA

Marcia Denine, WHNP-BC
Clinical Coordinator, Co-Director
Health Awareness Services
Marlboro, MA

Nancy Gardner Dirubbo, FNP-C, WHNP-C, FAANP
Director, Founder
Laconia Women's Health Care
Laconia, NH

Kate Green, MS, RN, CNM
Clinical Assistant Professor, Nursing
University of Massachusetts-Amherst
Amherst, MA

Yolanda R. Hill, MSN, FNP-BC
Family Nurse Practitioner
Specialist Occupational Health
Medicine and Occupational Health–
ExxonMobil Corporation
Baton Rouge, LA

Karen Kalmakis, NP, APRN-BC
Assistant Professor
School of Nursing
University of Massachusetts
Amherst, MA

Cathy R. Kessenich, DSN, ARNP
Professor of Nursing
University of Tampa
Tampa, FL

Rebecca Koeniger-Donohue, PhD, APRN-BC, WHNP-BC
Associate Professor, Nursing
Simmons College, School of Health Sciences
Boston, MA

Deborah Lipkin, MS, FNP-BC
Nurse Practitioner
Harvard Vanguard Medical Associates
Burlington, MA

Preface

The majority of individuals who seek health care are women. As the baby boomers begin to age, even more and more women will seek professional care. With health care reform, renewed emphasis is being placed on the knowledgeable assessment of women to provide preventative care. In today's rapidly changing health care climate, advanced practice clinicians are being viewed as a group of providers who are well qualified to care for health issues related to women. Additionally, the scope of their practice is broadening to include more advanced clinical skills and procedures. *Advanced Health Assessment of Women: Clinical Skills and Procedures, Second Edition*, brings together clear and concise factual information related to the health assessment of women.

This text provides an enhanced definition to the role and clinical skills of providers, including physician's assistants (PAs), nurse midwives (CNMs), and nurse practitioners (NPs). These practitioners will play a vital role in managing the health of women in a variety of settings, including internal medicine, family practice, and specialty areas such as women's health care or infertility centers.

Some of the procedures described in this manual are quite advanced and are appropriate only within certain practice settings. It must be remembered that advanced practice clinicians are under a heavy mandate to practice within the scope of legal and professional mandates, as well as a personal comfort level, when considering performing advanced techniques and procedures. Consult your state licensing board if in doubt about the legality of performing any of the procedures described. The scope of practices varies among NPs, PAs, and CNMs, in relation to educational programs, practice settings, and geographical location, and state laws and regulations. The text provides guidance so that each practitioner may become increasingly aware of when to practice independently, when to comanage, when to consult, and when to refer.

Many of the assessment skills, techniques, and procedures described are fast becoming routine to the advanced practice clinician.

Practitioners are educated in a variety of different ways, with differing approaches within today's conventional medical model. College curricula provide basic content for the beginning practitioner, but most curricula offer little in relation to advanced assessment and practice. This text is designed to fill that gap.

This second edition of *Advanced Health Assessment of Women: Clinical Skills and Procedures* offers an integrated and unique approach to the health care of women. It goes beyond content commonly found in texts related only to health assessment. It provides an excellent resource to link theory to clinical practice, using critical thinking skills. This manual is practical and user-friendly. It provides detailed descriptions, enhanced by tables and figures, to clearly describe these advanced skills. The assessment of many aspects of care related to women is outlined, with sample assessment forms integrated throughout.

An outline format was chosen because this clear and concise format allows the information to flow in a logical sequence without one having to wade through unnecessary jargon. Where techniques are explained, a comprehensive list of equipment necessary for each technique or procedure is given as well as information on patient preparation and recommended follow-up. The entire text is enhanced with a plethora of boxes, figures, and tables. The casual format offers easy access to pertinent information.

The different techniques and procedures were selected because they are within the expanding scope of the practitioner's experience but are often not described in assessment books. This manual delineates strategies that are on the leading edge in the expanded role of the advanced practice clinician. Obviously, one cannot expect to learn the technical aspects from simply reading about them. This manual provides a foundation for and an understanding of the rationale behind the assessments and procedures described. It is a good idea to observe a new procedure first and then to be supervised for as many times as it takes to feel comfortable. Always carefully read manufacturers' recommendations that accompany any instrumentation you might use, in addition to the information found in this text. This manual is not meant to dictate how procedures should be performed or to supply a strict recipe for techniques and procedures. It does, however, provide a clear starting point for developing guidelines specific to each individual's clinical style and practice setting.

The text begins with a comprehensive review of the basic anatomy and physiology of women. A complete understanding of the complexities of the menstrual cycle and normal vaginal flora, as examined at the cellular level, is imperative for accurate understanding and diagnoses of conditions that affect women.

The health history chapter discusses elements of a comprehensive, developmentally relevant, health history, with a unique approach to the physiologic, psychological, and sociocultural components involved. Advanced health history techniques are detailed in which interaction is viewed as an equal partnership between provider and patient. Critical issues related to the assessment of HIV infection are summarized. The basic techniques of the physical examination—with a focus on the gynecologic exam—are outlined, with possible clinical alterations listed for each area assessed. Evaluation of the breast includes basic techniques with a current section on how to examine the augmented breast (an explanation not commonly found in traditional health assessment books).

Two new chapters have been added to Unit 2 that are relevant and timely. The first is assessment of vulvar pain, which addresses the diagnoses of vulvodynia and vestibulitis. Obesity is becoming a national epidemic. This new chapter explores the assessment of obesity and Body Mass Index (BMI).

Information provided in the vaginal microscopy chapter is the most comprehensive description of the interpretation and evaluation of the wet mount available in any current text. In the Papanicolau smear chapter, recommendations for interpretation and follow-up of an abnormal Pap smear are outlined. Current information on the Thin-Prep is included. New guidelines are included.

The chapter on urinalysis offers a fresh look at an old test. Differential diagnosis of gynecologic versus urologic conditions is always challenging in women. This chapter contains an in-depth analysis of the components of urinalysis, and a step-by-step explanation of urine microscopy—a skill every advanced practice clinician should feel comfortable with. Concerns of older women are addressed in the comprehensive new sections on menopause and urinary incontinence.

Two newly emerging techniques that are becoming an integral part of assessment of women are sonohysteroscopy and bone densitometry. The various machines are described and interpretation of results is clearly explained.

Up-to-date information on emerging topics such as *BRCA* gene testing is provided. Content on *BRCA* gene testing will help to identify those women at risk and to provide the clinician with skills necessary to help a woman choose whether or not to be tested.

The infertility section presents guidelines for the assessment, evaluation, and management of the woman who is unable to conceive.

Controversies and clinical dilemmas are explained. Techniques of semen analysis, sperm washing, and artificial insemination are clearly delineated.

Another unique section of this text is the chapter on pessary insertion. Such descriptive information is not found in any comparable text. As baby boomers age, the incidence of genital prolapse, often accompanied by incontinence, is increasing. Today pessaries offer a viable alternative to urologic surgery. The fitting of pessaries requires patience, knowledge, and experience. Advanced level clinicians are in a key position to assume care of this rapidly expanding population of women.

This text contains critical information regarding the woman at risk. A nationally tested questionnaire is included to help identify the victim of violence and abuse. Management and follow-up of the rape victim is included.

Technical skills related to insertion of various contraceptive devices are outlined. Characteristics such as the advantages and disadvantages, mechanisms of action, and contraindications of each device are necessary to educate the woman in making an informed decision regarding her contraceptive management. The technique of fitting and follow-up care is outlined in detail. New information on the technique of insertion and removal of Implanon and use of the FemCap is clearly described, with figures for clarification. The Intrauterine Contraception chapter has been expanded to include the Mirena.

In the final section, the more advanced techniques are explained. Performing endometrial biopsy surgery requires skill and practice. It is also important to understand the indications for biopsy study, the implications, and interpretation of the results. The chapter describes the necessary equipment and walks the practitioner through each step. Mastering the technique of acrochordonectomy, or the removal of skin tags, will please many patients bothered by unsightly skin tags. New information on how to perform a cystometrogram is important in diagnosing the cause of urinary incontinence.

Advanced Health Assessment of Women offers a variety of clinical tools to enhance content. Feel free to use any information provided and adapt it to your organization. End-of-chapter appendices contain a special patient education series that may be used and/or adopted for use by your practice.

It is our hope to offer some real guidance to students and practitioners. The content reflects an extensive review of current literature, integrated with our years of clinical experience and teaching.

Experts in various women's health forums have generously shared their expertise as contributors and reviewers.

Helen A. Carcio
Mimi Clarke Secor

Acknowledgment

Thanks to my husband Frank, and sons Marc, Ben, and CJ, who are willing to share their mother with a computer. It wasn't always easy but it is certainly always rewarding.

Helen A. Carcio

Thanks to Helen for all her support as I ventured into coauthoring my first book with her. I also want to thank my husband Mike, daughter Katherine, and my mom for their understanding and support throughout this long and arduous process. It was a most interesting and rewarding experience.

Mimi Clarke Secor

We gratefully thank Margaret Zuccarini, Executive Editor, Nursing, and Pamela Lankas, Production Editor, for their professionalism, knowledge, and invaluable support through the lengthy publication process. You were both always extremely responsive to all our questions and concerns.

We both thank Springer for their special dedication to educating nurse practitioners and to their commitment to women's health care.

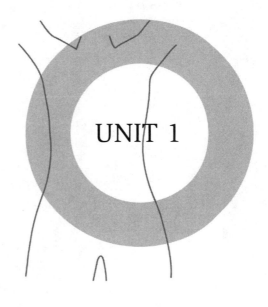

UNIT 1

Female Reproduction

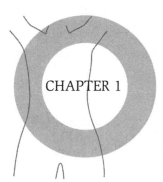

CHAPTER 1

Anatomy and Physiology of Female Reproduction

Helen A. Carcio

I. **Female reproduction explained.**
   A. In the female, the urinary and reproductive systems are completely separate, unlike in the male.
   B. The internal female reproductive organs are located in the lower pelvis and are safely tucked inside the bony pelvis, behind the pubic bone.
   C. External genitalia collectively include the mons pubis, the labia majora, the labia minora, the vestibule, the clitoris, and the vaginal orifice (Figure 1.1).
   D. The structures of the peritoneum are listed and compared in Table 1.1.

II. **Ovaries.**
   A. Description.
      1. Each ovary lies in a depression in the lateral pelvic wall, on either side of the uterus.
      2. Ovaries are small and almond shaped.
      3. The ovaries vary considerably in size among women but

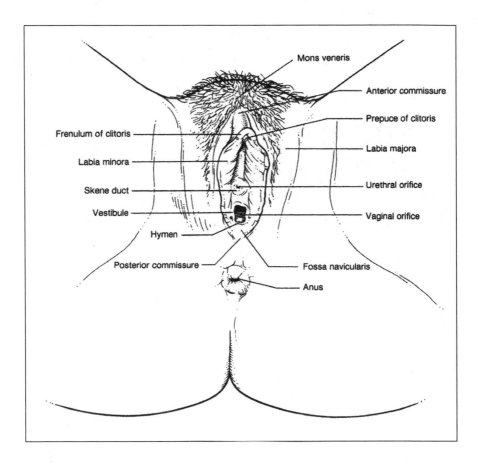

Figure 1.1 External female genitalia.

usually measure between 3 and 5 cm long, 1.5 and 3 cm wide, and 1 and 1.5 cm thick—about the size of a thumbnail.

4. They are pinkish white to gray.

5. They are not directly attached to the uterus and tubes. The ovaries lie suspended in a strong, flexible structure called the *round ligament*, which anchors them to the uterus.

6. The uterine tubes, which consist of the oviducts and the fallopian tubes, are not directly connected to the ovaries. They open to the peritoneal cavity area near them.

B. Function.

Table 1.1   **Structure, Functions, and Purposes of the Organs of Female Reproduction**

Structure	Function	Purpose
External genitalia	Sensitive to touch and external stimulation	Sexual arousal and sensation of orgasm
Vagina	Passage for intercourse Provides space for containment of sperm Excretory outlet for the uterus Becomes birth canal during the birthing process	Organ of copulation
Cervix	Fibrous, muscular band that holds bottom of uterus closed and keeps fetus inside during pregnancy	Major source of mucus production during the menstrual cycle
Uterus	Organ of menstruation	Fertilized egg implants here Maintains and protects developing fetus until birth Contracts during labor to birth the neonate
Fallopian tubes	Transport of sperm upward Transport of the egg downward	Location of fertilization of the egg Carries the egg to the uterus
Ovaries	Maturation and development of eggs Ejection of eggs Secrete hormones, including estrogen, progesterone, and testosterone	Produce eggs during ovulation

1. The ovaries house the female sex gametes.
2. The ovaries are counterparts to the testes in the male, in that they secrete sex hormones, estrogen, progesterone, and testosterone.
3. The ovaries produce an ovum (egg) during ovulation in response to hormonal stimulation.

III. Fallopian tubes.
   A. Description.
      1. The fallopian tubes extend outward from either side of the

body of the uterus and act as a connecting tunnel between the ovary and the uterus.

2. They are approximately 13 cm (5 in), rubbery, and less than half the diameter of a pencil (.05–1.0 cm).
3. They have two layers—inner and outer serous layers—that surround the layers of involuntary muscle.
4. The fallopian tubes are narrow and muscular (acting as oviducts) and lined with cilia.
5. They consist of four sections.
   a. Interstitial section, which lies within the uterine wall.
   b. Isthmus.
      (1) The isthmus is the narrowest section closest to the uterus.
      (2) It opens into the cavity of the uterus.
      (3) It has a thick muscular wall.
   c. Ampulla.
      (1) The ampulla is the longest section, about two thirds of the total length.
      (2) It widens progressively to the wide distal opening in the infundibulum.
      (3) It is thin walled.
      (4) It is the site of fertilization.
   d. Infundibulum.
      (1) The infundibulum is the fimbriated end that lies in close proximity to the ovary.
      (2) Fingerlike projections at the ends of the tubes are the *fimbriae*, which sweep over the ovary, scoop up the egg, and propel it toward the inner ampullae.
B. Function.
   1. Transports the sperm and the egg (Box 1.1).
      a. The inner wall of the fallopian tubes is lined with cilia, which are hairlike projections.
      b. It is believed that the beating motion of these cilia transports the fertilized egg along the tube to the uterus, where the egg is implanted.
      c. Muscle contractions in the fallopian tube assist in moving the egg along its journey, much like in intestinal peristalsis.
      d. Fallopian tubes have the unique ability to transport the egg in one direction and the sperm in the opposite direction.
   2. Collects the egg.

Transport of the Egg by the Fallopian Tubes   **BOX 1.1**

Egg is released during ovulation
↓
Egg is scooped up by petals of fimbriae
↓
Egg enters the tube at the infundibulum
↓
Fertilization occurs in the ampullae
↓
Ampullae transport fertilized egg (ovum) in the direction of the uterus (tube progressively narrows from the flared tips)
↓
Muscle contractions and ciliary action in the tube help propel the egg
↓
Egg enters the uterus from the isthmus
↓
Implantation of the egg in the wall of the uterus
↓
Pregnancy

      a. The cilia on the fimbriae have adhesive sites that help navigate the egg into the fallopian tube.
      b. Near the time of ovulation, the fimbriae bend down in proximity to the ovaries.
      c. The swooping motion of the petals sweeps up the egg.

IV. The uterus.
    A. Description of the uterine corpus, or uterine body.
      1. The uterus is shaped like an inverted pear.
      2. The uterus is hollow, thick walled, and muscular, lying between the bladder and the rectum.
      3. The size and the shape of the uterus vary.
        a. Length—7.5 cm (3 in.).
        b. Width—5 cm (2 in.).
        c. Depth—2.5 cm (1 in.)—a little smaller than a fist.
      4. The uterus consists of two sections, roughly divided in the middle at the isthmus.
        a. Upper portion.
          (1) The corpus—the main body.
          (2) The fundus—the dome-shaped portion located at the point at which the fallopian tubes enter the uterus.
        b. Lower narrower portion—the cervix.

5. The uterus is mobile and expands readily to accommodate a developing fetus.
6. The uterine artery is the main source of blood for the uterus.
7. The uterus is supported by the levator ani muscle and eight ligaments.
8. Major ligaments that help the uterus remain supported in mid position are the elastic broad ligaments, which act as "guide wires."
9. The position of the uterus within the pelvis varies (Figure 1.2).
   a. Anteverted/anteflexed—tilted toward the bladder.
   b. Retroverted/retroflexed—tilted toward the rectum.
   c. Midposition—found less frequently.
   d. Positions do not affect fertility.
10. Relationship of the uterine body to the cervix.
    a. Anteflexed—the anterior surface bends toward the cervix.
    b. Retroflexed—the posterior surface bends toward the cervix.
11. Consequently, a uterus can commonly be anteverted (tilting toward the front) and anteflexed (the anterior portion bent).
12. The uterus is a freely movable organ suspended in the pelvic cavity and actual placement varies as the woman changes position.
13. The wall of the uterus consists of three layers.
    a. Perimetrium—the serous external peritoneal covering.
    b. Myometrium—the middle muscular layer.
    c. Endometrium—the inner layer of the cavity.
       (1) The endometrium is controlled hormonally.
       (2) It is involved with menstruation or development of the placenta.
B. Description of the uterine cervix.
   1. The uterine cervix is visible and palpable in the upper vagina and is a knoblike structure.
   2. It is smooth, shiny, and pink.
   3. It is firmer to palpation than the uterine corpus because there is more connective tissue. (It feels like the tip of the nose.)
   4. It is covered by two types of epithelium.
      a. Squamous epithelium.
         (1) The squamous epithelium is pink and shiny.
         (2) It is contiguous with the vaginal lining.
      b. Columnar epithelium.

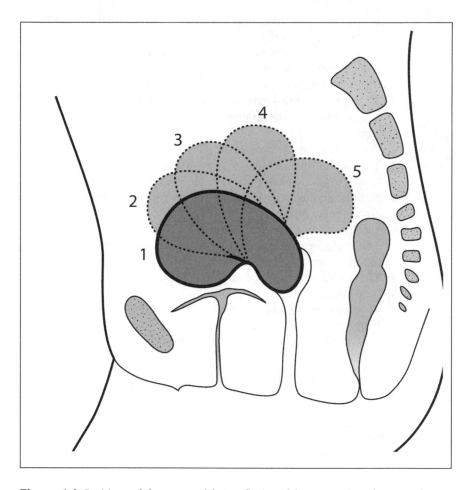

Figure 1.2 Positions of the uterus. (1) Anteflexion. (2) Anteversion, the normal position. (3) Midposition. (4) Retroversion. (5) Retroflexion.

      (1) The columnar epithelium is deep red.
      (2) It is an extension of the lining of the endocervical canal.
   5. The cervical opening, the *external os*, connects the vagina to the endocervical canal, which connects to the body of the uterus.
   6. The size of the external os varies.
      a. The external os is a tiny, round opening in women who have not given birth vaginally.

      b. It is open, slitlike, and irregular in women who have had children vaginally.

      c. It becomes tight and tiny in postmenopausal women because of a decrease in estrogen levels.

C. Description of nabothian cysts.

  1. The surface of the external cervix normally has endocervical glands that secrete mucus in response to hormonal stimulation.

  2. The ducts can become obstructed and cystic.

  3. The extent of obstruction varies from a few tiny cysts to large cysts covering the entire cervix.

  4. Nabothian cysts are common; however, infection may increase their number.

D. Description of endocervical canal.

  1. The endocervical canal is open at both ends, connecting the external os to the internal os.

  2. The endocervical canal is about 2 to 2.5 cm (1 in.).

  3. It is lined by columnar epithelium.

  4. The *ectocervix* is the cervical portion extending outward from the external cervical os.

      a. Anterior lip—the portion above the cervical os.

      b. Posterior lip—the portion below the cervical os.

  5. The *endocervix* is a narrow column, extending upward from the external os to the internal os of the uterine endometrium.

E. The cervical epithelium is composed of squamous and columnar epithelia.

  1. Squamous epithelium.

      a. The squamous epithelium is smooth, shiny, and pink.

      b. It covers the ectocervix.

      c. It has four layers, similar to the skin (Figure 1.3).

         (1) Basal layer—lies within the thin basement membrane. This layer has one or two cell layers.

         (2) Parabasal layer. This layer has three or four cell layers.

         (3) Intermediate layer. This layer is thicker than the parabasal and basal layers.

         (4) Superficial layer. This layer is composed of mature cells that continuously shed. It is the thickest layer.

         (5) The response to estrogen levels and presence of inflammation or infection of these four layers varies. (See chapter 23.)

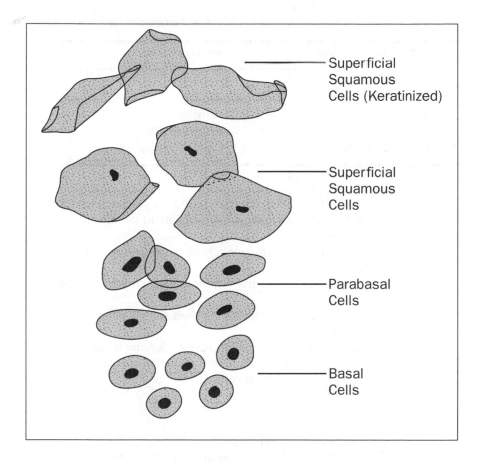

Figure 1.3 Layers of squamous epithelium.

2. Columnar epithelium.
   a. The columnar epithelium is dark red and granular.
   b. It lines the endocervical canal.
   c. It secretes mucus.
3. Squamocolumnar junction or transformation zone.
   a. This junction is the boundary between the squamous and columnar epithelia.
   b. Squamous metaplasia occurs naturally as columnar epithelium is changed to squamous epithelium. (It is differentiated.)
   c. This area of metaplasia is the area of endocervical cells,

• *Table 1.2*   **Comparison of Fertile and Nonfertile Cervical Mucus**

Ovulatory Fertile Mucus	Nonovulatory Mucus
Clear to slightly cloudy	Opaque
Abundant	Scant
Stretchy, like raw egg white	Nonstretchy
Slippery	Rubbery
Dries without residue	Leaves white flakes when dry

which is critical to sample during the routine Pap smear because it is particularly susceptible to neoplastic changes.
    d. The location of this junction varies with hormonal variation.
        (1) In adolescents, the junction is visible on the external cervix.
        (2) The junction extends up the canal as estrogen levels decrease.
    e. It is termed *eversion, ectropion,* or *ectomy* if visible on the ectocervix as a granular, red, well-circumscribed area.
   F. Cervical mucus—changes in response to hormonal variations (Table 1.2).

V. Vagina.
   A. Description of the vaginal canal.
     1. The vaginal canal is a fibromuscular canal about 7.5 cm (3 in.).
     2. It is located between the rectum, posteriorly, anterior to the urethra.
     3. It is lined with squamous epithelia arranged in folds called rugae, extending from the cervix to the vestibule.
     4. It extends from the vaginal opening on the outside of the body to the uterus.
     5. The muscular coat of the vagina is much thinner than that of the uterus.
     6. The uterine cervix enters and protrudes into the upper vagina, causing the formation of deeper rings around the cervix, called *fornices.*
     7. The vagina can stretch and contract easily during intercourse or delivery.

  8. It is usually pinkish red.
  9. It does not contain any mucus-secreting glands.
      a. It is moistened by cervical secretions.
      b. Additional fluids percolate into the vagina from other fluid compartments during sexual arousal.
  10. The blood supply of the vagina is carried by the vaginal branches of the uterine artery.
  B. The function of the vagina is as a passageway.
      1. Menstrual flow to exit the uterus.
      2. Fetus to be expelled from the uterus.
      3. Sperm to travel toward the egg.
  C Vaginal ecology.
      1. The epithelium contains large amounts of glycogen.
      2. Normal bacterial florae of the vagina consist of *Lactobacillus,* which metabolizes the glycogen.
      3. Lactobacilli produce lactic acid.
      4. Lactic acid helps maintain the vaginal pH as acidic, thus decreasing bacteria. (See chapter 8 for further explanation.)
  D. Hymen.
      1. The hymen is located at the outer opening of the vagina.
      2. It is a folded membrane of connective tissue.
      3. It may nearly occlude the vaginal opening in women who have never had sexual intercourse or who have never used tampons.
  E. Bartholin glands.
      1. The Bartholin glands are two small, bean-shaped glands.
      2. They secrete a mucousal substance that helps lubricate the vaginal canal.
      3. They are located on either side of the vagina, deep in the labia minora.
  F. Fornix.
      1. The fornix is a deep ring that posteriorly surrounds the cervix where it protrudes through the upper vagina.
      2. It is comparatively thin walled and allows the ovaries and the uterus to be felt with palpation.
      3. May act to pool semen after ejaculation, allowing a "time-release" effect as the sperm intermittently swim through the cervix.

VI. Pelvic support.
  A. All the internal reproductive organs are supported in a slinglike fashion by ligaments that are covered by peritoneal folds.

B. The pelvic and urogenital diaphragms provide support for the perineum.
  1. The pelvic diaphragm.
      a. The pelvic diaphragm contains the levator ani and coccygeus muscle.
      b. It forms a broad sling within the pelvis that swings forward at the pelvic outlet to surround the vagina and the rectum as a form of sphincter.
      c. The pubovaginalis is the actual sphincter that acts as a sling for the vagina. It is the main muscular support of the pelvic organs.
  2. The urogenital diaphragm.
      a. The urogenital diaphragm is the triangular area between the ischial tuberosities and the symphysis pubis.
      b. It contains urethral striated sphincter muscles, trigone fascia, and the inferior urogenital trigone fascia.
      c. It provides support for the lower urethra and the anterior wall of the vaginal canal.

VII. Uterine ligaments.
  A. Broad ligaments.
  1. The broad ligaments are two wormlike structures extending from the lateral margin of the uterus to the pelvic walls, dividing the uterine cavity into anterior and posterior compartments.
  2. Cardinal ligament.
      a. The lower portion of the cardinal ligament is composed of dense connective tissue that is firmly joined to the supravaginal portion of the cervix.
  3. The broad ligaments support the vagina and prevent uterine prolapse.
  B. Round ligaments.
  1. The round ligaments are fibrous cords.
  2. They attach to either side of the fundus, just below the fallopian tubes.
  3. They extend through the inguinal canal and end in the upper portion of the labia minora.
  4. They aid in holding the fundus forward.
  C. Uterosacral ligaments (two).
  1. The uterosacral ligaments are cordlike structures.
  2. They extend from the posterior cervical portion of the uterus to the sacrum.

3. They help support the cervix.
   a. The uterovesical ligament is a fold of peritoneum that passes over the fundus, extending to the bladder.
   b. The rectovaginal ligament is a fold of peritoneum that passes over the posterior surface of the uterus.

VIII. Associated pelvic organs.
   A. Bladder.
      1. Location.
         a. The bladder is located anteriorly in the pelvis, immediately posterior to the pubic symphysis.
         b. The upper surface is rounded and is covered by the peritoneum of the anterior wall of the pelvis.
         c. Posteriorly, it passes on to the uterus at the junction of the cervix and corpus.
         d. When the bladder is empty, usually the uterus rests on its superior surface.
   B. Urethra.
      1. Description.
         a. The urethra is a small tube 2.5 to 5.0 cm long.
         b. It is 2 to 8 mm wide.
      2. The orifice lies between the labia minora, anterior to the vaginal opening and posterior to the clitoris.
      3. The urethra opens into the vaginal vestibule, about 2 cm posterior to the clitoris.

CHAPTER 2

The Reproductive Cycle

Helen A. Carcio

I. **Reproductive cycle.**
   A. The female reproductive cycle is regulated through the highly co-ordinated functions of the brain, the hypothalamus, the pituitary, the ovaries, and the uterus.
   B. Each component must be in communication with the others to stimulate or suppress one of the other hormones.

II. **Hormonal influences explained.**
   A. Two hormones affect the female reproductive tract. These hormones are directly concerned with gonadal function and, therefore, are classified as gonadotropic hormones.
      1. Follicle-stimulating hormone (FSH) stimulates the development of the follicles in the ovary, which leads to the ripening of the follicle, ovulation, and the secretion of estrogens.
      2. Luteinizing hormone (LH) stimulates the maturing follicle before its rupture.
      3. FSH stimulates the first part of the ovarian cycle; LH, together with FSH, influences preovulatory enlargement, ovulation, and development of the corpus luteum (Box 2.1).
   B. The ovary, under the influence of the gonadotrophic hormones, secretes two hormones: estrogen and progesterone.

Hormonal Influences in Embryo Development   **BOX 2.1**

Oocytes recruited and mature in the follicular phase
(under influence of FSH)
↓
Dominance of one follicle
↓
Grows and matures while others regress
↓
Final maturation of the dominant follicle (under influence of LH)
↓   ↓
Ovulation occurs   Estrogen increases
↓   ↓
Egg fertilized in fallopian tube   Endometrium proliferates
↓   ↓
Egg transported to uterus   Secretory endometrium forms
(under influence of progesterone)
↓
Implantation of the embryo
↓
Secretion of human chorionic gonadotropin (hCG)
↓
Stimulates corpus luteum
↓
Increases production of estrogen and progesterone
↓
Maintains pregnancy

FSH: follicle-stimulating hormone; LH: luteinizing hormone.

1. Basic function of estrogen.
   a. Estrogen produces all the physical characteristics of a mature female.
   b. It helps prepare the endometrium of the uterus for implantation by a fertilized egg.
   c. It helps regulate the production and release of FSH and LH by the pituitary gland.
   d. It intensifies the effects of progesterone.
   e. Together with FSH, it helps promote the growth and development of the primary follicle.
2. Basic function of progesterone.
   a. After ovulation, progesterone prepares the uterus for pregnancy by promoting the growth of secretory endometrial cells.
   b. If pregnancy occurs, progesterone acts to maintain the pla-

centa and inhibits uterine contraction to prevent abortion of the embryo.

III. **Ovarian cycle.**
  A. Basics of the ovarian cycle.
    1. During hormonal stimulation, the ovary undergoes many changes that result in the development and release of an ovum and in the formation of the corpus luteum.
    2. The ovarian cycle consists of the follicular phase, ovulation, and the luteal phase.
  B. Follicular phase explained.
    1. At birth, each ovary contains about 400,000 primordial egg cells (oocytes).
    2. These oocytes have a large nucleus with clear cytoplasm surrounded by theca and granuloma cells.
      a. Oocytes secrete fluid to create the ovarian blister.
      b. Theca cells are the primary source of circulating estrogens.
      c. Granuloma cells are the source of estrogens in the follicular fluid.
    3. A *primordial follicle* comprises an egg cell and its surrounding cells.
      a. The production of primordial follicles stops around the time of birth of the fetus.
      b. The primordial follicles are considered permanent cells.
      c. Additional eggs are not produced throughout the woman's lifecycle.
    4. At the time of puberty, about 30,000 primordial follicles remain, which will either mature into eggs or disintegrate in the approximately 30 years of active ovarian activity between puberty and menopause.
    5. In normally ovulating women, one egg will mature within a follicle each month, totaling between 300 and 400 eggs during the reproductive years.
  C. Ovulation explained.
    1. As the egg matures and the fluid pressure increases, the egg and the follicle are naturally moved toward the outside of the ovary.
    2. The mature egg and the follicular fluid are now called a *graafian follicle.*
    3. At some point, the graafian follicle thins to the outside edge of the ovary and ruptures into the area outside of the ovary.

Table 2.1   **Comparison of Nomenclature for the Various Phases of the Reproductive Cycle**

	Predominant Hormone	Ovarian Cycle	Endometrial Cycle	Menstrual Cycle
Days 1–14	Estrogenic phase	Follicular phase	Proliferative	Menstrual (days 1–7)
Days 14–28	Progestational phase	Luteal phase	Secretory	Premenstrual (days 21–28)

4. The fimbriated edges of the fallopian tube draws the egg toward the tube.
   D. The luteal phase explained.
   1. Development of the corpus luteum.
      a. After ovulation, the spot at which the egg ruptured transforms itself.
      b. The cells remaining in the follicle become filled with yellow material, and the follicle is now called the *corpus luteum.*
   2. The development of the corpus albicans.
      a. About 8 days after ovulation, the corpus luteum reaches full maturity.
      b. It slowly begins to evolve into a white body called the *corpus albicans.*
   3. If conception and pregnancy occur, the corpus luteum increases in size and governs hormonal requirements during gestation, particularly for the first 4 months.
   4. The principal hormone secreted by the corpus luteum is progesterone.
   5. If conception does not occur, the progesterone secreted by the corpus luteum controls the postovulatory phase of the menstrual cycle for about 2 weeks.

IV. **The endometrial cycle.**
   A. Basics of the endometrial cycle.
      1. This section refers to cyclic changes in the *endometrium,* which comprises the cells lining the uterus.
      2. The endometrial cycle is broken into three phases: proliferative, secretory, and ischemic (menstruation).
      3. These cycles correspond directly to phases that are occurring in the ovary (Table 2.1).
   B. The proliferative phase explained.

1. At the end of menstruation, the endometrium is thin and considered ischemic.
2. Within the second week of the cycle, hormonal production of estrogen increases and the endometrium becomes thicker.
3. The cells undergo proliferative growth and become taller as the glandular cells become deeper and wider.
4. This thickness can increase up to eight times.
5. Glands of the endometrium become more active, secretory, and nutritive.
6. At the same time, the follicles (i.e., theca cells) are producing more follicular fluid containing estrogen, which further primes the uterus.
7. The proliferative phase is also called the *follicular phase* or *estrogenic phase* (to signify that the predominant hormone at this time is estrogen).

C. The secretory phase explained.
1. The secretory phase comprises the last 2 weeks (days 14–28 after ovulation).
2. After the egg is released from the follicle, the cells of the corpus luteum secrete progesterone, which governs the second half of the endometrial cycle.
3. Under the influence of progesterone and estrogen, the endometrial glands grow even more fluid-filled and congested.
4. The blood supply of the endometrium increases, and the lining becomes filled with vacuoles and reservoirs that contain nutrient fluids.
5. The vascular arterioles become more spiral, twisted, and looped back, allowing for a nutritive layer if conception should occur.
6. Other names for this phase are *luteal* (referring to the ovary), *progestational* (referring to the dominant hormone), and *premenstrual* (see Table 2.1).

D. Menstruation explained.
1. If conception does not occur, the function of the corpus luteum wanes and levels of progesterone and estrogen decrease.
2. The lining of the endometrium becomes ischemic and cell degeneration occurs.
3. As further cell degeneration occurs, the cells rupture, bursting small arterioles.
4. The deteriorated endometrium sloughs off the uterine wall and passes through the vagina.
5. Menstruation allows the endometrial wall to be rebuilt with

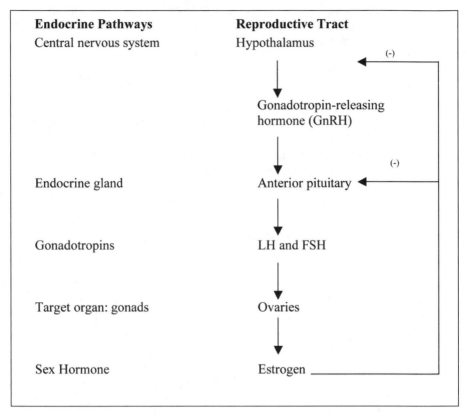

Figure 2.1 Feedback mechanism of the hypothalamic-pituitary-ovarian axis. Estrogen inhibits both the hypothalamus and the anterior pituitary.

each monthly cycle, ensuring a fresh new lining for each possible conceptus.

   6. This phase is called the *ischemic phase* or *menstruation.*

V. **Hormonal regulation and feedback mechanisms (Figure 2.1).**

   A. Each ovarian and endometrial cycle is regulated through the
   complex interaction of hypothalamic, pituitary, and ovarian hormones secreted in varying concentrations throughout the cycle.

   B. To integrate the system, various feedback mechanisms organize
   the sequencing of hormones.

   C. Within the hypothalamus, which is connected to the pituitary by
   a network of vessels called the *hypothalamic–hypophyseal (pitu-*

itary) portal system, gonadotropin-releasing hormone (GNRH) is secreted.

D. GNRH moves down the portal system to control the secretion of FSH, LH, and gonadotropin from the anterior pituitary.

E. FSH is active in mid cycle and controls the release of the ovum; LH is active in the luteal phase.

F. The hypothalamus is influenced by changes in neural and cerebral environments.

G. Prostaglandin also influences the cycle by influencing receptors in the hypothalamus.

H. At the start of each menstrual cycle, the pituitary secretes larger amounts of FSH, which, together with LH, promotes the maturation of several ovum follicles.

　　1. The emission of LH and FSH in combination promotes the secretion of estradiol, the most active estrogen and the primary estrogen of younger women.

　　2. Blood levels of estradiol begin to increase, and these increasing levels of estradiol provide negative feedback on the hypothalamic-pituitary secretion of FSH.

　　3. The level of FSH begins to decrease, but FSH continues to work on the follicle in combination with LH to ripen one follicle.

I. On approximately Day 12 (about 2 days before ovulation), most of the follicles that have ripened—except one—begin to degenerate or undergo atresia.

J. The follicle that is most mature continues to grow, and in turn, estrogen activity increases markedly.

K. Increasing amounts of estrogen secreted at this time promote secretion of GNRH (positive feedback), which causes LH and FSH to be released from the pituitary.

L. This LH spike provides the final stimulus for maturation of the follicle, and ovulation takes place within 1 to 2 days.

M. Changes in estrogen levels before ovulation prepare the cervical mucus to allow sperm to migrate up the reproductive tract.

N. Changes in mucus.

　　1. During the period immediately after menstruation, the mucus in the cervix is thick, scanty, and opaque.

　　2. Around the time of ovulation, the mucus becomes much thinner, clear, and stretchable to allow the passage of sperm.

　　3. *Spinnbarkeit,* or stretchability of midcycle mucus, provides a good clinical assessment of cyclic changes (see chapter 27).

      4. Table 1.2 in chapter 1 compares ovulatory with nonovulatory mucus.

O. After ovulation.

      1. The ruptured follicle becomes a corpus luteum, which is supported by LH.

      2. The corpus luteum begins to secrete progesterone, and by Days 19 to 21, progesterone secretion is at its maximum to prepare for implantation.

      3. Increased progesterone levels after ovulation inhibit the secretion of FSH and LH (negative feedback).

P. If implantation occurs, another hormone produced by the chorionic villi of the conceptus/trophoblast called *human chorionic gonadotrophin* (hCG; the hormone assayed in pregnancy tests) converts the corpus luteum into a corpus luteum of pregnancy to maintain its function to support the developing pregnancy.

Q. If pregnancy does not occur, the corpus luteum deteriorates, progesterone levels decrease markedly, and, without hormonal support, the endometrium begins to degenerate and slough off as menstrual flow.

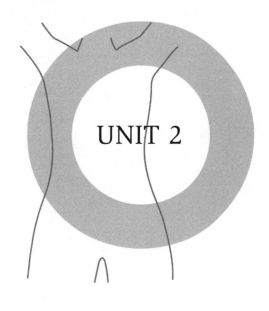

UNIT 2

Health Assessment

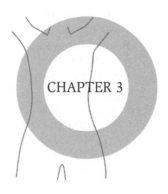

CHAPTER 3

The Health History

Helen A. Carcio and Paula Brooks

I. **The health history risk assessment.**

II. **Definition of sexual health.**
A. *Sexual health* is defined as the integration of somatic, emotional, intellectual, and social aspects of sexual beings in ways that are positively enriching and that enhance personality, communication, and love.
B. It is multidimensional and involves sexual attitudes, behavior, practices, and activity.
C. Its definition incorporates the whole person, including sexual thoughts, experiences, and values about being male or female. The three key elements of sexual health include
   1. A capacity to enjoy and control sexual and reproductive behavior in accordance with a personal and social ethic.
   2. Freedom from fear, shame, guilt, false beliefs, and other psychological factors that inhibit sexual response and impair sexual relationships.
   3. Freedom from organic disorders, diseases, and deficiencies that interfere with sexual and reproductive functions.

III. **Elements of a comprehensive, developmentally relevant sexual health assessment.**
A. Interviewing to gather information about a patient's sexual

history is an art requiring a grace and skill that can only come with practice.
B. Sexuality underlies much of whom and what a person is, and it is an inherent, ever changing aspect of life from birth to death.
C. The goal is to help a patient remember, identify, and verbalize.
D. The sexual assessment must include a physiologic, psychological, and sociocultural evaluation, as well as elements that focus on age-related issues.

   1. The physiologic component: Data should be gathered regarding the client's sexual response cycle (i.e., excitement, plateau, orgasm, and resolution) and any alterations in those phases. Also ask about
     a. Attempts to conceive.
     b. Previous high-risk pregnancies.
     c. Previous postpartum difficulties.
     d. Contraceptive choices and any associated problems.
     e. Data relating to past and present illnesses, surgeries, and medications.

   2. The psychological component: A woman's view of herself as female incorporates concepts of gender identity; the sense of having characteristics customarily defined as feminine, masculine, or both; and body image. Data should include
     a. The client's self-concept and body image.
     b. Client's view of the self as a sexual being.
     c. Level of confidence in ability to function sexually.
     d. Past and current psychiatric problems or illnesses, including anxiety and depression.
     e. Information about use of psychotropic medications.
     f. Satisfaction with current relationship.
     g. History of sexual abuse.

   3. The sociocultural component: A women's view of herself as female can be defined by her sociocultural upbringing and environment. Data should include
     a. Information about the client's perceptions of sex-appropriate roles for men and women in relationships and her perception of her ability to fulfill those roles competently.
     b. Information about the client's religious affiliation and beliefs.
     c. Information about the client's ethnic and cultural belief system.
     d. The woman's sources of sexual education, when she received it, and her reactions to the information. It is al-

ways important for the health care provider to assess whether the information that the client received was correct and accurate.

E. Age-related issues.

  1. Toddler and preschool child: Toddlers are able to identify themselves as "I'm a girl" or "I'm a boy," but they cannot integrate gender identity into their self-concept until they are 3 or 4 years of age, when they are able to understand that sex is a permanent condition.

    a. Children at this age are extremely curious. Assist parents in giving children the message that they and their bodies—including its sexual parts—are valuable and important.

    b. Family is the most important source of learning about sexuality issues in this age group, and the parents' attitudes and behaviors begin to shape feelings about sexuality.

    c. Provide parents with information about "normal" sexual behavior, and emphasize which developmental tasks are expected at approximate ages.

    d. Assist the parents in defining limits of appropriate and inappropriate behavior (e.g., it is not acceptable for a 3-year-old girl to discuss with a stranger on the bus the fact that she and her mother have vaginas but that her father and brother have penises).

    e. Stress the importance of teaching the child about appropriate and inappropriate touching from other people.

    f. Always assess for sexual abuse in all children in any health assessment.

  2. School-aged child: School-aged children continue to have a high level of curiosity about sexuality, their bodies, and their environment, and, because they are aware of the pleasure stimulation gives, may actively seek sexual arousal.

    a. Masturbation and sex games are typical, and both homosexual and heterosexual encounters are commonly seen.

    b. By the time a child reaches school age, or about 8 years of age, he or she begins to understand the significance of sexuality. This is an important time for the clinician to start discussing pubertal changes with parents and to encourage parents to discuss these changes with their child.

    c. The same principles of inclusiveness and freedom from assumptions apply when taking a family history of a pediatric patient. A mother or father may be homosexual. The parent or parents may live alone, in a group house with

other men or women, with the family of his or her origin, or with a partner.
3. Adolescence: Awareness and changes in sexual feelings occur during adolescence.
   a. It is a time of developing a capacity for sexual intimacy, sexual curiosity, and experimentation.
   b. Adolescents are fitting their sense of sexual being into their evolving self-image and personal identity.
   c. They are learning about their bodies' sensual and sexual responses to stimulation and are developing a sense of the moral significance of sexuality. The sexual history that is gathered from adolescents is designed to
      (1) Collect information.
      (2) Give the adolescent permission to ask questions and receive reliable information regarding issues of sexual concern.
         • Reinforce privacy and confidentiality.
         • Communicate an aura of comfort with the client; create an atmosphere that is free of prejudice; and avoid imposing one's values.
         • Assist the adolescent in feeling validated and comfortable revealing concerns and asking questions.
         • Ask questions that give the message that you expect the client is changing and is aware of and curious about these changes (e.g., "How are you feeling?" "How's your body?" "Do you notice that you are getting taller?" (see Section XL).
         • Ask questions to give the message that you care about the client's feelings ("How does that make you feel?" "Do you wonder sometimes about what is happening to your body?").
         • Always listen thoughtfully and carefully to the client's input, and respond positively by answering the client's questions as fully as possible while being calm, friendly, and open.
      (3) Allow the health care provider to incorporate sexuality-specific education as a normal component of anticipatory guidance.
         • Always give appropriate and factual information.
         • Offer complete, accurate information conveyed in an open, professional manner.
         • Assist the adolescent in understanding the physical,

emotional, and psychological changes of puberty, and inform the client of the true risks associated with premature sexual activity.

- Ask questions to give the message that sexual changes are as expected and normal as other body changes ("Have you noticed your breasts getting any bigger?").
- Sexually transmitted diseases and vaginitis occur most frequently during the reproductive years and reach peak incidence during adolescence and young adulthood. For this reason, it is necessary for a health care provider to offer services, education, and counseling.
- Reinforce that sexual activity under the influence of alcohol or drugs can lead to unsafe sexual practices and the risk of unwanted intercourse, pregnancy, and sexually transmitted diseases.

4. Early adulthood and the reproductive years (21–40 years of age): This is a critical period during which developmental tasks include achieving maturity in a sexual role and in the relationship tasks started in adolescence.
    a. Many of the problems experienced by this age group in terms of sexual relationships involve poor communication between partners.
    b. Major concerns in this age group include
        (1) Balancing careers.
        (2) Raising children.
        (3) Nurturing and maintaining relationships.
        (4) Experiencing pregnancy, the postpartum period, and lactation.
        (5) Dealing with infertility.
    c. Assess use of safe sexual practices (monogamy, condom use), discuss family planning and contraceptive choices, and address fertility concerns.
    d. Assist in facilitating communication between sexual partners, to teach clients about sexuality, and to clarify any misconceptions by providing information about sexual behavior, sexual activity, and sexual response.
    e. Provide information about intercourse, good hygiene practices, and foreplay, and to reinforce the practice of health promotion activities (i.e., breast self-examinations, yearly Pap smears).

5. Middle adulthood (41–65 years): This is a critical period for expanded sexual freedom and major physiologic changes.
   a. The primary tasks of mid life and later years are
      (1) Reappraisal, which includes a review of past and present accomplishments.
      (2) Reassessment of goals and life direction.
      (3) Redirection of energies or rededication to life's goals.
   b. Most women have established their careers and families. The children are often grown, and responsibilities of the mother may be decreased. More time can now be spent focusing on herself and her partner.
   c. Women during this period experience menopause (around the age of 50 years in the United States). Many fear the loss of sexual attractiveness and capacity.
   d. Health problems of either partner can be a major source of concern during these years.

IV. **Advanced health history techniques.**
   A. The interview: The gynecologic interview is primarily for gathering information. For many women, this may be the woman's sole source of preventive health care. Therefore, the purpose of this visit is fivefold.
      1. Provides information to develop problem lists, diagnoses, and plans.
      2. Screens for other existing or potential health problems.
      3. Provides general health maintenance and prevention of illness.
      4. Establishes a relationship between the care provider and the patient.
      5. Sets a tone for the entire visit and for subsequent visits.
   B. Patient–practitioner interaction is an equal partnership.
      1. Each partner contributes expertise.
      2. The provider has knowledge about health and health care in general.
      3. The patient has knowledge about her history and her body.
      4. When a practitioner expresses respect for what the patient brings to the encounter, the setting and implementation of common goals become possible.
         a. Expressing respect through verbal communication: This begins with the introduction
            (1) Always go into the waiting area to call the patient rather than having the receptionist bring the patient into the examination room. This allows the patient to meet the practitioner for the first time while the pa-

tient is fully dressed. This sets a more personal tone and promotes a feeling of equality in the patient–practitioner relationship.

(2) Determine how each wants to be addressed. Many practitioners establish relationships with patients on a first-name basis. This is both equal and personal. However, others may find this disrespectful. Ask the patient how he or she wants to be addressed (e.g., first name, last name, Ms., Mrs., or Miss). Some practitioners are most comfortable being called Ms., Mrs., Miss, or Mr.; consequently, the patient should be addressed in an equivalent manner.

b. Expressing respect through nonverbal communication, including facial expressions, eye contact, posture, and, when appropriate, touch

(1) Smiling: When appropriate, smiling conveys warmth and caring.

(2) Eye contact: Maintaining eye contact by frequently looking up from writing or waiting to write until the end of a conversation sends a message of interest. A practitioner who continually looks down at the chart or stares off into space establishes social distance.

(3) Posture: Sitting up in one's seat or leaning toward the patient creates an impression of interest.

(4) Touch: Touching may or may not be appropriate. Be aware that touch has meaning; use it to instill trust rather than distrust. In our culture, handshaking is always a respectful form of physical contact. However, other cultures find touching intrusive. Be aware of cultural norms, and use this information to guide your practice.

c. Expressing respect through the environment: When possible, try to positively manipulate the environment.

(1) Use round tables or couches and chairs rather than sitting behind a desk to conduct the interview. This eliminates the feeling of authority emanating from the behind-the-desk posture.

(2) Ensure privacy by shutting the doors and pulling the curtains. If this is not possible, at least ensure "psychological privacy" by using a soft voice and avoiding any interruptions.

5. Be aware of your own sexual biases: To provide adequate sexual health care, the health care provider must

      a. Be aware of his or her own sexual biases.

      b. Be comfortable with his or her sexuality.

      c. Have a genuine desire to help the client.

      d. Understand that personal barriers may prevent clinicians from comfortably addressing sexual issues.

          (1) It is critical to address any barriers and not make assumptions about a woman's sexual behavior, feelings, or attitudes.

      e. Continually monitor personal responses to detect negative or embarrassed feelings that may easily be conveyed to the client.

  6. Setting the stage.

      a. Choose a private location where the client is comfortable, and assure her that the information will be held in strict confidence.

      b. Sufficient time must be given to build trust and develop a rapport before soliciting information that the client may consider highly personal or intimate.

      c. Avoid obtaining a sexual health history when the client is experiencing an acute health problem.

      d. Obtain permission to ask questions in this potentially sensitive area: "I would like to ask you some questions about your sex life. I don't mean to embarrass you and it's okay if you'd rather not answer some of them. May I begin?"

  7. Begin with open-ended questions: Ask open-ended questions at the beginning of the interview and at the beginning of each of its sections.

      a. This gives the practitioner a chance to assess the language used by the patient and reveals the concerns that are most important to the patient.

      b. More pointed questions can then be asked to specify the conditions that are important for the practitioner to know about.

  8. Avoid using excessive medical terminology: Language must be understood clearly by both the provider and the client.

      a. Make sure that both you and the client know the meaning of the terms used.

      b. Sometimes, it may be helpful to use technical and nontechnical words in the same question: "Have you ever had hypertension—high blood pressure?"

  9. Avoid euphemisms: Inclusive language should be used while taking the patient history and going through the review of systems.

    a. Follow a standard procedure, ask every patient the same questions, and make no assumptions.

    b. Avoid wording such as "slept with."

    c. Use gender-neutral terms to refer to significant others, such as "partner" or "spouse."

    d. Frame inclusive questions when asking about sexual activity, but when the questions are pertinent to the complaint or work up, make inclusive questions about the sexual activity as specific as possible.

    e. Rather than using the words "coitus" and "intercourse," or the even more vague "sexual activity" or "sexual relations," inquire about "oral sex," "anal sex," and "vaginal intercourse (or) sex."

    f. If the client does not understand, describe the behavior being asked about (e.g., "Have you ever taken a man's penis into your rectum or mouth?").

    g. Most practitioners are uncomfortable discussing sex, particularly specific sexual acts. The only way to overcome such discomfort is through routine exposure.

10. Universalizing: Universalizing should be used only in appropriate situations.

    a. Prefacing questions with phrases such as "Many people" or "Research shows that" may make the client feel more comfortable when answering sensitive questions.

    b. Do not presume a client is heterosexual because the patient discusses an opposite-sex spouse or has children.

    c. Sexual orientation and sexual behaviors encompass a broad spectrum; the astute clinician recognizes that outward appearances may not be definitive.

    d. Do not assume that a woman who identifies herself as a lesbian is having sex only with women.

    e. Avoid labels that the patient does not use. For example, people who might acknowledge same-sex sexual behavior may not identify themselves as homosexual.

11. Move from simple to complex items: Always begin the interview with least threatening material and explain to clients the purpose of the questions. This approach will help build trust and rapport.

    a. A general guideline is to begin with questions about the individual's sexual learning history, such as childhood sexual education; then proceed to personal attitudes and beliefs about sexuality; and finally, assess actual sexual behaviors.

V. Special approaches to sexual health history.

A. A thorough sexual health history is the cornerstone of accurate diagnosis and identification of health risk factors and lays the foundation for health promotion. There are three basic types of sexual health histories:

    1. Initial or comprehensive history: A comprehensive sexual history is a detailed history that encompasses all aspects of sexual information about the individual, as well as his or her family of origin, siblings, and significant relationships.

        a. The initial or comprehensive history includes information concerning

            (1) Each phase of sexual development.

            (2) Body image.

            (3) Learned attitudes.

            (4) Feelings relating to sexuality.

            (5) Sexual debut.

            (6) Sexual orientation.

            (7) Range of sexual behaviors.

        b. The purpose of this type of history is to create an accurate and complete account of the patient's health status.

        c. It is a lengthy process that may not be accomplished at the first visit or with a single interview.

    2. A well-interim history: This history focuses on in-depth family and lifestyle information and is used to form the basis of health maintenance and health promotion.

    3. A systematic or problem-focused history: This type of history is obtained when the patient presents with a specific symptom. The focus is to gather information regarding the patient's current health problems and any confounding health factors.

        a. The systematic history focuses on the presenting symptom or assessment of specific behaviors, such as the risks for becoming pregnant or the acquisition of sexually transmitted diseases.

        b. Problem-oriented sexual histories: These histories are shorter, more direct, and specific to the immediate issue.

            (1) Indications that make it necessary to conduct the problem-focused pelvic examination:

                • Information obtained from the history, with or without symptoms.

                  ○ Maternal diethylstilbestrol (DES) exposure.

○ Multiple (contemporaneous or serial) sexual partners.
○ Unexplained infertility.
• New or recurrent sentinel symptoms.
○ Change in character, frequency, regularity, or duration of menses.
○ Midcycle, postcoital, or postmenopausal vaginal bleeding.
○ Lower abdominal pain or swelling, especially when it is unilateral.
○ Painful sexual intercourse (dyspareunia).
○ Vulvar or vaginal pruritus.
○ Change in quantity or character of vaginal discharge.
○ Urinary incontinence.
○ Burning or pain on urination (dysuria), with or without diagnosed urinary tract infection.
○ Lower back pain or any symptoms that bear consistent relationship to menstrual cycle.
○ Unexpected onset of menarche or menopause.
○ Bilateral lower limb edema (unexplained).

VI. **The reproductive health history.**
  A. Preconception care and counseling: The goal of preconception counseling is to optimize the health of the woman and the health of her potential infant. To reach this goal, the National Institutes of Health expert panel recommends that preconception counseling begin prior to 1 year before conception of a planned pregnancy. (For further information see chapter 7 on prenatal assessment.)
    1. Preconception assessment data: Includes history, physical examination results, and laboratory data.
      a. History.
        (1) A complete medical, social, reproductive, and family history must be obtained.
        (2) Information should be specific to the client's family, medical, reproductive, drug history, and human immunodeficiency virus (HIV) risk factors.
        (3) Nutrition and lifestyle choices should also be evaluated.
        (4) The use of a comprehensive screening tool, such as

the Sample Prenatal Genetic Screen, can be useful
(Appendix 3.1).
   b. Physical examination.
      (1) A complete physical examination with pelvic assess-
          ment should be performed, along with a Papanicolaou
          (Pap) smear, cultures for gonorrhca and chlamydia,
          and a wet smear evaluation.
   c. Laboratory testing.
      (1) Rubella titer and antibody screen.
      (2) Serology for syphilis.
      (3) Complete blood cell (CBC) count with indices.
      (4) Blood type and Rh.
      (5) Random blood sugar.
      (6) Urinalysis.
      (7) If sickle cell disease or thalassemia is a concern, he-
          moglobin electrophoresis should be performed.
      (8) Screening for viral diseases, such as HIV, hepatitis, cy-
          tomegalovirus (CMV), or toxoplasmosis, should be
          encouraged.
2. Client education and counseling.
   a. Menstrual cycles and basal body temperature (BBT): Ad-
      vise client to keep accurate record of her menstrual and
      ovulation cycles to help establish gestational dating (see
      chapter 26 on ovulation assessment).
   b. Exercise and nutrition.
      (1) Vitamin and mineral supplements.
      (2) Folic acid supplementation.
      (3) Ideal weight before conception.
      (4) Exercise program to improve cardiovascular status
          and impart a feeling of overall well-being.
      (5) Balanced diet.
   c. Avoidance of teratogens: Warn the client that potential te-
      ratogens can be related to occupation and lifestyle (Appen-
      dix 3.2). These teratogens can include:
      (1) Cleaning solutions.
      (2) Hair coloring and perms.
      (3) Photography solutions.
      (4) Radiation.
      (5) Chemicals used in processing food and textiles.
      (6) Drugs, including prescription, over-the-counter, and
          recreational drugs.
   d. Affirmation of pregnancy decision: Stress that the couple
      needs time to affirm the decision to attempt pregnancy.

e. Readiness for parenthood: Assess the couple's social, financial, and psychological readiness for pregnancy and commitment to parenthood.

f. Identification of unhealthy behaviors: Assist the couple in identifying and altering unhealthy behaviors such as
   (1) Smoking.
   (2) Alcohol consumption.
   (3) Drug use—prescription, over-the-counter, and illegal drugs.

g. Treatment of medical conditions: Ensure that medical conditions that may jeopardize the pregnancy outcome are evaluated. Refer the couple to a specialist as needed.

h. Identification of genetic risk (Appendix 3.1).
   (1) Indications for genetic counseling.
      • Women who are pregnant or are planning pregnancies and will be 35 years of age or older at delivery.
      • Couples or individuals who have had a previous fetus or child with a genetic disorder, birth defects, or mental retardation.
      • Individuals who have or are suspected to have a genetic disorder.
      • Individuals who have a parent with a genetic disorder.
      • Couples or individuals with a family history of a genetic disorder, birth defects, mental retardation, learning disabilities, cancer, or other conditions.
      • Families with members who have been diagnosed with the same mental or physical condition.
      • Couples or individuals with a history of pregnancy loss or miscarriages, or with unexplained infertility.
      • Individuals who are known carriers of a genetic disorder.
      • Couples or individuals of specific ethnic backgrounds known to have a higher incidence of certain disorders.
      • Women who were exposed during or before pregnancy to teratogenic drugs, infections, x-ray studies or radio therapy, or occupational hazards.
      • Couples who are first cousins or close blood relatives.
      • Women planning to undergo amniocentesis or chorionic villus sampling.
      • Women with abnormal findings at fetal ultrasonography.

- Women with abnormal results on prenatal screening tests.
  i. Preconception classes: Where appropriate, refer the couple to community adult educational resources for preconception classes, such as
    (1) March of Dimes.
    (2) Prenatal, pregnancy, birth, and after childbirth classes.
    (3) Parent training and sibling relations classes.
    (4) Cardiopulmonary resuscitation (CPR) classes.
    (5) Couple to Couple League.
    (6) Pursuing Parenthood class.
    (7) Parent Encouragement Program, which offers classes on parenting, marriage, and families.
  j. Laboratory tests: Order all appropriate laboratory tests, evaluate the results, and discuss the findings and their implications with the client.
  k. Appropriate vaccinations.
    (1) Rubella. If the client is not immune, administer the vaccine and advise the client to wait 3 months before attempting conception.
    (2) Tetanus.
    (3) Hepatitis.
  l. Special dietary needs: If the client has special dietary needs (vegetarian, cultural, diabetes, overweight, underweight), refer her to a dietitian. Women are highly motivated to improve their nutritional status when planning a pregnancy.

VII. **Techniques for screening for sexual abuse.**
   A. Screening for sexual abuse is imperative when obtaining any health assessment. (For specific guidelines, see chapters 18 and 19 on sexual abuse.)

VIII. **HIV risk assessment.**
   A. HIV is transmitted by the exchange of infected body fluids, including blood and semen. High-risk behaviors include
      1. Sexual activity: Unprotected intercourse with multiple partners. Homosexual men are at greatest risk, but all sexually active people are at risk depending on the risk factors of, and number of, sexual partners.
      2. Intravenous (IV) drug abuse.
      3. Persons who received blood products before 1985. Highest

risk is for those who received blood transfusions between 1975 and March 1985.
   4. Hemophiliac clients who received pooled plasma products.
   5. Children of HIV-infected women.
   6. Health care workers (e.g., those at risk for accidental needle sticks).
B. Questions to include.
   1. Are you a health care worker? Have you ever been stuck by a contaminated needle?
   2. Do you have sex with men, women, or both?
   3. How many partners have you had in the past year?
   4. Have you had intercourse without a condom? When did you start using condoms?
   5. Have you performed oral sex on a man or a woman without a barrier (such as a dental dam, plastic wrap, or a condom)?
   6. Have you been treated for a sexually transmitted disease?
   7. Do you smoke cigarettes, drink alcohol, or use other drugs?
   8. Have you had unprotected sex while under the influence of alcohol or other drugs?
   9. Have you had sexual partners who are at high risk for HIV (e.g., those who have a high-risk sexual history or needle-use history)?
   10. Do you, or have you in the past, injected drugs?
   11. Have you shared hypodermic needles, other drug equipment, or other skin piercing or cutting instruments with another person (for injection drug use, steroid use, vitamin injection, tattooing, body piercing, or scarification)?
   12. Do you use crack cocaine? If yes, have you had sex in crack houses?
   13. Have you received a tattoo from an unlicensed tattoo artist or when you were not sure that the needle used had been properly sterilized?
   14. Did you, or do you, receive any blood transfusions, or have you undergone surgery (most important between 1978 and 1985)?
C. Components of the history when assessing an HIV-positive individual (Appendix 3.3): The patient with HIV infection requires an initial evaluation, ongoing psychosocial support, and medical assessment. A complete history is needed, and questions should be directed to gather information specifically about HIV-related illnesses, vaccination history, history of sexually transmitted diseases, and assessment of HIV transmission category (please refer

to section IX for sample questions to ask to obtain this information). The history should include

1. Medical history, including information on cardiovascular disease; pulmonary disease; gastrointestinal disease; renal disease; neurologic disease; cancer; endocrine disease; ear, nose, and throat disease; liver disease; skin disease; chickenpox or shingles; viral hepatitis; bacterial infections; gynecologic problems; exposure to tuberculosis; and psychiatric treatment (outpatient or inpatient treatment).

2. Current medications and treatments: Over-the-counter drugs, vitamins, and, especially, immunosuppressive therapy (e.g., in an asthmatic patient who intermittently requires corticosteroids).

3. Identification of when a patient's acute HIV illness occurred, which may be helpful in determining the patient's prognosis.

   a. At least half of all HIV-positive patients may report a history of acute HIV infection, which presents clinically as a mild to severe mononucleosis-like illness lasting 1 to 2 weeks.

   b. The incubation period (time from exposure to onset of illness) for the acute syndromes may range from 5 days to 3 months but is usually 2 to 4 weeks.

   c. Symptoms include fever, diaphoresis, malaise, myalgia, arthralgia, pharyngitis, retro-orbital headaches, and, in some patients, lymphadenopathy or aseptic meningitis.

   d. Other less common manifestations of acute HIV infection include a history of polyneuropathy, brachial neuritis, and odynophagia with esophageal ulcers.

4. Common HIV-related illnesses: Oral candidiasis (thrush), persistent diarrhea, varicella zoster (shingles), oral hairy leukoplakia, *Pneumocystis carinii* pneumonia, recurrent bacterial pneumonia (in 12 months), cryptococcal meningitis, toxoplasmosis, Kaposi's sarcoma, candidal esophagitis, disseminated *Mycobacterium avium* complex, CMV infection, and tuberculosis.

5. HIV-related symptoms: Fever; night sweats; changes in sleep pattern; changes in appetite; weight loss; stomach pain; vomiting; diarrhea; skin rashes or lesions; oral thrush or ulceration; painful swallowing; swollen lymph nodes; unusual headaches; difficulty thinking; chest pain; cough; shortness of breath; numbness or tingling in hands or feet; muscle

weakness; changes in vision; and changes in neurologic function or mental status.

6. Vaccination history: Measles/mumps/rubella (MMR), last tetanus booster, hepatitis B, and pneumococcal vaccine.

   a. Tuberculosis history should include information on any known exposure to tuberculosis, date of last purified protein derivative (PPD) test, history of positive PPD test result. If positive, was prophylaxis given? If yes, what was the duration and type?

7. Sexually transmitted diseases: Information about possible contact with syphilis, gonorrhea, genital herpes, chlamydia, condyloma (warts), gastrointestinal parasites, hepatitis B, and trichomoniasis. The history should also include

   a. Questions about where the patient has lived and traveled.

   b. Questions about current sexual practices (type and number of sexual partners). Specifically, a sexual history should be taken to assess the patient's current sexual practices and to determine whether sexual partners are aware of the patient's possible HIV status and have been tested for HIV.

   c. Questions about the types of contraception used.

   d. Questions about past or present IV drug use.

   e. Questions about behaviors that might lead to further transmission of HIV.

8. Drug use: Active IV drug users should be asked about their drug-using practices; their source of needles; whether they share needles and, if so, with whom.

9. Psychosocial history.

   a. Depression is common among HIV-infected patients, and the history should include questions that focus on changes in

      (1) Mood.

      (2) Libido.

      (3) Sleeping patterns.

      (4) Appetite.

      (5) Concentration.

      (6) Memory.

   b. Patients should also be asked specifically about whom they have informed of their HIV status, how they have been coping with the diagnosis of HIV infection, and what types of support they have been receiving.

   c. It is important to know about the patient's family, living situation, and work environment and how these have been affected by the diagnosis of HIV infection.

10. Assessment of the patient's level of awareness about HIV infection and treatment.
    a. Evaluate the patient's educational needs, and determine the form that such support might take.
    b. Assessment of patient education should include information on safer sex guidelines, use of condoms and spermicide, and safe versus unsafe practices.
    c. Drug use and abuse must be discussed and must include issues of needle sharing, the use of bleach, and drug treatment options.

IX. **Sample questions and screening tools.**
   A. General initial history.
      1. Sexual activity: When were you last sexually active? Have you had sex in the past few months?
      2. Sexual orientation: Are you intimate with males, females, or both?
      3. Number of partners: How many sexual partners do you or did you have? How long have you been with your current partner? Quantify the number and sex of sexual partners over the past few months or years.
      4. Types of sexual activity: Do you or did you have vaginal, anal, or oral sex? If anal or oral, ask "Do you give it or receive it, or both?"
      5. Pregnancy and contraception: Do you desire to become (make your partner) pregnant? Is it possible that you are (she is) pregnant now? What are you doing to prevent pregnancy?
      6. Sexually transmitted diseases: Do you have vaginal discharge, itching, or pain on urination? Do you have any sores or lumps? Have you or any of your partners ever been treated for a sexually transmitted disease? Which one? How long ago? Do you or any of your partners have risk factors for HIV or acquired immunodeficiency syndrome (AIDS), such as blood transfusions, IV drug use, frequent sex with multiple partners or strangers, sex for money or drugs?
      7. Protection from sexually transmitted diseases: Do you or did you use a condom or other protection during sex or when you have had sex in the past? If no, ask: Why not? Do you ever have sex without protection? How recently?
      8. Violence and abuse: Have you ever been hurt or abused by your partner? Have you ever been raped? If the answer is "yes," assess the situation.

9. Satisfaction: Is sex satisfying for you? If no, ask: Why not?
10. Sexual concerns: Do you have any problems with or concerns about your sexual function?

B. Comprehensive adolescent sexual history.

1. Background data: Age (birth date); parents' ages; parents' religion; parents' educational levels; parents' occupations; parents' marital status; amount of affection in relationship (parent to parent); feelings toward parent or parents.

2. Childhood sexuality: What were your parents' attitudes about sexuality when you were a child? In what way did your parents handle nudity? Who taught you about sex? From whom did you learn about sex play, pregnancy, intercourse, masturbation, homosexuality, venereal disease, birth? When do you first recall seeing a nude person of the same sex? Of the opposite sex? How often did you play doctor–nurse or engage in other sex play with another child? Tell me about any other sexual activity or experience that had a strong effect on you.

3. Adolescent sexuality: How old were you at your first period? Onset of breast development? When did pubic hair appear? What were the characteristics of onset of menstruation (age, regularity of periods; initially, now)? What hygienic method do you/did you use (pads, tampons)? How were you prepared for menstruation? By whom? What were your feelings about early periods? Later periods? Have you had unusual bleeding?

4. Body image: How do you feel about your body? What about your breasts and genitals? How much time do you spend nude in front of a mirror?

5. Masturbation: How old were you when you began? What were others' reactions to your masturbation? What methods do you use? What are your feelings about masturbation? Do you fear that you are overdoing it?

6. Necking and petting: How old were you when you began? How often? How many partners do you currently have?

7. Intercourse: How often have you had intercourse? How many partners? How often do you initiate sex? How often are you currently having sex? How often have you had oral sex?

8. Contraceptive use: What kind of contraceptives have you used? What are you using now?

9. Homosexuality: What does it mean to you to be homosexual? How many homosexual persons have you known? How often have you had homosexual feelings? Have you and how

often have you been approached? How often have you had homosexual experiences? What kinds of experiences? What were the circumstances?

10. Seduction and rape: When have you seduced someone sexually? When has someone seduced you? Have you been raped? Have you raped someone? How often have you forced someone to have sex?

11. Incest and abuse: What kinds of touching did you receive in your home? From your mother? Father? Brother? Sister? Other relatives?

12. Prostitution: What feelings do you have about prostitution? Have you ever accepted money for sex?

13. Venereal disease: How old were you when you learned about venereal disease? Have you ever had a venereal disease? Gonorrhea? Syphilis?

14. Pregnancy: Have you ever been pregnant? At what age? How was the pregnancy resolved—miscarriage, abortion, adoption, marriage, single parenthood?

15. Abortion: What are your feelings about abortion? Have you had an abortion? If yes, at what age? What were your feelings? What about your feelings now? What about your feelings immediately afterward? What about your feelings after 1 year?

C. Content areas of reproductive health history for adolescent females.

   1. Menarche.

     a. Age of onset.

     b. Duration of flow: How many days do your periods usually last?

     c. Frequency: How often do you have your periods? Do you keep track of them by using a calendar?

     d. Date of last normal menstrual period (LNMP): When was the date of your LNMP?

     e. Dysmenorrhea: During your periods, do you ever have cramps? If so, does it affect your activities or school attendance? Do you use any remedies and medications? What is the name of the drug, the dosage, and the frequency of ingestion?

   2. Sexual activity.

     a. Age of sexual debut: Have you had in the past or are you currently having sex? If so, at what age did you have your first sexual experience? (Some youths may not have initiated intercourse and are seeking services before sexual debut [volitional or coerced]). Has anyone ever touched you on any part of your body where you did not want to be touched? (Issues of past sexual abuse or date rape by an acquaintance may be important areas of discussion.)

b. Sexual orientation: Who do you find yourself most attracted to, men or women, or both? (Allows youth to respond to feelings of attraction and does not connote a behavior such as actually having intercourse with a same-sex individual.) Have you ever had sex or been sexually intimate with a person of your sex?

c. Frequency of coitus: How often do you have sex? Once a month? Once a week? Twice a week? (Allow adolescents a range of choices.) What was the last episode of intercourse?

d. Number of sexual partners: How many partners have you had in the past 2 months? How many in the past year? How many since you first started having sex? Have you had prior sexual contact with a sexual partner or intravenous drug user?

e. Sexual practices: Include questions that involve a full range of sexual expression, including activities such as kissing, touching, masturbation (solo or mutual) to oral, vaginal, and anal intercourse. To counsel youth regarding safer sex practices, the clinician must be aware of the teen's entire repertoire of behaviors.

f. Sexual pleasure: Is having intercourse or sex pleasurable for you? Are you satisfied with your sexual life the way it is now? Do you think your partner is satisfied?

3. Contraceptive use.

a. Current method of birth control used: It may be helpful to list the choice of specific methods (e.g., foam, condoms, withdrawal or "pulling out," birth control pill). Ask the teen the frequency with which she uses a method (e.g., never, sometimes, always). Ask whether she has any perceived or real side effects from using a specific method. Ask whether a condom is used with new partners.

b. Communication skills regarding use of contraception: Are condoms or other barrier methods used as a method of fertility control or to prevent the transmission of sexually transmitted diseases?

4. Obstetric and gynecologic.
   a. Number of pregnancies: List the exact number and out-
      come, including number of live births and spontaneous
      and therapeutic abortions.
   b. Recent gynecologic procedures: Dilation and curettage
      (D & C), recent abortion, complications after the
      procedure.
   c. History of pelvic inflammatory disease: When did the dis-
      ease occur, and where was it treated? Did you have inpa-
      tient or outpatient management?
5. Sexually transmitted diseases.
   a. History of previous sexually transmitted disease: Type,
      date, type of treatment. Was your partner treated?
6. Drugs.
   a. Onset, duration, and frequency of use: Ask about the use
      of cigarettes, alcohol, or illicit drugs. Ask about intrave-
      nous or injection drug use. Inclusion of this information
      is essential in the assessment of behaviors that may place
      the client at risk for HIV infection.
7. Partner.
   a. Partner involvement: Is the adolescent female's partner in-
      volved in the visit today? Was there prior discussion re-
      garding contraception or other topics?
   b. Male partner sexually transmitted disease assessment:
      Ask whether the male partner has any symptoms of infec-
      tion. Include symptoms of urethritis (discharge or dys-
      uria), any open sores, or warts on the genital region.
8. Support system.
   a. Parents and friends: Who is aware of your sexual activity?
      Have you experienced any potential negative effects re-
      garding disclosure of your behavior to parents or friends?
      Have you had any support?
D. Adolescent sexual problem history.
   1. Have the adolescent describe the sexual concern, problem, is-
      sue, or difficulty: How do you feel about discussing this
      problem? How long have you had it? When did this problem
      begin? What do you think caused you to have this problem?
      What might be contributing to this problem? What kinds of
      things have you done to treat or solve this problem? What
      health professionals have you seen? What, if any, medica-
      tion have you taken or are you taking? Have you talked to a
      friend or relative? Have you read any books to solve this
      problem? What books?

APPENDIX (3.1)

Sample Prenatal Genetic Screen

1. Will you be 35 years or older when the baby is   Yes ❐   No ❐
   due?

2. Have you or has the baby's father or anyone
   in either of your families ever had any of the
   following disorders?
   Down syndrome (mongolism)   Yes ❐   No ❐
   Other chromosomal abnormality   Yes ❐   No ❐
   Neural tube defect, spina bifida   Yes ❐   No ❐
   (meningomyelocele or open spine), anencephaly
   Hemophilia   Yes ❐   No ❐
   Muscular dystrophy   Yes ❐   No ❐
   Cystic fibrosis   Yes ❐   No ❐
   If yes, indicate the relationship of the affected person
   to you or to the baby's father:

3. Do you or does the baby's father have a   Yes ❐   No ❐
   birth defect:
   If yes, who has the defect and what is it?

4. In any previous marriages, have you or has the   Yes ❐   No ❐
   baby's father had a child, born dead or alive,
   with a birth defect not listed in Question 2?
   If yes, what was the defect and who had it?

5. Do you or does the baby's father have any close   Yes ❐   No ❐
   relatives with mental retardation?
   If yes, indicate the relationship of the affected person
   to you or to the baby's father: Indicate the cause, if known:

6. Do you or does the baby's father or a close relative   Yes ❐   No ❐
   in either of your families have a birth defect, any
   familial disorder, or a chromosomal abnormality
   not listed above?
   If yes, indicate the condition and the relationship of the
   affected person to you or to the baby's father:

7. In any previous marriages, have you or has the   Yes ❐   No ❐
   baby's father had a stillborn child or three or more
   first trimester spontaneous pregnancy losses?

8. Have either of you undergone a chromosomal   Yes ❐   No ❐
   study?
   If yes, indicate who and the results:

9. If you or the baby's father is of Jewish ancestry,   Yes ❐   No ❐
   have either of you been screened for Tay-Sachs
   disease?
   If yes, indicate who and the results:

10. If you or the baby's father is Black, have either of   Yes ❐   No ❐
    you been screened for sickle cell trait?
    If yes, indicate who and the results:

11. If you or the baby's father is of Italian, Greek, or   Yes ❐   No ❐
    Mediterranean background, have either of you
    been tested for beta thalassemia?
    If yes, indicate who and the results:

12. If you or the baby's father is of Philippine or South-   Yes ❐   No ❐
    east Asian ancestry, have either of you been tested
    for alpha thalassemia?
    If yes, indicate who and the results:

13. Excluding iron and vitamins, have you taken any   Yes ❐   No ❐
medications or recreational drugs since being preg-
nant or since your last menstrual period? (Include
nonprescription drugs.)
*If yes, give name of medication and time taken
during pregnancy:*

Environmental Exposure History Form

1. Have you ever worked at a job or a hobby in which you came in contact with any of the following by breathing, touching, or ingesting (swallowing)? If yes, please place a check beside the name.

Acids	Ethylene dichloride	Rock dust
Alcohols (industrial)	Fiberglas	Silica powder
Alkalies	Halothane	Solvents
Ammonia	Isocyanates	Styrene
Arsenic	Ketones	Talc
Asbestos	Lead	Toluene
Benzene	Manganese	TDI (toluene
Beryllium	Mercury	diisocyanate)
Cadmium	Methylene chloride	or MDI (methy-
Carbon tetrachloride	Nickel	lenediphenyl
Chlorinated naphthalenes	PBBs	diisocyanate)
Chloroform	PCBs	Trichloroethylene
Chloroprene	Perchloroethylene	Trinitrotoluene
Chromates	Pesticides	Vinyl chloride
Coal dust	Phenol	Welding fumes
Dichlorobenzene	Phosgene	X-rays
Ethylene dibromide	Radiation	Other (specify)

2. Do you live next to or near an industrial plant, commercial business, dump site, or nonresidential property?

3. Which of the following do you have in your home? *Please circle those that apply.*

Air conditioner	Electric stove (gas or oil?)
Air purifier	Wood stove
Central heating	Humidifier
Gas stove	Fireplace

4. Have you recently acquired new furniture or carpet, refinished furniture, or remodeled your home?

5. Have you weatherized your home recently?

6. Are pesticides or herbicides (bug or weed killers; flea and tick sprays, collars, powders, or shampoos) used in your home or garden, or on pets?

7. Do you (or any household member) have a hobby or craft?

8. Do you work on your car?

9. Have you ever changed your residence because of a health problem?

10. Does your drinking water come from a private well, city water supply, or grocery store?

11. Approximately what year was your home built?

If you answered *yes* to any of the questions, please explain.

APPENDIX **3.3**

Summary of Critical Issues in the HIV Initial History

HIV testing.

When did the patient first have a positive test result for HIV?

Where was the first test conducted that resulted in positive HIV status?

What was the reason for being tested?

Does the patient have documentation of a positive enzyme-linked immunosorbent assay (ELISA) and Western blot test results?

Has patient ever had a negative HIV test result?

What is the patient's usual source of health care?

What is the patient's most recent CD4 cell count (if known)?

Medical history.

Cardiovascular disease

Pulmonary disease

Gastrointestinal disease

Renal disease

Neurologic disease

Cancer

Endocrine disease

Ear, nose, and throat disease

Liver disease

Obstetric and gynecologic illness

Skin disease

Chickenpox or shingles (varicella)

Psychiatric treatment

HIV-related illnesses.

Oral candidiasis (thrush)

Persistent diarrhea

Varicella zoster (shingles)

Oral hairy leukoplakia

Pneumocystis carinii pneumonia

Recurrent bacterial pneumonia (in 12-month period)

Cryptococcal meningitis

Toxoplasmosis

Kaposi sarcoma

Candidal esophagitis

Disseminated *Mycobacterium avium* complex

Cytomegalovirus (CMV) infection

Tuberculosis

Invasive cervical cancer

Other HIV-related illnesses

Vaccination history.

Measles-mumps-rubella (MMR)

Last tetanus booster

Hepatitis B

Hepatitis A

Pneumococcal vaccine

Tuberculosis history.

Any known exposure to *M. tuberculosis*

Date of last purified protein derivative (PPD) test

History of positive PPD test result?

If yes, was prophylaxis given?

If yes, duration and type.

Sexually transmitted diseases.

Syphilis

Gonorrhea

Genital herpes

Chlamydia (nongonococcal urethritis [NGU] or cervicitis)

Condyloma (warts)

Gastrointestinal parasites

Hepatitis B

Trichomoniasis

Pelvic inflammatory disease (PID)

Gynecologic history.

Has the patient ever been pregnant?

If yes, how many:

Full-term pregnancies

Premature births

Miscarriages or abortions

Living children

Have there been any pregnancies since the patient has learned of her HIV status?

What was the beginning date of the client's last menstrual period.

Was the last menstrual period normal?

Is the patient pregnant now?

If yes, was a prenatal care referral made?

Does the patient use a birth control method?

If yes, specify what type.

When was the patient's last Pap test? Was it normal?

Medication.

Current medications and treatments (include over-the-counter drugs and vitamins).

Habits.

Does the patient smoke or has the patient smoked in the past? (Inquire about quantity.)

Does the patient use alcohol or has the patient used alcohol in the past? (Inquire about quantity.)

Does the patient use drugs or has the patient used drugs in the past? (Specify what type and the quantity used.)

HIV transmission category.

Homosexual contact

Heterosexual contact

Injection drug use

Transfusion recipients (dates and location)

Hemophilia

Unknown

Patient education.

Safe-sex guidelines (condoms, spermicide); safe versus unsafe practices.

Is the patient sexually active?

If yes, is the partner or partners aware of the patient's status?

Have the partner or partners been tested for HIV?

If so, were the results positive? (Inquire about drug use [needle sharing, bleach]).

Was treatment referral offered?

Review of systems.

Has the patient had any of the following symptoms in the last 3 months?

Unexplained weight loss

Swollen lymph nodes

Night sweats

Fevers

Unusual headaches

Changes in appetite or sleep pattern

Trouble thinking

New skin rash or spots on the skin

Sores or white spots in the mouth

Pain when swallowing

Chest pain, cough, or shortness of breath

Stomach pain

Vomiting or diarrhea

Numbness or tingling in the hands or feet

Muscle weakness

Changes in vision

CHAPTER 4

The Physical Examination

Helen A. Carcio

I. **A complete physical examination is an integral part of the health assessment of women. Components of the examination include assessment of:**
   A. The thyroid gland.
   B. Body habitus, including fat and hair distribution.
   C. Breast examination (see chapter 6).
   D. Abdominal examination.
   E. Pelvic examination.

II. **The examination of the thyroid gland. Thyroid dysfunction can cause irregular menses, anovulation, and infertility.**
   A. Anterior approach: Examiner stands in front of the patient.
      1. The woman is asked to extend her head and neck slightly.
      2. As the woman swallows, using your finger pads, palpate below the cricoid cartilage for the isthmus of the thyroid.
      3. Ask the woman to flex her head and neck slightly forward to her right. This relaxes the sternocleidomastoid muscles, enhancing palpation.
      4. Place right examining thumb on upper portion of the left lobe, and displace the gland to anatomic right, while hooking the tips of the index and middle fingers of left hand behind right sternocleidomastoid muscle, and palpate deeply in front of the muscle with left thumb for the right lobe.

    5. Reverse and repeat procedure for the left side.

    6. The isthmus may be palpable, but the thyroid gland itself is usually not visible or palpable.

  B. Posterior approach.

    1. Examiner stands behind the patient, who is seated.

    2. Instruct patient to slightly flex her chin toward her chest.

    3. Place fingerpads of both hands around the patient's neck.

    4. Palpate the isthmus by placing fingerpads in the midline of the neck, below the cricoid cartilage.

    5. Compare the right and left lobes by sliding your fingerpads laterally, below the cricoid cartilage, on either side of the tracheal rings.

    6. Ask the patient to tilt her head to the left as you displace the right lobe to the left (medially) with the right hand.

    7. Palpate the left lobe as patient swallows using the fingerpads of the left hand.

    8. Reverse the procedure to examine the right lobe.

  C. Thyroid-stimulating hormone (TSH) testing is indicated if

    1. Anomaly of the thyroid gland is palpated.

    2. In the presence of associated signs or symptoms.

    3. During an infertility work-up as indicated.

    4. If galactorrhea is present or hyperprolactinemia is suspected. (Hypothyroidism is present in 3 to 5% of women with hyperprolactinemia.)

  D. Note.

    1. Motion of isthmus as the woman swallows. Thyroid tissue rises with swallowing; this movement is noticeable with an enlarged gland

    2. Compare lobes for contour, consistency, or tenderness as the patient swallows.

  E. Normal findings.

    1. The thyroid gland is usually not palpable.

    2. The isthmus may be felt as a band of tissue that obliterates the tracheal rings.

    3. No nodules or enlargement of the lobes should be felt.

III. The breast examination (see chapter 6).

IV. Abdominal examination.

  A. A thorough abdominal examination should precede the gynecologic examination and includes assessing any palpable masses or tenderness, including inguinal lymph nodes.

  B. Conducting the abdominal exam before the gynecologic examination often helps reduce some of the anxiety associated with having the gynecologic examination and may serve to "break the ice." Make sure hands are warm!

C. Position.

  1. Supine, with examiner on right.

  2. Closely monitor the woman's expressions for signs of discomfort.

D. If the woman is ticklish, begin examination with her hand under the examiner's hand.

E. Inspect the abdomen for diastasis recti.

  1. Is there a separation of the abdominal rectus muscles from pregnancy, multiparity, congenital weakness, or marked obesity?

     a. Ask the patient to raise her head and hold it above the pillow for 5 seconds, tensing the abdominal muscles.

     b. Note the location and length of any midline separation between the contracted muscles.

     c. Abdominal muscles should be tight together.

F. Inspect the contour and shape of the abdomen.

G. Observe for the presence of striae.

  1. Striae are lines seen after normal skin has been excessively stretched.

     a. Linea alba from the stretching of the skin from pregnancy.

     b. Purple lines associated with Cushing's disease.

H. Palpate the lower abdomen for tenderness in the presence of pelvic pain.

I. Palpate the inguinal lymph nodes.

  1. The nodes may be enlarged in the presence of herpes simplex virus.

     a. Note size, shape, mobility, consistency, temperature, and tenderness of the nodes. Refer for any hard, immobile nodes.

     b. Nodes are soft and tender in a patient with herpes.

V. The pelvic examination explained.

A. The approach.

  1. The approach to the gynecologic examination must be systematic, thorough, and carried out in a calm, relaxed manner. Encourage the woman to give verbal feedback throughout the examination.

  2. The pelvic examination should follow other parts of the

physical examination in order to allow the woman time to become comfortable with the examiner. However, sometimes the woman is so anxious that it is best to proceed with the examination first to "get it over with."

3. Ask the patient to empty her bladder before the examination.

4. Determine whether this is her first pelvic examination. A woman undergoing a first pelvic examination is far more anxious than a woman who has undergone the examination previously. (Also remember that anxiety can increase if any previous pelvic examination was not a positive experience.)

5. Observe for signs that indicate increased anxiety as the client assumes the supine position. For example, the patient:
   a. Holds or wrings hands.
   b. Covers eyes or has eyes shut.
   c. Places hands on shoulders.
   d. Places hands over pelvis.
   e. Places hands on thighs.
   f. Places hands so she can hold the table.

6. Explain each aspect of the examination thoroughly before and as it is performed in order to reduce the woman's level of anxiety. Always be as gentle as possible.
   a. Explain the rationale for each aspect of the examination, and provide information about what a woman might feel during the examination. (e.g., "you might feel some pressure when I insert my fingers into your vagina").
   b. Suggest coping strategies to deal with any stress the woman may be experiencing.
   c. Encourage patient to progressively relax different body parts or to try taking deep breaths and exhaling slowly at any point during the examination that she might feel tense.
   d. May teach how to use statements to herself such as "I know this is uncomfortable but I will be fine."
   e. Reassure her that you will stop anytime she becomes uncomfortable.

7. It is often a good idea to offer an "educational" pelvic examination, by explaining about the techniques used, the sensations that the patient may feel, and the function of body parts examined.

8. Offer the patient a mirror (a telescoping handled type is best) so she can view her vulvar area. Such measures help

Table 4.1   **Alternatives to the Traditional Pelvic Examination**

Alternative Examination	Reason
Bimanual examination without use of speculum	Only indicated for patients at low risk Perform a bimanual examination Digitally locate cervix Slide cotton swab adjacent to finger Rotate the swab over cervix several times Preliminary data support efficacy despite lack of endo-cervical component
Ultrasound	Virginal woman at low risk Can identify other problems such as uterine fibroids or ovarian cysts
Sedation	Recommended for the disabled woman who cannot tolerate the examination; may use: 2–8 mg/kg ketamine, 0.2–0.4 mg/kg midazolam

patients feel more in control at a time when they may feel especially vulnerable and apprehensive.

    a. Some women are very interested in seeing their cervix, whereas others are not interested or are even "turned-off."

  9. The woman should be encouraged to give verbal feedback throughout the examination so that the examiner can be informed of any maneuvers that cause particular discomfort. This feedback will help maximize the client's cooperation and minimize anxiety regarding the examination.

 10. Explain that the whole examination should take no longer than a few minutes.

 11. Acknowledge that the woman may feel rather awkward, but she should not experience any pain unless certain conditions are present such as herpes.

 12. May offer alternative to the traditional pelvic examination (Table 4.1).

 13. Table 4.2 summarizes common pelvic examination problems.

 B. Draping.

  1. The issue of draping can be left to the woman.

  2. If draping is used, the drape should cover the patient's lower abdomen and thighs.

  3. The drape should be depressed in between the knees in

Table 4.2 **Common Pelvic Examination Problems and Interventions**

Pelvic Examination Problem	Interventions
Extreme anxiety	Step-by-step desensitization, relaxation techniques, deep breathing, Kegel then bear down, antianxiety meds, counseling
Inability to insert speculum due to discomfort	Use Pederson or small speculum, or Use a small swab to collect samples for Pap, STIs, wet mount, deep breathing Consider urine testing for STIs
Inability to insert speculum due to dryness	Palpate introital tissues, or palpate cervix before speculum insertion Apply scant lubricant to tip of speculum
Inability to insert speculum due to small and/or tight introitus	Use small, Pederson speculum or nasal speculum, Kegel and bear down, or use dacron swab, encourage deep/slow breathing
Inability to visualize cervix	Palpate cervix before speculum exam, move speculum side to side (shimmy), change angle slightly, instruct patient to bear down, try larger speculum, open wider
Vaginal walls impede visualizing cervix	Apply condom over speculum (cut off tip) Use larger blade speculum like Graves or Clinton Graves, open wide Guttman or "Snowman" lateral vaginal wall retractor
Inability to view cervix because of extreme posterior position	Use large, extra long speculum, open wide Like "Clinton Pederson" style Palpate cervix before Push down on suprapubic area Instruct patient to bear down Lift hips, spread thighs, knee stirrups
Speculum comes out unless clinician holds it	Seek an assistant to hold the speculum while you collect specimens, remove speculum, then prepare tests
Patient unable to tolerate speculum in situ secondary to anxiety and/or pain	Collect samples, remove speculum, then prepare tests. Remember, samples are stable on sampling tools
History of sexual abuse and extreme phobia of pelvic exams—with or without vaginismus	Co-manage with a specialized counselor Use step by step desensitization program May not be able to complete a pelvic exam for several visits (may take months or years)

Mimi Clarke Secor © 2009.

Advantages of the Sitting Position During a Pelvic Examination	**BOX 4.1**

More comfortable for the patient
Relaxes the rectus and abdominal muscles
Increases eye contact
Allows the woman to hold the mirror more easily
Enables her to feel less vulnerable

order to allow the patient and examiner an opportunity to see each other's faces.

    4. It often helps to have the sheet draped so that the corner forms a triangle between the legs.

C. Position: The patient should be asked to assume a comfortable li-thotomy position on the examination table.

    1. For some women, the semisitting position is often preferable to the supine. Advantages of this position are summarized in Box 4.1.

    2. Position the patient's legs in the stirrups, with buttocks slightly overhanging the end of the table.

    3. The patient should be asked to keep her knees widely separated and her buttocks flat on the table. Women tend to push against their heels in the stirrups, unknowingly raising the buttocks off the table and tightening. Remind the patient to take the pressure off her heels.

    4. The woman's hands should be across her chest or at her sides. These positions help enhance abdominal relaxation.

D. Equipment.

    1. A good light, either freestanding or attached to a plastic speculum.

    2. Vaginal speculum (metal or plastic).

    3. Water-soluble lubricant (not always necessary).

    4. Supplies for the Pap smear and cultures as indicated. Note: Gloves should be worn throughout the examination and afterward when handling any equipment used. Some authorities recommend double gloving.

VI. Inspection of the external genitalia.

    A. Some comments.

        1. Examination of the external genitalia is conducted before the internal speculum and bimanual examinations.

2. The examiner should sit on a stool at the end of the table facing the client.
3. Position the light to obtain maximum illumination of the peritoneum.
4. Inspection begins by viewing the suprapubic and inguinal regions superiorly, then progressing inferiorly to include the clitoral hood, clitoris, urethral meatus, vaginal introitus, fourchette, and posteriorly, the anal and sacral areas.
5. Visual inspection of the genitals is also conducted in a medial to lateral fashion, from the vaginal introitus laterally to the labia minora, labia majora, and upper and inner thigh regions. A thorough visual inspection also includes gentle palpation as needed to view overlapping tissues.
6. A saline-moistened cotton-tipped applicator may also be used to separate overlapping skin surfaces (and to assess for areas of tenderness) and is particularly helpful in examining the labia and introital and hymenal structures.
7. Always remember to touch the thigh gently before actually touching the genitals.

B. Assess the mons pubis to determine the dermatologic condition of the pubic hair and underlying skin.
   1. Note general hygiene, hair distribution, and any lesions.
   2. Normal findings: Clean, coarse pubic hair extending in an inverse triangle, with the base over the mons pubis. No lesions should be present.
   3. Clinical alterations.
      a. Dirty-appearing hair shafts from pediculosis.
      b. Localized inflammation at the base of the hair shaft caused by folliculitis.
      c. Scaly epidermal plaques from psoriasis.
      d. Sparse hair associated with hormonal problems or advancing age.
      e. Racial variations.
         (1) Blacks. Shorter hair that is more tightly coiled.
         (2) Asians, Native Americans, and Alaskan Natives. Hair is generally sparser.
      f. *Phthirus pubis* (lice) or their eggs (nits). Bites seen as small red maculopapules.

C. Tanner staging.
   1. Pubic hair growth begins between 8 and 14 years of age.
   2. Staging should be assessed in adolescent girls as an assessment of the maturity of the pituitary-ovarian axis. It should be performed as routinely as possible.

D. Quantify the signs of androgen excess.

(a) few and scattered elements not thickly grown or settled

1. *Hirsutism* is defined as the presence of hair in a location where hair is not commonly found in women. Hair varies due to ethnic and racial factors.
2. Hair morphology and distribution should be graded. The most functional and widely used instrument is the Farriman-Galloway (F-G) scale, which semiquantitatively grades hair growth in nine body areas.
3. Cinical alterations.
   a. More than 10% of adult women have hair that extends up the abdomen to the umbilicus. This distribution is usually associated with racial variations.
   b. Absent or scant hair distribution may indicate endocrine dysfunction.
   c. Mild hirsutism associated with polycystic ovarian syndrome (sideburns, chin, chest, and lower abdomen).

E. Inspect the vulva for genital lesions.
   1. Note cysts, warts, chancres, ulcerations, and areas of hyperpigmentation.
   2. Normal findings: Labia majora are hair-covered epidermal surfaces; labia minora are pink, glistening mucosal surfaces. Hart's line is present.
   3. Clinical alterations.
      a. Nontender, firm nodules of sebaceous cysts.
      b. Micropapillomatosis labialis.
         (1) Can be differentiated from condyloma, in which multiple papillae converge toward a single base, each finger-like papillomatous projection having its own base.
         (2) Often related to chronic infections such as trichomonas or candidiasis.
      c. Wartlike protrusion singly or in clusters from condyloma acuminatum or condyloma latum.
      d. Genital warts.
      e. Round, clear umbilicated vesicles of molluscum contagiosum.
      f. Nontender chancre with a well-demarcated border from primary syphilis.
      g. Chancroid.
      h. Single or clustered, tender vesicles or ulcerations of genital herpes.
      i. Irregular, nontender hyperpigmented lesions related to carcinoma of the vulva.
      j. Genital mutilation associated with certain cultures.
      k. Varicosities associated with pelvic congestion (pregnancy).

F. Inspect the vulva for discoloration and pigmentation.

1. Normal findings: Pink with varying shades of white, brown and red, depending on racial characteristics.
   a. Usually the same color as the skin covering the external parts of the rest of the body.
   b. Color due to fine network of superficial blood vessels located just below the thick epidermal layers of the skin, and the amount of melanin.
2. Clinical alterations.
   a. Redness or erythema occurring in response to inflammation.
      (1) A reddened vulva with no specific lesions suggests extensive vaginal discharge that is irritating the delicate vulvar skin.
      (2) Dilatation of blood vessels and edema occur in such inflammatory conditions as Candida infection, seborrheic dermatitis, and psoriasis.
   b. Dark or pigmented lesions usually caused by increase in the amount or concentration of melanin.
      (1) Dark lesions require biopsy study to exclude the diagnosis of malignant melanoma.
      (2) Most dark lesions are either harmless freckles or nevi.
      (3) Routinely monitor nevi because of their potential to develop into melanoma.
   c. White lesions are related to:
      (1) Decreased vascularity.
      (2) Depigmentation (decrease in melanocytes in the basal layer).
      (3) Changes in the keratin in the presence of moisture. (The presence of water turns the keratin white, as if a hand or foot was soaked in water for 10 to 20 minutes.)
      (4) Common conditions that cause white lesions are lichen sclerosus and squamous hyperplasia.
G. Examine the external genitalia for any bruises which might indicate sexual assault.
H. Examine the clitoris.
   1. Note the size.
   2. Normal findings: Round, pink erectile tissue under the fourchette. Approximately 2 cm (0.75 inch) in length and 0.5 cm in width.
   3. Clinical alterations.
      a. Enlargement in masculinizing conditions, excess testosterone secretions, and use of testosterone-containing medications.

       b. Atrophy to the point of disappearance with lichen sclerosis.

I. Inspect the urethral orifice.
    1. Note erythema or purulent discharge.
    2. Normal findings: Pink tissue without discharge.
    3. Clinical alterations.
        a. Caruncle associated with estrogen deprivation is seen as a small red protrusion through the orifice. It resembles a polyp.
        b. Prolapse of the urethral mucosa, which forms a swollen red ring around the urinary meatus. The condition is often associated with menopause.
        c. Leaking of urine associated with stress incontinence.

J. Examine the vaginal orifice.
    1. Note presence of discharge, hymen, and bulging of vaginal tissue or cervix through the orifice.
    2. Normal findings: Small amount of white to clear discharge; intact hymen or hymenal remnant surrounding the orifice; no bulging.
    3. Clinical alterations.
        a. Discharge secondary to vaginitis or cervicitis.
            (1) Perform wet mount evaluation on any discharge present (see chapter 10 on Vaginal Microscopy).
        b. Thick, pink membrane overlying the vaginal orifice from an imperforate hymen.
        c. Anterior bulging of vaginal tissue through the orifice from a cystocele.
            (1) A cystocele is the prolapse of the bladder against the anterior vaginal wall.
            (2) It is generally related to the weakening of vaginal and pelvic support by childbirth.
            (3) It is aggravated by obesity.
        d. Posterior bulging of the vaginal tissue from a rectocele.
            (1) A rectocele is the prolapse of the rectum against the posterior vaginal wall. It is generally related as above.
    4. It is sometimes useful to draw a diagram of any anomalies.

K. Inspect perineum and anus.
    1. Posterior skin of the perineum between the vaginal introitus and the anus should appear smooth.
    2. If woman had an episiotomy, a scar may be visible.
    3. Note any skin tags, fissures, or hemorrhoids in anal area.

VII. Palpation of the external genitalia.
  A. Some comments.

1. Avoid startling the patient, by telling her when she will be touched and where.
2. Palpation of the external genitalia is conducted using a gentle approach, and if tenderness is elicited, a cotton-tipped applicator may be used to assess more specifically the location and severity.
3. Placing the finger beneath the urethra along the anterior vaginal wall may help identify the presence of a urethral diverticulum or express any material that might be present in the Skene's glands.
4. During palpation of the introitus, obese and parous patients may also be asked to perform a Kegel contraction followed by a Valsalva maneuver to assess tone and laxity of the pelvic musculature and to detect any degree of cystocele or rectocele.
5. Avoid excessive "fingering" of the genitalia, which otherwise might be interpreted as sexual.

B. Assess Bartholin's glands and Skene's glands.
   1. Technique. Insert index finger into the vagina with thumb remaining outside on the posterior portion of the labia majora. Press thumb and index finger together at the 5 and 7 o'clock positions of the lateral labia minora.
   2. Note any swelling, masses, discharge, or tenderness.
   3. Normal findings: Skene's and Bartholin's glands are normally not palpable. The surface should be homogenous, nontender, and without discharge.
   4. Clinical alteration. Varying degrees of enlarged gland from a Bartholin's cyst. Marked warmth and tenderness may indicate an abscess.
   5. If discharge is present, a gonorrheal culture (GC) should be performed because gonorrhea may cause a Bartholin's abscess.

C. Assess paraurethral gland and urethra.
   1. The technique: Insert the gloved hand slowly into the vagina, palm upward. Exerting upward pressure, remove finger, milking the urethra
   2. Note discharge from the urethra or paraurethral glands, or any tenderness.
   3. Normal findings: Negative discharge.
   4. Clinical alteration: Purulent discharge related to gonococcal or chlamydial urethritis.

D. Evaluate vaginal wall support.

1. Technique: Spread the vaginal orifice with thumb and forefinger, and ask patient to bear down. Assess any degree of prolapse. You may also ask woman to cough.
2. Note any anterior or posterior bulging of the vaginal wall. Some leakage of urine from the urinary meatus may also be noted during this maneuver.
3. Normal finding: No protrusion through the vaginal orifice.
4. Clinical alterations.
   a. Anterior bulging of vaginal tissue in varying degrees through the introitus indicating a cystocele or cystourethrocele.
   b. Posterior bulging. A rectocele will balloon upward toward the introitus during the Valsalva maneuver.
   c. Cervix visible at the opening, which may indicate a uterine prolapse
E. Assess vaginal tone.
   1. Place two fingers into the vagina, and ask the woman to tighten her vaginal muscles or to squeeze the examiner's fingers.
   2. Examiner should feel upward pressure on the fingers.
   3. Normal findings: Maintains tension for 3 seconds.
   4. Clinical alteration. Impaired strength due to
      a. Vaginal deliveries (traumatic or multiple).
      b. Older age, particularly with decreased estrogen levels in women not receiving hormone replacement.
      c. Neurologic impairment such as multiple sclerosis.
   5. Impaired tone may cause urinary or fecal incontinence.

VIII. The bimanual examination.
A. Special considerations.
   1. Any pelvic mass detected during the bimanual examination should be described in terms of its position, motility, consistency and size in centimeters.
   2. It is very important for the patient to relax completely because voluntary guarding of the abdominal musculature will prevent effective palpation of any pelvic organs.
   3. Controversy exists regarding which portion of the pelvic examination should be performed next. Many clinicians believe that the bimanual examination should precede the speculum examination. There are many advantages (Box 4.2).
      a. This technique helps facilitate the insertion of the

Advantage of Performing the Bimanual
Examination Before the Speculum Examination

**BOX
4.2**

Able to use woman's own vaginal secretions for lubrication
Facilitates insertion of the speculum
Eliminates use of messy gels
Clues the examiner to palpated anomalies that require further inspection
Perceived by the patient as less invasive
Helps the inexperienced clinician determine the position of the cervix in
order to make insertion of the speculum and location of the cervix easier

speculum, because the woman's own vaginal secretions
can be used as a lubricant, thus eliminating the use of
messy gels.

b. Water applied to the gloved hand may be used in place of
a lubricant.

c. Once any anomalies are palpated, they can be thoroughly
inspected during the speculum examination. Most lesions
are better palpated than visually inspected within the
deep folds of the vagina.

d. When the bimanual examination is performed before the
speculum examination, the clinician can better determine
the position of the cervix, which makes the speculum insertion easier for both the patient and the clinician.

e. Gentle palpation may be perceived as less invasive to the
woman than inserting the speculum first.

f. A disadvantage of this technique is the possibility of mixing cervical and vaginal flora together, altering the accuracy of any subsequent vaginal microscopic analysis.

4. The bimanual examination involves using both hands, with
one inside the vagina and the other hand palpating the pelvic structure through the abdominal wall.

5. It is very important that the patient be relaxed during the bimanual examination because guarding and tightening of the
abdominal muscles will greatly alter the examiner's ability to
palpate the underlying structures beneath the rigid
musculature.

6. A metal speculum can be warmed by keeping it on a heating
pad or running it under warm water.

7. Some clinicians touch the blades of the speculum to the inside of the client's thigh before insertion to let the client

Advantages and Disadvantages of the Plastic (Disposable) Speculum

BOX 4.3

Advantages of the Plastic Speculum
Provides an unobstructed view of the vaginal walls through its clear blades
Eliminates the need to warm the speculum
Reduces patient anxiety because clear plastic is generally less "threatening" to patients than metal
More comfortable due to the rounded edges of the speculum blades
Can attach to a light source
If attached: enhances illumination of the cervix and vaginal walls
If attached: reduces risk of contamination of lamp from adjusting an external light source
Disadvantages of the Plastic Speculum
Accumulation of medical waste that needs to be disposed of
The speculum can break—it should not be used with obese or restless patients
A click occurs during the opening and closing of the blades that may startle the patient

know what it feels like and to be sure that the temperature is comfortable.

8. A virginal orifice easily admits a single examining finger. Modify the technique so as to use the index finger only. Should the orifice be too small, a single finger in the rectum can be used for a fairly accurate bimanual examination. Be sensitive to the invasiveness of the procedure.

9. Box 4.3 lists the advantages and disadvantages of using a plastic speculum.

B. Technique. Stand between stirrups.

1. Insert the index and middle fingers of your gloved hand, exerting firm pressure primarily downward. (The thumb should be abducted, with the ring and little finger flexed into the palm.)

C. Palpation of the cervix: The cervix should be palpated by sweeping the fingers around the protruding knob in the area of the fornices. Move knob back and forth.

1. The cervix should normally be able to be moved without discomfort.

2. Note depth and angle of the cervix.

   a. Should the cervix be markedly tilted to the right or left, or fixed, endometriosis or adhesions (or both) should be suspected.

3. Note size, shape, and consistency (like the tip of the nose).
4. Note any palpable lumps.
5. Clinical alterations.
   a. Presence of cervical motion tenderness (CMT), which is indicative of pelvic inflammatory disease.
   b. A fixed cervix due to endometriosis or a tumor displacing it.
   c. Small lumps associated with nabothian cysts.
   d. Prominent anterior lips from maternal use of diethylstilbestrol (DES).
   e. An anterior pointing cervix suggests a retroverted uterus.
   f. A posterior pointing cervix suggests an anteverted uterus.
   g. Projection of the cervix into the vagina more than 3 cm (1.2 inches) may indicate a pelvic or ovarian mass.
D. The vagina should be carefully palpated for tenderness, lesions, masses, or foreign bodies (e.g., forgotten tampons).
E. Palpation of the uterus.
   1. Some comments.
      a. The uterus is sometimes difficult to palpate effectively.
      b. It may not be palpable in an obese woman or in one whose abdominal muscles are tense and rigid.
      c. If the uterus is not palpable in a thin, relaxed woman, it may be absent, or tipped posteriorly (retroverted).
   2. The technique.
      a. Place the abdominal hand on the abdomen, midway between the umbilicus and the symphysis pubis.
      b. Insert the first and second fingers of the other hand into the vagina, with the palmar surface facing anteriorly.
      c. Apply firm pressure on the posterior surface of the cervix to ballot the uterus into the lower abdomen, raise the cervix upward against the abdominal palpating hand, and try to grasp the uterus between the two hands. Assess the uterus with the abdominal hand (Figure 4.1).
   3. Note anteflexed, retroflexed, anteverted, or retroverted position.
      a. The uterus is normally anteverted and slightly anteflexed.
      b. If it is retroverted and immobile, suspect endometriosis.
      c. A retroverted uterus is not palpable during a bimanual examination (Figure 4.2).
   4. Consistency, size, and shape.
      a. Mobility.
         (1) It should be normally mobile in the anteroposterior plane.

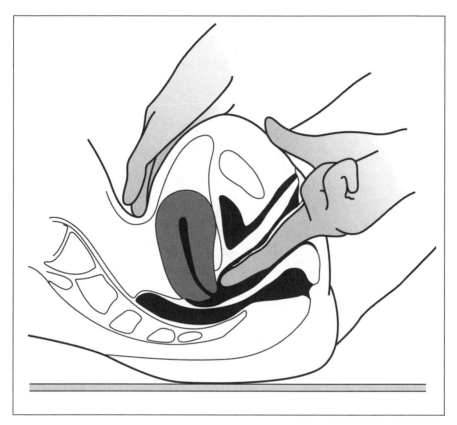

Figure 4.1 Bimanual palpation of an anteverted uterus. (Gray, R. H. [1980]. *Manual for the provision of intrauterine devices [IUDS]*. Geneva: World Health Organization.)

      (2) It has limited mobility in the transverse plane because it is held by the cardinal ligaments.

      (3) Immobility in the anteroposterior plane suggests scar tissue due to previous pelvic inflammatory disease, endometriosis, or surgery.

   b. Tenderness.

   c. Palpable masses.

   d. Normal findings: Smooth, firm surface; mobile, without tenderness of masses.

   e. Clinical alterations.

      (1) Soft enlargement from an intrauterine pregnancy.

      (2) Tenderness of the uterus suggesting possible infection, endometriosis, or pregnancy.

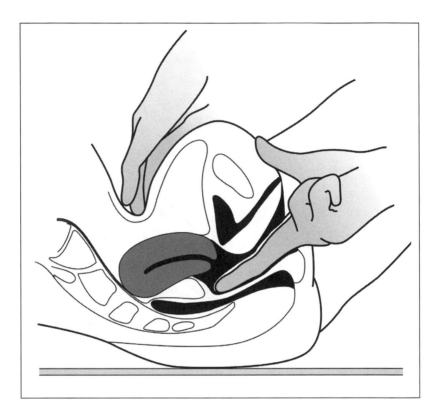

Figure 4.2 Bimanual palpation of a retroverted uterus. The examiner is unable to palpate the body of the uterus between the vaginal and abdominal examining fingers. (Gray, R. H. [1980]. *Manual for the provision of intrauterine devices [IUDS].* Geneva: World Health Organization.)

       (3) An irregular, firm uterus is related to the various shapes and positions of fibroids (Figure 4.3).
       (4) An immobile, tilted uterus is associated with endometriosis or an abdominal mass.

IX. Palpation of the ovaries and fallopian tubes.
    A. Some comments.
       1. The ovaries are small (the size of a thumbnail) and difficult to assess, particularly in the presence of extra adipose tissue or muscle rigidity. In endometriosis, the ovaries may be located behind the uterus, making them difficult to assess.
       2. The ovaries should not be palpable in postmenopausal

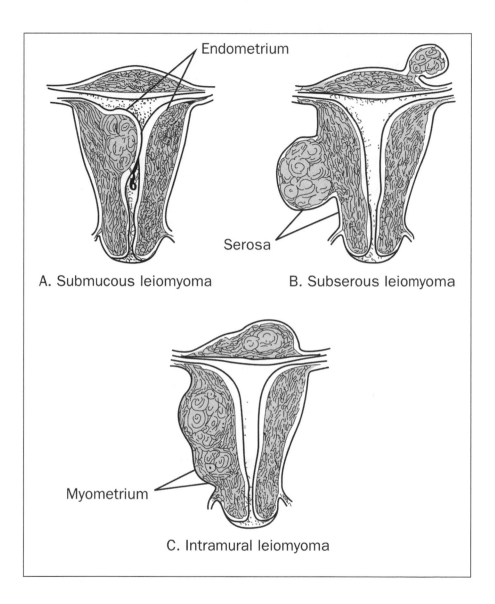

Figure 4.3 Appearance of uterine fibroids. (A) Submucous leiomyoma. (B) Subserous leiomyoma. (C) Intramural leiomyoma.

women; if they are palpated, they should be considered abnormal and should be investigated.

3. Advise the patient that there may be a fleeting sensation of discomfort when the ovaries are palpated.
4. The fallopian tubes are normally not palpable. If they are enlarged, the examiner should suspect salpingitis or an ectopic pregnancy.

B. The technique.
1. The ovaries are evaluated by first locating the vaginal fingers to either the right or left sides of the lateral fornix.
2. Move the abdominal hand to the lower abdominal quadrant on the same side as the internal hand.
3. Apply firm and steady pressure, beginning medially to the anterior iliac crest. Sweep your abdominal hand inward toward the vaginal hand and down to the mons pubis
4. Repeat the procedure on the opposite side.

C. Note.
1. Size, tenderness, and masses.
2. Location.
3. Thickening or enlargement.

D. Normal findings.
1. Ovaries may normally be tender.
2. The fallopian tubes should be nonpalpable and nontender.

E. Abnormal findings.
1. Enlarged, cystic ovaries are related to polycystic ovarian syndrome.
2. Enlarged ovary owing to an ovarian cyst or ovarian cancer. If the condition is suspected, a pelvic ultrasound should be ordered to confirm the diagnosis.
3. Palpable tubes. The tube may feel like fibrous bands, suggesting previous salpingitis or endometriosis.

X. **Rectovaginal examination.**
A. Instruct client to bear down when the finger is inserted into the rectum, then relax and continue to inhale and exhale slowly. The exam is usually uncomfortable and is considered invasive.
B. Technique.
1. After applying a new glove, insert one lubricated, gloved finger rectally and one gloved finger vaginally, palpating the rectovaginal septum.
2. Insert the fingers as far in as possible.
3. With the other hand on the abdomen, push the uterus as posteriorly as possible.

    4. Palpate the posterior surface of the uterus and the rectal wall with the internal fingers.

    5. Note any masses, tenderness, hemorrhoids, or the presence of a retroverted uterus.

C. Guaiac assessment for occult blood.

    1. Take stool adhered to the examining glove and wipe on the appropriate section of the test paper.

    2. Place one to two drops of developing solution over sample.

    3. Wait 30 seconds.

    4. A positive response is the appearance of a blue or dark green color.

D. Flexible sigmoidoscopy screening.

    1. Colon cancer is the second most common cause of death from malignant disease in the United States.

    2. When individuals become symptomatic, most tumors have spread beyond the bowel.

    3. Early screening for asymptomatic colorectal cancer is important.

    4. Suggest screening of average-risk women from 50 years of age every 3 to 5 years.

    5. High-risk women include those with advancing age, a diet high in fat, or a family history of colon cancer.

    6. Recommend screening of high-risk women from 40 years of age every 2 years.

    7. Education is critical.

XI. The speculum examination.

A. Some comments.

    1. The diameter and tone of the introitus influences the size and type of the speculum that is selected.

    2. Select a speculum size that will be comfortable for the patient while allowing optimal viewing of the cervix

    3. If a metal speculum is used, it should be warmed or lubricated with tap water.

    4. Commercial lubricants may interfere with the Pap smear, cultures, and vaginal microscopy tests.

    5. The patient should be told that the speculum will be inserted. Showing the patient the speculum before it is inserted often lessens anxiety during the procedure. (However, it may increase anxiety in others.)

B. Choice of speculum. Either a plastic or metal speculum may be used.

1. Plastic speculums can be purchased with an attached light. This feature greatly enhances visualization because it allows direct illumination of the vaginal vault.

C. Technique.

1. Using your nondominant hand, spread the labia with index and middle fingers while applying downward pressure at the lower margin.
2. This helps avoid pinching or dragging the labia into the introitus as the speculum is inserted.
   a. Some examiners suggest a woman bear down at this point as it eases insertion of the speculum, and consequently increases the patient's comfort.
3. Hold the speculum at an angle during insertion. This places the long blades parallel to the longitudinal slit of the vaginal opening.
4. The speculum is next gently directed downward toward the sacrum, while putting downward pressure against the peritoneum until it is fully inserted.
5. Gradually open the blades, and bring the speculum back to the horizontal position as the cervix comes into view. This technique reduces the risk of irritating the sensitive urethral tissues.
   a. If the visible vaginal wall is rugated, the speculum is probably anterior to the cervix; if the visible wall is smooth, it is probably placed posterior to the cervix.
6. Be careful not to pinch the labia or pull on any pubic hair.
7. Sometimes, a side-to-side movement of the blades will help you visualize the cervix.
8. Small adjustments in speculum angle may also be helpful.
9. The bimanual examination, if previously performed, will help you know where to direct the speculum and locate the cervix.
10. The blades may be held open by either tightening the screw of a metal speculum (be careful not to catch any pubic hair) or by clicking the plastic blades into an open position.
    a. There is no need to secure the blades wide open. It is sometimes more comfortable for the patient if the blades are held partially open for the short time during which the vagina and cervix are inspected.
11. The vaginal canal is inspected as the speculum is removed. This is enhanced with a lighted plastic speculum.

D. Inspection of the vagina.

1. Note the quantity, quality, color, and odor of any vaginal discharge.
   a. A vaginal pH, whiff test, and a wet mount are recommended for all women who are concerned regarding their fertility and for complaints of a change in vaginal discharge in order to confirm the presence of normal vaginal flora, and to detect any vaginal infections or estrogen deficiencies (Ch. microscopy).
   b. Abnormal flora can interfere with the movement of sperm that is deposited in the vagina.
   c. Research suggests that bacterial vaginosis (BV) and streptococcus may be linked to preterm labor and many gynecologic problems.
   d. It is now recognized that lactobacilli-dominant flora is important for all women of reproductive age, including those who are attempting pregnancy. A culture for gonorrhea or chlamydia may be indicated if the wet mount shows an abundance of polymorphonuclear white blood cells.
2. The vaginal mucosa should be examined as the speculum is slowly rotated and withdrawn from the vagina. This is facilitated by use of a clear plastic speculum. Special attention should be given to any lesions that were palpated earlier.
3. Note any abnormal alterations.
   a. Presence of rugae (mucosal folds). Rugae indicate a good estrogen effect. In a woman with low estrogen levels, the mucosa will be thin, atrophic, and without rugae.
   b. A spatula or cotton-tipped applicator is used to collect a lateral vaginal wall sample to assess pH, perform a whiff test, and prepare the wet mount.
   c. Cervical mucus may alter the pH and wet mount reading, so it should be avoided, if possible.
E. Visualization of the cervix. If discharge obscures the view, gently remove it by using a large cotton swab or rectal probe. Culture any unusual discharge. Pay special attention to any anomalies previously palpated. Note:
   1. Size and shape of the cervical os.
      a. Normal findings and clinical alterations.
         (1) Slit associated with vaginal delivery.
         (2) Lacerations from a tear during a precipitous delivery.
         (3) An oval os is found in nulliparous women.
         (4) A tiny os, which may be partially obliterated, may be

Table 4.3   **Conditions Affecting the Cervix**

Condition	Symptoms Identified During Assessment
Nulliparous cervix	Os is small and either round or oval. Covered by smooth epithelium.
Parous cervix	Slit-like appearance.
Cervical polyp	Small berry-like protrusions. Usually arise from the endocervical canal becoming visible when they protrude through the cervical os.
Nabothian cyst	Vary in size, can be single or multiple. Appear as translucent nodules on the cervical surface. Often caused by chronic cervicitis.
Ectropion	An extension of the endocervical columnar epithelium onto the ectocervix. Often seen with increased estrogen production such as pregnancy or birth control pills.
Erosion	Friable tissue surrounding os from an infected ectropion. Might be first evidenced by bleeding with a Pap smear.

found in menopausal women who are not taking hormone replacement therapy.

2. Characteristics of the cervix such as friability, or lesions.
   a. A friable cervix may be related to a cervical infection such as chlamydia or vaginitis.
   b. Lesions of Bartholin's cysts appear smooth, round, small, yellow, and raised.
   c. A wartlike excoriation is associated with cervical cancer. (Cervical cancer is usually not visible in the early stages.)
3. Cervical surface.
   a. A cervical erosion is a denuded area of squamous epithelium with a clearly defined but slightly irregular border.
   b. Varying amounts of squamous epithelium are visible on the ectocervix, depending on the patient's age and hormonal status.
   c. Conditions affecting the cervix are listed in Table 4.3.
4. Cervical mucus. Evaluate for quality and quantity including clarity, opacity, and mucus. Perform a wet mount, if indicated (see chapter 10).

Signs of Diethylstilbestrol (DES) Exposure **BOX 4.4**

Cockscomb: Prominent anterior portion of the cervix
Collar: Flat rim or hood surrounding the posterior cervix, covered with columnar epithelium
Pseudopolyp: Lypoid appearance of cervix resulting from circumferential groove, thickening of stroma of anterior or posterior endocervical canal
Hypoplastic cervix: Cervix less than 1.5 cm in diameter
Other: Columnar epithelium that covers most of the cervix; may extend to the vaginal wall

5. Signs of DES exposure (Box 4.4).
6. Color of the cervix. It is normally pink but may have a bluish hue in early pregnancy or increased vascularity.
7. Schiller's test.
    a. If suspicious lesions are noted, paint the cervical surface with Lugol's solution. Normal tissue will take up the stain. Abnormal tissue will appear whitish pink.
    b. Use of this test has been replaced by colposcopy.
    c. The disadvantage is that it is nonspecific; normal areas such as a cervical erosion may not pick up the stain.

XII. On completion of the pelvic exam, the woman:
   A. Should be given verbal reassurance and offered tissues with which to wipe herself. A pad should be given if any bleeding is present.
   B. Provide the woman privacy to dress then return to complete the visit. Allow ample time to address any questions arising from the examination.
   C. At this point, information obtained from the comprehensive health history is combined with findings related to the physical examination.
   D. The resulting assessment will help guide the course of the evaluation process.
   E. All factors should be clearly reviewed with the woman.
   F. Review timing of the results of any testing done.
   G. Document findings clearly and accurately (Box 4.5).
   H. Arrange for any follow-up or additional testing.

Charting a Normal Pelvic Examination (Sample)

BOX 4.5

External genitalia: Normal distribution of pubic hair. No lesions or growth. No deformities or discoloration. No masses or discharge from the Bartholin's glands or urethra.

Vagina: Pink; rugated without bulging; clear mucus discharge without odor; good muscle tone.

Cervix: Pink, intact, no lesions; no cervical motion tenderness.

Uterus: Anterior; firm without enlargement, tenderness, or masses; motile.

Adenexae: Ovaries palpated without tenderness of masses.

Rectovaginal: No fissures, masses, or fistulas.

CHAPTER 5

Assessment of Vulvar Pain

Deborah Lipkin

I. **Vulvar pain explained.**
   A. Vulvar pain is a syndrome of neuropathic pain, sexual dysfunction, and psychological disability.
      1. There are multiple theories and anecdotes, but comparatively little evidenced-based medicine.
      2. The most successful treatment involves a multimodal approach of one or all of the following: medical management of identifiable underlying conditions, management of pain, psychological support, sexual therapy, and physical therapy.
   B. Demographics.
      1. In the late 1880s, Skene identified "excessive sensitivity" of the vulva, but it was not until the early 1980s that vulvar pain was covered in the literature.
      2. A 2003 study revealed that 1,280 (16%) of 8,000 women 18 to 64 years of age reported a history of chronic burning, knifelike pain, or pain on contact, with or without itching, that lasted for at least 3 months or more.
      3. Incidence may be much higher. Women are reluctant to disclose their symptoms because of embarrassment, shame, lack of response from multiple clinicians, or well-meaning clinicians who do not have the knowledge to manage or correctly assess these conditions or who diagnose by phone.
   C. Presentation.

| *ISSVD Terminology and Classification of Vulvar Pain* | **BOX 5.1** |

A) Vulvar Pain Related to a Specific Disorder
   1) Infectious (e.g. candidiasis, herpes, etc.)
   2) Inflammatory (e.g. lichen planus, immunobullous disorders, etc.)
   3) Neoplastic (e.g. Paget's disease, squamous cell carcinoma, etc.)
   4) Neurologic (e.g. herpes neuralgia, spinal nerve compression etc.)

B) Vulvodynia
   1) Generalized
      a) Provoked (sexual, nonsexual, or both)
      b) Unprovoked
      c) Mixed (provoked and unprovoked)
   2) Localized (vestibulodynia, clitorodynia, etc.)
      a) Provoked (sexual, nonsexual, or both)
      b) Unprovoked
      c) Mixed (provoked and unprovoked)

Reprinted with permission from ISSVD (2003).

---

    1. Pain may range from mild to severe and debilitating; it may be chronic, intermittent, provoked, or unprovoked.
    2. It may involve other systems; that is, the urinary tract or the bowel.
    3. Pain may be described as sharp, burning, aching, or itching.
  D. Classification.
    1. In 2003, the World Congress of the ISSVD (International Society for Study of Vulvovaginal Disease) revised the classification of vulvar pain disorders (Box 5.1).
    2. There are two major divisions:
      a. Pain with a known cause
      b. Pain without underlying, recognizable disease
    3. In either case, pain might occur spontaneously or develop as a result of physiologic provocation. Further classification of vulvodynia recognizes generalized pain and local pain, both of which may be provoked, unprovoked. or mixed.
  E. Pelvic floor dysfunction.
    1. Many women with vulvar pain are likely to have contractile characteristics of the pelvic floor musculature. This becomes a secondary source of pain.
    2. It is common for women to have no awareness of the tension held within the pelvic floor; they can contract their mus-

Causes of Vulvar Pain	**BOX 5.2**

Infection (i.e., recurrent yeast)
Genetic factors
Immune factors
Neuropathway involvement
Injury or trauma:
      Laser treatments
      Early and frequent
      intercourse
      Atrophic vaginitis
      Oral contraceptives started
      at 16 years of age or
      younger and taken for
      more than 3 years
      Dermatosis
      Dermatitis
      STI
      Metabolites
      Childbirth
      Cryotherapy, other
      treatments causing
      inflammatory conditions
      Chemotherapy

cles when asked to "Kegel," but they are unable to release or "drop down" the muscles of the pelvic floor.

F. Box 5.2 summarizes causes of vulvar pain.

G. What causes the sensation of pain? There are several theories, including the following:

　1. Vulvodynia may be caused by increased numbers of intraepithelial nerve fibers, causing the thresholds for temperature and pain to be lowered, increasing blood flow and erythema.

　2. Vestibulodynia: May be due to nociceptors (C-nerve fibers) or neuropathic pain.

　　a. Trauma or chronic inflammation of C-nerve fibers may cause the inflammatory cytokines that surround them to fire repeatedly.

　　b. Mechanoreceptors develop allodynia (pain elicited by non-painful stimuli) secondary to central sensitization. Neuropathic pain is caused by injury to the sensory nervous system itself.

II. **Assessment of a woman with vulvar pain.**

"My yearly Pap is very painful; please use your smallest speculum."
"I can't use tampons because they hurt too much."
"I cannot have sex anymore."
"I have a disgruntled vagina."
"I scratch my vulva all night long."
"I've had yeast infections/BV for years."
"It hurts to wear jeans."
Or worse, "My doctor told me to drink more wine, this is all in my head."

A. History: The patient history may be the most critical piece of the diagnostic tool kit.
   1. A patient with vulvar pain presents with some of the symptoms listed in Box 5.3.
   2. Symptoms: May be provoked or unprovoked: burning, itching, stabbing, throbbing, associated with intercourse or touch.
       a. Was onset gradual or was there one precipitating event?
       b. How long have the symptoms been present and are they constant/intermittent/cyclic?
       c. What are the characteristics of the symptoms? Descriptions might include itching, burning, soreness, sharp, stabbing, prickly, raw, irritated.
       d. Is the location general or very specific? In other words, is the pain located over the whole vulva; only at the introitus, anus, or perineum; or elsewhere?
       e. Is the pain provoked or unprovoked?
       f. Are there associated skin symptoms, such as bumps, rash, cracks, splitting/fissuring?
       g. Are there associated vaginal symptoms, such as discharge or bleeding?
       h. Which other systems have associated symptoms in particular, urinary tract, bowel, dermatologic, or other gynecologic complaints?
       i. Use of a pain scale will be helpful, especially for reassessment after treatment.
       j. What treatment methods have been tried? What helps? What makes it worse?
   3. Gynecologic history.
       a. Gravida/para, types of deliveries.
       b. Menstrual history.

      c. Contraception.

      d. Menopausal symptoms.

      e. History of abnormal Papanicolaou (Pap) smear.

      f. History of sexually transmitted infections.

      g. Sexual history, current partner, duration of time with current partner.

      h. History of yeast or bacterial vaginosis.

      i. Genital injury or trauma.

      j. History of sexually transmitted disease (STD).

      k. Orgasm: Is the client able to achieve orgasm? Has she ever achieved an orgasm?

    4. Review of systems, may reveal a constellation of other, related disorders or autoimmune dysfunction.

      a. Urinary symptoms, especially frequency, urgency, bladder pain.

      b. Gastrointestinal symptoms, especially constipation.

      c. Dermatologic symptoms.

      d. Family history of vulvovaginal symptoms or disorders.

    5. Medications: A number of medications may cause vulvar lichenoid processes.

    6. Allergies.

B. Examination: When a woman has vulvar pain, the utmost of gentleness and delicacy is necessary for an examination.

    1. External inspection.

      a. Mons pubis: Note hair distribution and any fissuring or cracking of the skin, especially at the natal cleft.

      b. Hair distribution over labia majora.

      c. Skin pigmentation: Several conditions may cause skin changes.

        (1) Lichen sclerosus may present with whitening, extending over the surfaces of labia minora and interlabial folds (commonly noted as a "keyhole" or "butterfly" pattern, surrounding the labia minora, the perineum and the anus.)

        (2) Postinflammatory hyperpigmentation is noted as a darkening of labia minora or interlabial folds and may also be noted in the vestibule.

        (3) Lichen planus may cause a reticular, lacy pattern.

      d. Normal architecture: Do the labia minora extend fully to the perineum or are they flattened posteriorly? Inflammatory conditions such as lichen planus and lichen sclerosus may cause resorption of the labia minora.

      e. Clitoris: Does the clitoral hood retract easily over the clitoris? Are the clitoral hood and clitoris scarred? Are they obliterated? Lichen planus and lichen sclerosus both can cause scarring and resorption.

    f. Are there any unusual lesions?

    g. Lichenification: In lichen sclerosus or lichen simplex chronicus this may appear as thickening of the skin, or there may be whitening.

    h. Is there notable inflammation?

    i. Are there any fissures? Lichen sclerosus or lichen simplex chronicus often present with fissuring at the perineum or interlabial folds. There may be increased skin-fold markings.

2. Palpation.

    a. Bladder.

    b. Inguinal nodes.

    c. Labia majora.

    d. Cotton swab examination in the vestibule. Cotton swab examination will produce allodynia, pain elicited by a stimulus that is not normally painful, and hyperpathia, when a stimulus causes greater pain than is expected.

3. Vaginal examination: Use of a virginal speculum is preferred.

    a. Assess discharge color, consistency and odor.

        (1) Yeast may present as white, thick discharge.

        (2) Bacterial vaginosis discharge may be off-white or gray with a fishy odor. It never causes vaginal mucosal inflammation.

        (3) Inflammatory vaginitis discharge may be yellow with a strong odor.

    b. Vaginal walls may be a normal pink or may be inflamed. There may be telescoping or strictures noted during bimanual examination.

    c. Note unusual fissures, lacy patterns, or lesions.

    d. Vaginal tone: Hypertonicity can be noted during speculum and manual examination; however, during manual examination, specific tender spots may be identified.

        (1) It may also be possible to assess involuntary pelvic floor spasms.

        (2) Vaginismus is very common in women with any type of pelvic pain.

    e. Wet mount and pH.

        (1) Inflammatory conditions may be assessed with use of

microscopy and pH, as they will often present with elevated pH, an increased number of white blood cells,
and presence of immature epithelial cells.

(2) These conditions include vaginal atrophy, desquamative inflammatory vaginitis, lichen planus, and trichomonas. Yeast typically presents with a normal pH;
however, *yeast is often* not observed by microscopy.
Bacterial vaginosis will present with elevated pH and
clue cells will be noted by microscope (see chapter
10, Vaginal Microscopy).

f. Yeast culture: Yeast is only observed 30% to 40% of the
time by wet mount; therefore, a culture is imperative; it
will also speciate, which will guide treatment.

g. Biopsy anything that is concerning. (See chapter 32, Vulvar Cancer and Biopsy.)

III. **Diagnosis: There may or may not be an identifiable cause of vulvar pain. The differential diagnosis may include:**

A. Vulvodynia: a spontaneous, generalized vulvar pain disorder,
which may or may not involve dyspareunia, that lasts for more
than 3 months.

1. Vestibulodynia: pain on touch in the vestibule for more than
3 months. It is nearly always associated with dyspareunia.

2. Clitorodynia: a localized form of vulvodynia, causing pain in
or around the clitoris. The pain is often associated with exci-
tation or orgasm.

3. Infectious conditions.

B. Yeast.

C. Herpes.

D. Trichomonas.

E. Inflammatory conditions.

1. Lichen sclerosus: This condition is 10 times more prevalent
in women than in men, is often associated with other autoimmune disorders, runs in families, and can occur any time
in life.

a. Lesions can be present on back/shoulders/wrists.

b. There is a 4% to 5% associated risk for squamous cell
carcinoma.

c. Typical presentation includes itching and the classic whit-
ening, dry, tissue-paper appearance; however, it can be
more subtle.

d. Diagnosed by biopsy only. "Vulvitis" is an acceptable diagnosis in the absence of biopsy confirmation.

  2. Lichen planus: Vulvar appearance can be reticular or lacy, with "Wickham's striae," or erosive (intensely bright red, tender mucosa, typically well demarcated).
     a. Similar to lichen sclerosus, this condition is also present elsewhere on the body.
     b. Lichen planus is diagnosed by biopsy. "Vulvitis" is an acceptable diagnosis in the absence of biopsy confirmation.
  3. Eczema/dermatitis: This is characterized by red patches, cracking, weeping excoriations, crust formation, and yellow scale. This may be associated with an irritant or allergic reaction.
  4. Lichen simplex chronicus: results from the "itch-scratch-itch" cycling of eczematous dermatitis. Skin may appear thickened, but there may also be excoriations.
  5. Desquamative inflammatory vaginitis (DIV). Also known as lichenoid vaginitis: This is a vaginal inflammatory condition presenting with profuse, yellow, vaginal discharge.
     a. Wet mount will reveal many white blood cells and parabasal cells.
     b. Discharge may or may not be irritating.
     c. DIV may be on a continuum of vaginal lichen planus.
  6. Atrophic vaginitis: Lack of estrogen may cause an inflammatory condition.
     a. Presentation may include elevated pH, profuse, yellow discharge; wet mount may reveal many white blood cells and parabasal cells.
     b. This condition is seen in postmenopausal women but also women using medroxyprogesterone (Depo-Provera™), breastfeeding mothers, women being treated with gonadotropin-releasing hormone agonists, and, occasionally, oral contraceptive users.
     c. Atrophic vaginitis cannot be distinguished from DIV or inflammatory vaginal conditions either clinically or microscopically.
F. Neoplastic conditions.
  1. Paget's disease: presents with pruritus as primary symptom; may be eczematous with well-demarcated raised edges.
  2. Squamous cell carcinoma: presents with pruritus as primary symptom; may appear as vulvar plaque, ulcer, or fleshy, nodular or warty mass.
G. Neurologic conditions.
  1. Postherpetic neuralgia: onset of pain, tingling or burning more than 4 months after the onset of herpetic lesions.

  2. Spinal nerve compression: Symptoms may include sharp pain or burning.
H. Anatomic/Structural conditions.
  1. Bartholin's gland: Glands located bilaterally in vagina at 4 and 8 o'clock. Pain associated with Bartholin's glands is typically caused by cyst or abscess.
  2. Unruptured or tight hymen: caused by incomplete degeneration of the central portion of the hymen.
  3. Postepisiotomy: Disruption of the nerve pathways may result in pain.
  4. Postsurgical: Disruption of the nerve pathways may result in pain.
I. Table 5.1 summarizes the assessment of the vaginal environment.

IV. **Management: Vulvovaginal complaints are often complex; rarely do they resolve simply. They may require frequent visits with varied trials of treatment before the woman's symptoms are stable and manageable. Psychological support is a cornerstone of all treatment: these women will need understanding and patience. Following is a list of possible options for treatment of vulvar pain and treatment for some of the many possible conditions that cause it.**
A. Comfort measures.
  1. Sitz bath/cool soaks.
  2. Cool packs.
  3. Avoidance of irritants (soaps, perfumed soaps, douching).
  4. Use of vaginal lubricants without preservative (olive oil is a good option).
B. Topical treatments for pain.
  1. 5% lidocaine; may be applied up to 5 times daily. It may cause burning or increase in pain. If this occurs, it should be compounded in a neutral base.
  2. Dyclonine: not commercially available, but can be compounded.
  3. EMLA: lidocaine/prilocaine combination cream.
  4. Doxepin: compounding is necessary.
  5. Baclofen/tricyclic antidepressant: compounded.
C. Dietary treatments: A small number of women have found it helpful to lessen or eliminate high-oxalate foods from their diet.
  1. These diets can be restricting, and it may be enough to add calcium citrate to bind oxalates and avoid the worst triggers.
  2. High-oxalate foods include but are not limited to
    a. Berries.

Table 5.1   **Assessment of Vaginal Environment**

	Condition of Vaginal Walls	Odor	Discharge Color	Epithelial Cells	WBC/ Epithelial Cell Ratio	pH	Clue Cells or Other
Normal	Normal, supple, pink	None	White	Mature appearance	1:1	3.8–4.2	None
Atrophic vaginitis	Smooth, pale *or* inflamed	May be strong	May be scant or yellow	Immature cells are typically present	> 1:1	Elevated	None
DIV/ lichenoid vaginitis	Inflamed	May be strong	Yellow	Immature cells are typically present	> 1:1	Elevated	None
Lichen planus	Inflamed, erosions may be noted	May be strong	Yellow	Immature cells are typically present	> 1:1	Elevated	None
Bacterial vaginosis	Normal	Fishy	Off- white, gray	Mature appearance	1:1	Elevated	Clue cells present
Yeast	May be inflamed	Yeast- like	White/ clumpy	Immature cells may be present	Often > 1:1	3.8–4.2	None
Tricho- monas	May be inflamed	May be strong	Yellow/ green, frothy	Immature cells may be present	Often > 1:1	Elevated	Tricho- monads present, no clue cells

WBC = white blood cell.

        b. Nuts.
        c. Legumes, including soy and soy products.
        d. Grains, especially wheat.
        e. Chocolate.
        f. Various vegetables.
    D. Treatment for yeast: After treatment of active infection, long-term weekly suppression may be necessary. Most patients will tolerate and can safely use fluconazole 150 mg weekly.

E. Treatment for herpes: long-term suppression with antiviral agents.

F. Treatment for *Trichomonas*: metronidazole.

G. Systemic treatment for pain.

　　1. Tricyclic antidepressants: Start at 10 mg, increase by 10 mg every 3 to 5 days as tolerated; may go as high as 150 mg. These medications can be remarkably helpful in reducing pain but may have significant side effects.

　　2. Anticonvulsant medications: Gabapentin—start at 100 mg, increase by 100 mg every 3 to 5 days, as tolerated; may go as high as 3,600 mg; may also be associated with significant side effects. A newer option is pregabalin, or Lyrica (Pfizer Inc.), which may be taken as 100 mg dosages three times a day, with potential for a higher dose.

　　3. Selective norepinephrine reuptake inhibitors: venlafaxine HCl and duloxetine HCl both have shown some ability to treat neuropathic pain.

H. Local treatment can include intralesional injections with lidocaine and steroids.

I. Treatment for inflammatory conditions.

　　1. Superpotent steroid: Clobetasol, halobetasol, or betamethasone diproprionate are the cornerstones of treatment for vulvar inflammation. They can be tolerated for long-term treatment because of the high mitotic rate of the vulvar skin. These medications are sometimes irritating and can be compounded.

　　2. Tacrolimus or other immunomodulary medications: These are nearly always irritating, and so are not first-line treatment. They should be used in minuscule amounts as the skin adjusts. Tacrolimus can be very effective in treating otherwise unresponsive lichen planus.

　　3. Systemic triamcinolone injections can be used for unrelenting disease.

　　4. Vaginal estrogen can be used for atrophic conditions.

　　5. Vaginal steroid suppository for DIV/lichenoid vaginitis: May begin with commercially prepared 25-mg suppositories (prepared for rectal use) inserted per vagina. If this is ineffective, may try 100-mg compounded hydrocortisone suppositories.

J. Treatment for vaginismus: Pelvic floor physical therapy with biofeedback has been shown to help a significant number of women.

V. Patient education and clinician resources.

A. Stewart, E. G., & Spencer, P. (2002). *The V book: A doctor's guide to complete vulvovaginal health.* New York: Bantam.

B. Glazer, H., & Rodke, G. (2002). *The vulvodynia survival guide: How to overcome painful vaginal symptoms and enjoy an active lifestyle.* Oakland, CA: New Harbinger Publications.

C. International Society for the Study of Vulvovaginal Disease: www.issvd.org

D. The National Vulvodynia Association: www.nva.org

E. The Vulvodynia Guideline: www.jigtd.com

F. The Vulvar Pain Foundation: www.vulvarpainfoundation.org

CHAPTER 6

Assessment of the Female Breast

Helen A. Carcio

I. **Basics related to examination of the female breast.**
   A. The examiner must possess a thorough understanding of the normal anatomy and physiology of breast structure to identify any anomalies.
   B. Physical examination of the breast by clinicians and self-examination is important for breast cancer detection. Breast cancer is not preventable; it is the early detection of breast cancer that is key to the patient's survival.
   C. The examination of the breast includes inspection and palpation of the breasts and palpation of the lymph nodes that drain the breast.
   D. Proper positioning of the patient and good lighting are key factors to inspection and palpation of the breast.
   E. It is important for the examiner to acknowledge the societal association of the breast with sexuality; this makes the assessment of the breast an emotionally uncomfortable examination for many female clients.
   F. Assessment of breast symmetry is essential; the client must have both breasts uncovered for comparison.
   G. Ideally, the breast examination should not take place

immediately before a woman's menstrual period, when the breast may be normally tender and engorged.

H. The breast examination provides the examiner with an excellent opportunity to demonstrate breast self-examination (BSE) and to reinforce teaching.

I. More than 1 million women in the United States have breast implants.
   1. There are limitations in detecting breast cancer in women with implants.
   2. Proper positioning techniques can be used to overcome these limitations.

II. Important statistics.

A. Statistics related to breast cancer are reliable and are particularly important to review with the patient. The incidence of breast cancer in women continues to increase.

B. American women have an 11% lifetime probability of development of breast cancer, which translates to one woman in eight being affected, with most of the risk occurring after the age of 50 years.

C. Breast cancer is the most common form of cancer in women (although lung cancer is steadily increasing) and the second greatest cause of death.

D. There are a distressing 46,000 deaths a year from cancer of the breast.
   1. The good news is that the cure rate in early disease has increased by 20%.
   2. This improvement is most likely related to improvements in methods of early detection and an increase in women's awareness of the importance of the clinical breast examination (CBE) and BSE.

E. Breast cancer is far more curable when the tumor is detected early.
   1. Tumor size less than 2 cm.
   2. Before the cancerous cells have left the breast and metastasized to other body regions.
   3. A recent study reported that women who performed a thorough BSE had a 35% decrease in advanced-stage disease.
   4. A 1-cm tumor with an average doubling time has been present for 6 or 7 years.

F. The likelihood of finding a tumor during CBE is 25 to 48%.

G. It is estimated that only 29% to 46% of women perform BSE on a monthly basis.

H. *The breast cancer death rate is decreasing.*
   1. The rate has dropped 2.2% since 1990.
   2. The rate has dropped 4.8% since 2001 in women older than 50 years of age.
   3. Early detection is the most likely cause.

III. Anatomy and physiology of the breast.
   A. Breast tissue.
      1. Each breast contains 12 to 20 major ducts that intertwine, with each duct opening at the nipple. Most breast cancers originate in these ducts.
      2. The breasts extend from the second or third rib to the sixth or seventh rib, and from the sternal edge to the anterior axillary line.
      3. Breasts consist of glandular tissue, fibrous tissue, ducts, fat, blood vessels, nerves, and lymph nodes (Figure 6.1).
         a. Glandular tissue is contained in the lobes.
         b. Fibrous tissue is the supporting tissue that lies between the glandular tissue.
      4. Each lobe is subdivided into 50 to 75 lobules, which drain into separate excretory ducts, which in turn drain into the nipple.
      5. These lobules in the peripheral breast tissue emerge at the nipple (the hub) like the spokes of a wheel.
      6. The lobules produce milk, and the ducts carry the milk to the areola.
      7. Each duct dilates as it enters the base of the areola to form a milk sinus, which serves as a reservoir for milk during lactation.
      8. Inframammary ridge: The ridge of fat on the lower portion of the breast is called the inframammary ridge. The breast tissue here is often more dense than the surrounding tissue. Muscle: There is very little muscle in the breast except for a small amount in the areola and the nipple, which causes the nipple to contract, facilitating the emptying of the milk sinuses.
      9. The areola and nipple.
         a. Dermal papillae contain sebaceous glands. The skin of the areola contains occasional hair follicles.
         b. Sebaceous glands on the areolar surface are the Montgomery tubercles.
      10. Tail of Spence: More than half the ducts are present in the

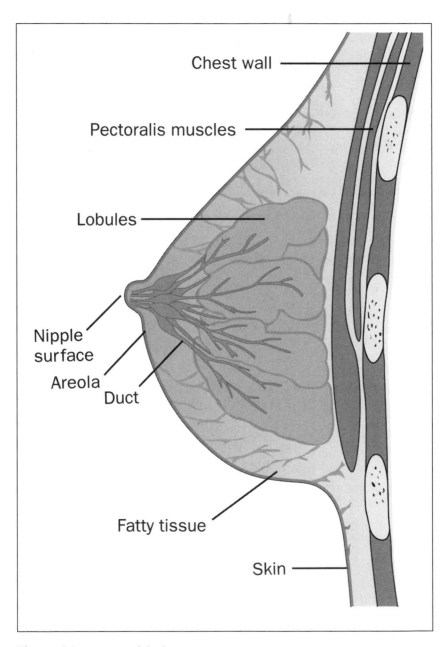

Figure 6.1 Anatomy of the breast.

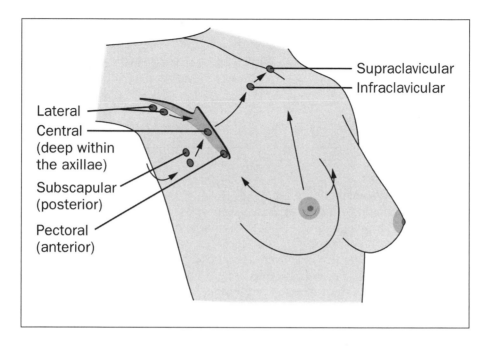

Figure 6.2 Arrows indicate direction of lymph flow.

upper, outer breast quadrant (divide the breast into four parts, with the nipple at the center).
   a. Breast tissue feels firmer in those areas.
   b. Breast cancer is more common here (many cancers arise from ductal tissue).
   11. Lymph nodes drain the area in and around the breast (Figure 6.2).
   12. The breast undergoes changes during pregnancy and lactation.

IV. Breast self-examination.
   A. BSE explained.
      1. Few women practice BSE regularly. This is due to many different factors (Box 6.1).
      2. Recent research suggests that BSE plays a small role in the detection of breast cancer.
      3. Women are more likely to practice BSE if they know what to look for. Health education is vital.

Reasons Why a Woman Might Not Perform   **BOX**
Breast Self-Examination (BSE)   **6.1**

Fear of finding a lump that is cancerous can actually be immobilizing.
She may not have the confidence that she can perform the BSE efficiently,
so why bother.
She may not really believe that performing BSE will ever result in detecting
a cancerous lump.
She may simply forget to perform it regularly.

---

    4. Women should report:
       a. New lumps or thickness of breast or underarm (axilla).
       b. Nipple tenderness or discharge or physical change (persistent soreness).
       c. Skin irritation such as a pucker, dimple, new crease, or fold.
       d. Warm, red, swollen breasts with skin resembling the skin of an orange (peau d'orange).
    5. Inform the woman that any firm lump that remains unchanged with cyclic variations is suspect and warrants a visit to her health care provider.
    6. In women who are disabled, primary caregivers or chaperones should be trained to perform BSE.
    7. Performing BSE provides the woman with a great opportunity to assume an active role in her own health care.
    8. BSE is an important screening tool for breast cancer because most breast lumps are discovered by the woman herself.
    9. Performing BSE is vital to discovering interval cancers, which are lumps that grow large enough to become palpable between annual CBEs.
   10. Point out that BSE should never act as a substitute for either CBE or mammography.
   11. A woman is more likely to detect breast cancer earlier if she practices routine BSE.
  B. The technique.
    1. The BSE is relatively easy to perform; however, because the area to be palpated is large, women often believe that the technique is complicated.
    2. Women must simply be informed that there is the overlying skin on the top, with the palpable ribs underneath. They must feel for the presence of any lumps or masses in between these structures.

3. If a woman learns how to identify and even count her ribs, she will develop a sensitivity to feel for any lumps or changes in breast tissue.
4. Educate the woman in the following:
   a. Keep the middle three fingers on the skin when palpating, varying the pressure as you palpate in dime-sized areas.
   b. Do not use the tips of your fingers, but use the pads because they have more sensitive pressure receptors.
   c. Use a systematic pattern: either circles or strips (the vertical up and down pattern seems to be the easiest to use).
   d. Be sure to cover the entire breast, beginning in the middle of the armpit, where there are many ducts.
   e. Move up and down in vertical strips (a finger's width) between the collarbone and the bra line, and progress across the breast to the middle of the hard bone of the sternum.
   f. Ask the woman whether she can count her ribs beneath the breast tissue.
   g. The average examination, depending on breast size and density, should take up to 10 minutes per breast. If it does not take the patient that long, she needs to reevaluate her technique.
   h. The examination can be performed in the shower, in the bathtub, lying in bed, or upright in front of the mirror

V. **A patient history relevant to the examination of the female breast must be gathered to assess for any risk factors (Box 6.2).**
   A. Age: The older a woman is, the more the risk for breast cancer increases.
   B. Menstruation: The fewer ovulatory cycles a woman has, the lower the risk for breast cancer, as well as ovarian cancer. It is important to assess:
      1. Age of menarche.
      2. Date of last menstrual period.
      3. Age at menopause.
      4. Number of years taking oral contraceptives or estrogen replacement agents.
   C. Family history of breast cancer (see chapter 14, *BRCA* Testing)
      1. Nearly 85% of woman diagnosed with breast cancer have no close relative with breast cancer.
   D. Childbearing: Nulliparous woman and those who gave birth to a first live-born child at age 30 years or older have a somewhat increased risk for breast cancer. Ask the client about

---

| *Risk Factors Associated With Breast Cancer* | BOX 6.2 |

Advancing age.
    Older than 40 years.
Family history.
    First-degree relative: mother, sister, daughter.
    Mother or sister has disease.
    Relative was premenopausal at time of diagnosis.
    Personal history of breast cancer or ovarian cancer.
Previous breast biopsy or benign breast disease.
    Atypical hyperplasia.
    Lobular neoplasia.
    Reproductive issues.
Estrogen exposure.
    First pregnancy at 30 years of age or older.
    Early menarche (before age 12).
    Late menopause (after age 55).
    Infertility or nulliparity.
    Never breastfed.
Hormonal treatments.
    Estrogen replacement therapy (controversial).
    Recent use (within 5 years).
    Long-term use.
    Oral contraceptive use (probably does not increase risk).
Dietary factors.
    Obesity (older than age 50)
    High-fat diet.
    Alcohol use (more than two glasses per day).
Lifestyle factors.
    Pesticide exposure.
    Smoking.
    Lack of exercise.
    Personal or family history of colon cancer.
Radiation therapy to the chest.

---

      1. Number of children.
      2. Age when children were born.
      3. Breastfeeding pattern (decreases risk somewhat).
   E. Breast self-examination.
      1. Evaluate when and how performed, as well as how often.
      2. Evaluate any findings by the client.
      3. Assess level of comfort.
   F. Discharge from nipple: Inquire about
      1. Onset, duration, amount, color, odor, consistency, and
         frequency.
      2. Whether it's bilateral, spontaneous, or provoked (e.g., by ex-

ercise or sexual activity). The examiner should be concerned if the discharge is spontaneous, unilateral, and persistent.

   3. Use of medications that may increase prolactin levels, such as birth control pills, steroids, or antidepressants.

G. Breast pain or lumps: Inquire about

   1. Onset, duration, quantity, quality, location (one or both breasts), radiation of pain, relation to menstrual cycle, and history of previous episodes.

   2. Presence of predisposing factors, such as menstruation, lactation, pregnancy, or history of fibrocystic disease.

   3. Presence of associated signs and symptoms, such as dimpling of the skin or discharge from the nipple.

H. Breast implants: Inquire about

   1. Year surgery was performed.

   2. Presence of any discomfort or tenderness in area of the implant.

   3. Acute or gradual onset of pain that may be related to a ruptured implant.

   4. Occurrence of any trauma in the area of the implant

I. Medications: Past or present use.

   1. Use of oral contraceptives.

     a. Duration.

     b. Type.

     c. Presence of complications or side effects.

     d. Reasons for discontinuing.

   2. Use of estrogen replacement therapy: Risk for breast cancer may be increased if estrogen replacement therapy is used for more than 10 years. Inquire about past or present use.

     a. Duration.

     b. Type.

     c. Reason for discontinuing.

     d. Concomitant use of progesterone.

J. Social habits pertinent to risk factors for breast cancer.

   1. High-fat diet.

   2. Alcohol intake. (Question whether patient consumes more than two drinks per day.)

   3. Smoking history (can be cofactor in the development of breast cancer).

K. Personal history.

   1. Personal history of cancer of the breast or other reproductive cancer.

   2. Pelvic surgery, including oophorectomy.

   3. Family history of breast cancer.

L. *BRCA* testing (see chapter 14): Ask about
   1. Rationale for testing.
   2. Results.
   3. If results were positive, was any special monitoring necessary?

VI. Inspection of the breasts.
   A. Position.
      1. The client should be seated, with arms at her side; she should be disrobed from the waist up.
      2. Begin inspection 3 ft from the client to fully inspect both breasts.
   B. Compare the breasts.
      1. Note size, symmetry, hair pattern, location, and contour.
      2. Normal findings.
         a. Breasts should be equal bilaterally; a slight asymmetry is common in adolescents.
         b. Breasts extend from the third to the sixth ribs, with the nipple and areola over the fourth or fifth rib; convex contour; sparse hair surrounds areola. (There may be racial variations.)
         c. Size of breasts varies with overall body weight, and genetic and hormonal influences.
         d. Flatter breasts are seen in geriatric clients (less fat).
      3. Clinical alterations.
         a. Marked asymmetry resulting from cysts, inflammation or tumor.
   C. Assess the breast skin.
      1. Note color, texture, venous pattern, temperature, and the presence of edema, dimpling or retraction, and lesions.
      2. Normal findings: Warm, smooth skin; silver striae; lighter color than exposed areas of skin.
      3. Clinical alterations.
         a. Edema and dimpling are often suggestive of breast cancer.
         b. Inflammation is often caused by mastitis, breast abscess, or inflammatory breast carcinoma.
         c. Retraction results from a benign or malignant tumor.
         d. Dilated superficial veins result from a benign or malignant tumor of the areolar area.
         e. The breasts are engorged in pregnancy and lactation, with dilated superficial veins.

D. Inspect the areolae and the nipples.
   1. Note size, shape, texture, pigmentation of the breast, direction, pigmentation of the nipples; also, note the presence of any discharge or supernumerary nipples.
   2. Normal findings.
      a. Symmetrically round or oval areolae.
      b. Pigmentation should be pink to dark brown, with roughened Montgomery's tubercles; nipples should be erect and the same color as areolae.
   3. Clinical alterations.
      a. Inversion (new onset) is often associated with breast cancer.
      b. Excoriation is often associated with Paget's disease.
      c. Areola is darkened during pregnancy.
E. Observe for milk lines.
   1. Origin: Breast tissue arises out of the ectoderm, extending along the lines from the axilla to the groin (Figure 6.3).
   2. Accessory or supernumerary mammary glands and nipples are sometimes found along these embryotic lines. Women may have thought that they were moles or fleshy warts.
   3. Supernumerary nipples are often found 5 to 6 cm below the normal nipples.
F. Observe breasts when the client is in the following positions:
   1. Sitting with both arms raised over head.
   2. Sitting with both arms pressed firmly on hips, flexing pectoral muscles.
   3. Sitting, leaning forward with arms outstretched, allowing breasts to hang freely.
   4. Supine with arm above head, on the side being examined. This stretching of the pectoral muscles pulls on breast tissue and exaggerates any dimpling or pucker or retraction.

VII. **Palpation of the breast.**
   A. Basics.
      1. In a very large breast, it is unlikely that anything but the most obvious lesions will be discovered. Mammograms should be performed yearly.
      2. The presence of adipose tissue affects the nodularity, density, and fullness of the breast.
         a. In a woman who has recently lost a considerable amount of weight, the breasts are lumpy because the cushion of fatty tissue is absent. The breasts may feel similar to tapioca pudding.

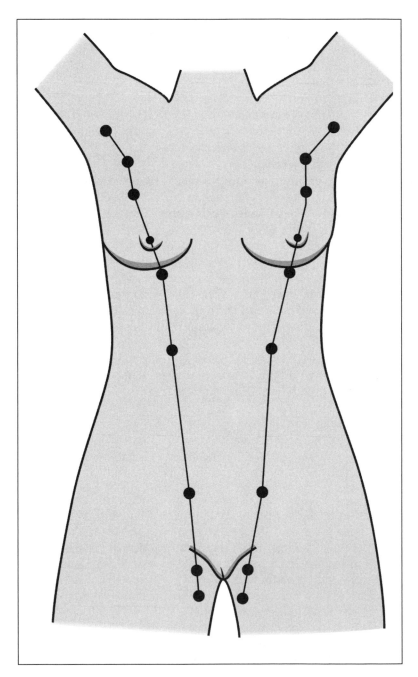

Figure 6.3 Milk lines. Possible sites of accessory breast tissue or supernumerary nipples, both of which may become more prominent during pregnancy and the puerperium.

    b. Women who are overweight have fuller breasts.

3. Three to 5 days before menstruation, the breasts become engorged, increasing in size. The CBE should not be performed during this time.

4. Wash hands with warm water before examination.

5. Placing a small pillow under the side to be examined flattens the breast tissue and distributes it evenly across the chest wall to facilitate the detection of masses or accessory breast tissue or supernumerary nipples, both of which may become more prominent during pregnancy and the puerperium.

6. If a woman reports a problem with one or both of her breasts, examine the unaffected side first to provide a baseline for comparison.

7. Palpation may be performed with one or two hands.

8. Lower the woman's arm to relax the pectoral muscles to best examine deep in the muscles in the area of the tail of Spence.

9. Sensory component of fingertips.

    a. Uses sensitive pressure receptors in the fingertips.

    b. With training, fingertips can detect most 3.0-mm tumors.

    c. The structure must be denser than the surrounding tissue.

10. Use powder if the patient's skin is moist with perspiration.

B. Palpate the four quadrants of the breast.

    1. Instructions to client: Observe how your breast is being examined so that you can use this technique at home. Describe any tenderness.

    2. Technique.

        a. The examiner should lubricate his or her fingers with lotion or soap and warm water or powder.

        b. Gently palpate the breast with the pads of the four fingers.

        c. Starting at the 12 o'clock position on the upper aspect of the breast, rotate finger pads in imaginary concentric circles or lines, toward the center of the breast, the areola, and the nipple.

        d. Do not lift fingers from the breast when moving from one section to another.

        e. In large-breasted women, use bimanual palpation, compressing the breast between hands.

        f. Next, palpate the breast with the client supine, with her arm above her head on the side being examined.

        g. Repeat for the other breast.

        h. Chart any anomalies. A diagram works best.

3. Note temperature; size (in centimeters), location, delimitation (borders of the mass), mobility, degree of fixation, and consistency (hardness) of any masses; and breast tenderness.
4. If a mass is present, assess for the retraction phenomenon:
   a. Elevate and mold the breast around the mass. Observe for any dimpling.
5. Normal findings.
   a. The breast should be warm, smooth, and elastic.
   b. No masses or discharge should be present; the breast is coarser and more nodular in a geriatric client.
   c. Generalized, uniform nodularity (may be increased in second half of cycle in a woman taking progesterone supplements).
   d. Increased density and nodularity in the area of the inframammary ridge (firm, crescent-shaped ridge of compressed tissue along the lower edge of the breast).
6. Clinical alterations (see Table 6.1, which compares different types of lumps).
   a. Nontender, mobile, smooth, well-delineated nodules associated with fibroadenoma.
   b. Nontender, immobile, or fixed nodule suggestive of breast cancer.
   c. Tender, multiple nodes in one or both breasts associated with chronic mastitis.

VIII. **Palpate the nipple and the areola.**
   A. Technique.
      1. Gently compress nipple between index finger and thumb.
      2. Repeat for other nipple.
   B. Note
      1. The amount, color, and odor of any fluid that is ejected from the nipple.
      2. Shape and consistency of nipple.
   C. Evaluation of the discharge. (See Table 6.2, which compares the various types of nipple discharge.)
      1. A guaiac test may be necessary to test for blood in the discharge.
      2. Cytologic examination of breast discharge.
         a. Compress the nipple, and express the discharge onto a slide.
         b. Spray with fixative, as with Papanicolaou (Pap) smear.
         c. A Pap test may reveal abnormal cells.

Table 6.1   **Comparison of Different Types of Breast Lumps ✔**

Characteristic	Fibrocystic	Fibroadenoma	Cancer
Age	25 to 55 years (rare after menopause)	Puberty to menopause (peak 20–29 years)	Older than 30 years of age Incidence increases with age
Number	Usually multiple, may be single	Usually single	Usually single; two primary lesions may occur in the same breast
Shape	Smooth, round, may be multilobular	Smooth, lobular, round	Irregular
Delimitation	Well circumscribed	Well circumscribed	Poorly delineated from surrounding tissues
Mobility	Mobile	Mobile	Limited mobility; fixed to surrounding skin or underlying tissue
Pain	Present, cyclic (second half of menstrual cycle)	Usually not painful	Usually nontender
Axillary involvement	None	None	May be present with regional metastasis to axillary lymph nodes
Nipple discharge	Absent	Absent	Often present

  3. If bilateral nipple discharge is present, suspect galactorrhea. Measure prolactin levels to check for a pituitary tumor.
 D. Normal findings: No discharge, except during lactation; nipple is erect.
 E. Clinical alterations.
  1. Unilateral, serous (egg white), or serosanguineous discharge is suggestive of intraductal papillomas.
  2. Clear, yellowish fluid is associated with chronic mastitis.
  3. Sanguineous or dark red discharge is associated with Paget's disease.

Table 6.2   **Comparison of Types of Nipple Discharge**

Types of Nipple Discharge	Description	Comments
Milky white, thin	White, thin	Lactation
Serous, thin, clear, and yellowish	Thin, clear (like the white of an egg) or yellowish	Suggests intraductal papilloma
Serosanguineous, thin	Thin, clear, and pink	Suggests fibrocystic changes or cancer
Bloody	Thick, opaque, and red	Suggests fibrocystic changes or cancer
Watery	Thin, clear, and colorless (rare)	Suggests cancer
Purulent	Thick, opaque, greenish or yellowish	Suggests infection

Note: Pap test should be performed on any nipple discharge.

4. Galactorrhea is associated with the use of tranquilizers, marijuana, and high estrogen levels.

IX. **Palpate lymph nodes.**
   A. Technique.
      1. Using the same rotating motion, gently palpate the supraclavicular and infraclavicular areas.
      2. Face the patient, abduct her right arm with your right hand, and place your left hand against the chest wall, high into the axilla.
      3. Rotate your hand, cup the examining fingers, and reach high into the axilla using gentle pressure to palpate the subscapular, central, pectoral, and lateral axillary nodes as the hand slides down the axilla.
      4. Support the woman's arm with the opposite hand. This approach relaxes the pectoralis muscle and permits careful evaluation of the axilla.
      5. Repeat for the opposite axilla. Repeat with the client supine with her arm over her head.
   B. Note location (which quadrant), size (in centimeters), shape, consistency, mobility, and tenderness of any nodes palpated. A diagram is helpful.
   C. Normal findings: None.

D. Clinical alterations.
   1. Nontender, hard enlarged lymph nodes are indicative of metastatic breast cancer.
   2. Lymphadenitis: Freely mobile 3 to 5 mm, associated with an infection of the client's hand or arm.
E. Refer any abnormal findings for further evaluation.

X. Physical examination of an augmented breast.
   A. Physical examination includes evaluation of both the natural breast tissue and the implant. The breast must also be examined for possible complications related to the implants.
   B. In both the upright and supine positions
      1. Assessment procedure when the woman is upright with arms at her side:
         a. Instruct the woman to elevate her arms over her head and then to place her hands on her hips and lean forward, flexing the pectoralis muscle when asked.
         b. Palpation of the natural breast tissue with the patient upright is often easier if she leans slightly forward.
         c. The breast tissue should be gently pinched or pulled away from the implants.
      2. Assessment procedure when the woman is in the supine position.
         a. The patient's arm should not be elevated above the head, but rather relaxed at her side to relax the pectoral muscles, making the implants more mobile and compressible.
         b. Contraction of the pectoralis muscle contracts the implant into a ball.
         c. Push the implant away from each wedge of tissue as it is examined.
            (1) Some implants are soft and easily displaced.
         d. Palpate the axillary and supraclavicular area for lymph nodes as described previously.
         e. Evaluate the implant for compressibility and mobility.
   C. Note the following elements of the implant:
      1. Contour.
         a. Flatness.
         b. Bulges.
         c. Indentations.
      2. Abnormal skin changes.
         a. Thickening.
         b. Lesions.

      c. Nipple abnormality.

   3. Compare the size of the breasts, observing the location of the augmentation scar.

   4. Determine whether the implants are visible.

   5. Observe for signs of capsular contraction or abnormal shape of implants.

   6. Assess the integrity of the implant by evaluating any capsular scarring or contraction.

      a. A ruptured implant may not be evident clinically.

      b. May feel firm or hard from silicone granuloma formation.

XI. Chart.

  A. Carefully document physical examination findings.

   1. A diagram is helpful because it graphically documents any suspected anomalies.

   2. Divide the breast into four quadrants by drawing two imaginary lines through the nipple at right angles to each other. Tail of Spence is an extension of the upper outer quadrant.

  B. Record: Breasts symmetric; normal contour; no dimpling, retraction, or erythema; nipples erect, no discharge; areola pink; firm, smooth, elastic breasts; no masses or palpable lymph nodes.

XII. Mammogram.

  A. Mammography explained.

   1. Radiographic examination of the breast.

   2. Only reliable means of detecting breast cancer before palpation.

  B. Mammography can pick up soft tissue densities not yet palpable, as well as calcifications that are too small to feel. BSE and CBE are complementary to mammography, and each test is performed to detect a mass missed by the other two.

  C. Indications.

   1. To obtain a baseline mammogram in women 40 years of age, or earlier if clinically indicated.

   2. To evaluate a lump or mass found during palpation of the breast by either the woman or the clinician.

   3. To screen a woman for breast cancer, particularly those at risk for development of breast cancer.

   4. To evaluate the breast for any abnormalities before initiating estrogen replacement therapy.

  D. Advantages.

   1. Easy to perform.

2. Eighty-six percent sensitivity for cancers (percentage of cancers detected by test as malignant or probably malignant).
3. Ninety percent specific for benign disease (percentage of benign disease detected by test as benign).
4. Positive predictive value for cancers is 95%.
5. Relatively inexpensive.

E. Disadvantages.
   1. Requires special equipment and trained personnel.
   2. Low sensitivity in women younger than 50 years of age because of the fat content of breasts.
   3. Uncomfortable for the woman.

F. Role of ultrasound.
   1. Used to distinguish between solid and cystic masses.
      a. If the mass is cystic, refer for possible aspiration.
      b. If solid, refer for needle localization biopsy.

G. Screening parameters as recommended by the American Cancer Society.
   1. Mammography.
      a. Baseline mammography by 40 years of age.
         (1) May start earlier if there is a strong family history of breast cancer, positive *BRCA* test results, fibrocystic disease (makes palpation more difficult), or breast augmentation.
      b. Mammography should be performed every year after 40 years of age.
      c. High-risk individuals. Mammography and magnetic resonance imaging (MRI) every year.
   2. Digital mammaography.
      a. Similar to traditional mammography but the system uses a digital receptor and computer.
   3. Clinical breast examination.
      a. Every 3 years between the ages of 20 and 40 years. (Many clinicians start earlier.)
      b. Every year for women older than 40 years of age.

H. Special findings.
   1. Microcalcifications.
      a. Tiny specks of calcium in the breast.
      b. Often found in areas of rapidly dividing cells.
      c. Appear benign.
      d. Subsequent mammography in 3 to 6 months.
      e. If the microcalcifications are clustered or in small group-

ings, refer the patient for needle localization biopsy or removal.
2. Macrocalcification.
   a. Calcium deposits are frequently associated with degenerative changes in the breast.
   b. Due to aging, old injuries, or inflammation.
   c. Usually benign.
   d. First appearance; subsequent mammography in 6 months.
   e. Stable—mammography should be performed every year.

XIII. Breast cancer risk assessment tool.
   A. For an excellent tool for screening women for breast cancer on a yearly basis go to: http://www.cancer.gov/bcrisktool/

Assessment of the Pregnant Woman

CHAPTER 7

Kate Green

I. **Initial prenatal evaluation.** The initial evaluation of a pregnant woman should include a thorough review of the patient's medical history and a careful physical examination. This visit is a good opportunity to screen for potential complications of pregnancy and to begin to establish a trusting relationship with the pregnant woman.

II. **Documentation of pregnancy.** Many practices require a positive pregnancy test result documented on the chart before the onset of the comprehensive initial prenatal evaluation, to verify the woman's pregnancy. Urine and serum pregnancy tests are based on levels of human chorionic gonadotropin (hCG), which is secreted into the maternal bloodstream and then excreted through the maternal urine.

A. Urine pregnancy tests.
   1. Accurate 95 to 99% of the time.
   2. Sensitive within 7 days after implantation.
   3. Possible for pregnancy to be detected before first missed period; however, this is not a certainty.
   4. The test is inexpensive, private, and easy to obtain over the counter.
   5. Use first morning void when possible because concentrated

117

urine improves the pregnancy detection rate (nearly equal to that of serum).
6. The test is specific for beta subunit of hCG, eliminating cross-reactivity with other hormones.
B. Serum qualitative or quantitative tests do not indicate pregnancy until levels rise above baseline values (may vary by laboratory, but usually around 25–30 mIU/dL).
   1. hCG is detectable in serum as early as 7 to 9 days after ovulation or just after implantation.
   2. During the first 3 to 4 weeks after implantation, the hCG level doubles every 2 days.
   3. The level should be 50 to 250 mIU/dL at the time of the first missed menstrual period.
   4. The level peaks at 60 to 70 days after fertilization, then decreases during the first half of pregnancy, after which it remains relatively constant throughout the remainder of the second half of pregnancy.
   5. Qualitative test results are read as positive or negative (false-positive results are rare).
   6. Quantitative beta-hCG is a radioisotope test performed on a blood sample to quantify levels of hCG. It is most useful when
      a. Serial testing is desired to monitor suspected ectopic pregnancy, molar pregnancy, or spontaneous abortion.
      b. Variable results from other tests are present.
   7. Must specify qualitative or quantitative test when ordering scrum hCG.
C. Progesterone levels.
   1. These levels remain constant through the first 9 to 10 weeks of pregnancy, unlike hCG.
   2. Nonviable pregnancies have much lower levels than normal pregnancies.
   3. Highly predictive of pregnancy outcome.
   4. Not routinely performed.
D. Signs and symptoms of pregnancy: The diagnosis of pregnancy is based on the following:
   1. Presumptive signs (Table 7.1 lists signs and symptoms).
   2. Probable signs.
   3. Positive signs.

III. Estimated date of confinement (EDC).
A. Obtain date of start of last menstrual period (LMP).

Table 7.1 Signs and Symptoms of Pregnancy

Presumptive signs	Description
Cessation of menses	Uterine lining does not shed. May have some spotting around the time of implantation.
Nausea, vomiting, "morning sickness"	Onset at 2 to 12 weeks' gestation, subsides 6 to 8 weeks later. Most severe on awakening.
Frequent urination	Bladder irritability from enlarging fetus pressing on bladder, causing reduced capacity.
Breast tenderness	Onset at 2 to 3 weeks' gestation, may be present throughout pregnancy. Soreness and tingling of breasts from hormonal stimulation.
Perception of fetal movement, or "quickening"	16 to 18 weeks' gestation, should be present until delivery. Sensation of "fluttering" or motion in abdomen perceived by the mother.
Fatigue	Common early in pregnancy. Usually resolves by 20 weeks' gesatation.
Skin changes	Abdominal striae and increased pigmentation from hormonal changes.

Probable signs	
Enlargement of the abdomen	Palpated abdominally above symphysis pubis at 12 weeks' gesatation.
Piskacek's sign	4 to 6 weeks' gesatation. Uterus asymmetric with soft prominence on side of implantation.
Hegar's sign	6 weeks' gestation. Palpable softening of lower uterine segment.
Goodell's sign	8 weeks' gestation. Softening of the cervix (changes from consistency of the tip of the nose to that of lips).
Chadwick's sign	6 to 8 weeks' gestation. Blue-violet hue from congestion seen on the vulva, vagina and cervix (particularly the vaginal opening).
Braxton Hicks contractions	May be felt as early as end of first trimester. Irregular, painless, intermittent uterine contractions.
Pregnancy test	Positive 7 to 10 days after conception.

(continued)

Table 7.1 *(continued)*

Positive signs	Description
Fetal heart	Ultrasound. Fetal heart motion by 4 to 8 weeks' gestation after conception. Doppler. Fetal heart sounds by 10 to 12 weeks after conception.
Movement	19 weeks' gestation. Mother may feel movement weeks earlier but it must be verified by examiner.
Visualization of the fetus	Ultrasound. Visualize fetus at 5 to 6 weeks' gestation. Rarely used to diagnose pregnancy, more frequently used to establish estimated date of confinement.

    1. Evaluate patient's surety on the date because EDC is based on the LMP.

    2. Conception usually occurs approximately 2 weeks after the LMP in a 28-day cycle.

B. Review of menstrual cycles.

    1. Frequency of menses: If the woman does not have a regular 28-day cycle, adjust EDC accordingly.

    2. Duration of flow.

    3. Question whether LMP was normal for the patient; if flow was exceptionally light or spotting only, the condition could be the result of syncytiotrophoblastic cells implanting in the endometrial lining at about the time the next menstrual cycle would have been expected. This process will cause a change in the EDC.

C. Accurate dating is imperative to allow for prenatal testing to be carried out at the appropriate time intervals.

    1. Nägele's rule: Estimated by adding 7 days to the first day of the LMP, and then 3 months are subtracted from that date.

    2. Obstetric wheels are available for calculation from many pharmaceutical companies.

    3. Clarification of terms.

        a. Pregnancy: 40 weeks (10 lunar months), or 280 days from LMP.

        b. Fetal calculation: 38 weeks or 266 days from conception.

D. Pregnancy tests are probable signs of pregnancy. Only auscultation of fetal heart tone, sonographic evidence, and fetal motion (according to some authorities) are positive signs of pregnancy.

IV. **Current identifying data: These items provide general information that is current and allow the woman to answer relatively uncomplicated questions comfortably, establishing a pattern for the rest of the interview. These items should include**
   A. Current name.
   B. Date of birth to screen for age-related complications.
      1. If the woman is older than 35 years of age, genetic counseling should be offered.
      2. Review the risk for chromosomal abnormalities relative to maternal age (Table 7.2).
   C. Current employment: Screen for occupational hazards to the health of the mother and the developing fetus.
   D. Partner's name, if involved with patient, or support person's name.
   E. Partner's employment.
   F. Household members.
   G. Race: Screen for race- and ethnicity-related disorders (see genetic assessment questionnaire, Appendix 7.1).
      1. Ethnic populations and carrier status.
         a. Black, some Hispanic, and Southeast Asian women may be at risk for sickle cell disease.
         b. Ashkinazi Jewish, French Canadian, Cajun, and Pennsylvania Dutch women may be at risk for Tay-Sachs disease.
         c. Mediterranean, North African, Middle Eastern and Asian women may be at risk for beta-thalassemia.
         d. Asian women may be at risk for alpha-thalassemia.
   H. Religion, if any.
   I. Educational level.

V. **Evaluate reactions to pregnancy: Pregnancy is the reason the woman has sought care, and it is the most important issue to her. It is wise to discuss early in the visit what her expectations are in relation to her pregnancy and to establish what care she is expecting. Additionally, the reactions of her partner and family should be explored.**
   A. Feelings about pregnancy: whether it was planned or unplanned.
   B. Plans for the pregnancy, including
      1. To keep the baby.
      2. To put the baby up for adoption.
      3. To terminate the pregnancy.

Table 7.2   **Risk for Chromosomal Abnormality (at Birth) at Various Maternal Ages***

Maternal Age	Risk for Down Syndrome	Total Risk for Chromosomal Abnormalities
20	1:1667	1:526
21	1:1667	1:526
22	1:1429	1:500
23	1:1429	1:500
24	1:1250	1:476
25	1:1250	1:476
26	1:1176	1:476
27	1:1111	1:455
28	1:1053	1:435
29	1:1000	1:417
30	1:952	1:385
31	1:909	1:385
32	1:769	1:322
33	1:602	1:286
34	1:485	1:238
35	1:378	1:192
36	1:289	1:156
37	1:224	1:127
38	1:173	1:102
39	1:136	1:83
40	1:106	1:66
41	1:82	1:53
42	1:63	1:42
43	1:49	1:33
44	1:38	1:26
45	1:30	1:21
46	1:23	1:16
47	1:18	1:13
48	1:14	1:10
49	1:11	1:8

*Because sample size for some intervals is relatively small, 95% confidence limits are sometimes relatively large. Nonetheless, these figures are suitable for genetic counseling.

C. Whether friends and family have been informed and their reactions.

D. Partner's response.

VI. Current physical symptoms: Include severity, when occurred, treatment or relief measures tried and their effectiveness. (Table

7.3 summarizes common complaints of pregnancy and their explanation.)

A. Nausea and vomiting (i.e., "morning sickness").
  1. Most common problem associated with pregnancy. Common in first trimester (70-85% of pregnant women); infrequently noted later.
  2. Unknown cause: Possible reaction to high levels of hCG.
  3. Frequent and consistent vomiting, dehydration, weight loss, electrolyte imbalance, poor appetite or food intake, or ketonuria may indicate hyperemesis gravidarum (0.5–2% of all pregnancies).

B. Breast tenderness (mastalgia).
  1. Related to increased levels of estrogen, progesterone, and chorionic somatomammotropin.
  2. Often, the first presumptive sign of pregnancy.

C. Abdominal pain or cramping.
  1. Commonly associated with round ligament pain.
  2. If present, should check for symptoms of impending miscarriage, such as bleeding, or for gastrointestinal disorders.

D. Vaginal discharge or bleeding.
  1. Discharge may be normal or may indicate genital tract infection.
  2. Heavy bleeding in pregnancy is abnormal and must be evaluated further. Consider
    a. Obtaining a sonogram.
    b. Obtaining quantitative hCG level for later comparison.
    c. Spotting may be normal and may indicate implantation of the blastocyst, resulting from invasive chorionic villi activity in the uterine lining. Spotting may occur at approximately the time a woman would have been expecting her menses if she were not pregnant.

E. Urinary frequency.
  1. Frequency may be normal due to uterine position in relation to maternal bladder in the first and third trimesters.
  2. If urination is accompanied by dysuria, it may indicate a urinary tract infection.

F. Headache: Must monitor for preeclampsia if persistent.

G. Nosebleeds: If they are mild, they are considered normal.

H. Fatigue.
  1. Very common in first trimester.
  2. Patients need reassurance that fatigue will lessen as the pregnancy progresses.

Table 7.3   Common Complaints During Pregnancy and Their Explanation

Common Complaint	Time in Pregnancy	Explanation and Effects on Woman's Body
No menses (*amenorrhea*)	Throughout	Continued high levels of estrogen, progesterone, and human chorionic gonadotropin after fertilization of the ovum allow the uterine endometrium to build up and support the developing pregnancy rather than to slough as menses.
Nausea with or without vomiting	First trimester	Possible causes include hormonal changes of pregnancy leading to slowed peristalsis throughout the gastrointestinal tract, changes in taste and smell, the growing uterus, or emotional factors. Women may have a modest (2–5 lb) weight loss in the first trimester.
Breast tenderness, tingling	First trimester	The hormones of pregnancy stimulate the growth of breast tissue. As the breasts enlarge throughout pregnancy, women may experience upper backache from their increased weight. There is also increased blood flow throughout the breasts, increasing pressure on the tissue.
Urinary frequency (nondisease)	First and third trimesters	There is increased blood volume and increased filtration rate in the kidneys with increased urine production. Due to less space for the bladder from pressure from the growing uterus (first trimester) or from the descent of the fetal head (third trimester), the woman needs to empty her bladder more frequently.
Fatigue	First trimester	Mechanisms not clearly understood.
Heartburn and constipation	Throughout	Relaxation of the lower esophageal sphincter allows stomach contents to back up into the lower esophagus. The decreased gastrointestinal motility caused by pregnancy hormones slows peristalsis and causes constipation. Constipation may cause or aggravate existing hemorrhoids.
Leukorrhea	Throughout	Increased secretions from the cervix and the vaginal epithelium, due to the hormones and vasocongestion of pregnancy, result in an asymptomatic milky white vaginal discharge.
Weight loss	First trimester	If a women experiences nausea and vomiting, she may not be eating normally in early pregnancy. (See Nausea previously described.)
Backache (nondisease)	Throughout, may increase third trimester	Hormonally induced relaxation of joints and ligaments and the minor lordosis required to balance the growing uterus sometimes result in a lower backache. Pathologic causes must be ruled out.

I. Heartburn.
   1. More common in late pregnancy.
   2. Related to increased pressure in abdomen and softening of pyloric sphincter.
J. Back pain.
   1. Common.
   2. Must discuss relief measure, such as good support bra, warm soaks, erect posture, and massage if no disease is noted during examination.
K. Quickening, if present (patient's first awareness of fetal movement).
   1. Assists in dating pregnancy.
   2. Quickening is usually not felt until approximately 20 weeks' gestation.
L. Skin changes may normally include
   1. Darkening of the areola.
   2. Linea nigra.
   3. Chloasma.
   4. Breast and abdominal striae from stretching of skin.
M. Ptyalism (excessive salivation).
   1. Reassure the patient that the problem is common and harmless.
   2. Attempts at treatment largely unsuccessful.
N. Absence of menses.
O. Constipation.
   1. Common.
   2. Probably related to steroid-induced suppression of bowel motility and compression of the intestine from the enlarging uterus.
   3. Aggravates hemorrhoids.

VII. **History since conception provides screening for agents that may increase risks for anomalies or miscarriage and risks for pregnancy outcomes for the pregnant woman and her baby.**
   A. Radiation exposure, including X-ray studies (even dental) without use of a shield (usually routinely used on women of childbearing age).
   B. Viral exposure.
      1. Includes rubella exposure.
         a. Rubella infection in pregnancy has a high rate of causing fetal malformations in early pregnancy; the risk decreases as the pregnancy progresses. Up to 50% if infected in the

first month of pregnancy, 20% in the second month of pregnancy, 7% in the third month, and 1 to 2% in the fourth and fifth months of pregnancy.
   2. Other "childhood illnesses" the woman has been exposed to since conception.
       a. Infection in pregnancy may cause varying complications or be entirely benign.
C. Fever.
   1. Include how high and when occurred.
   2. May provide a clue to first-trimester exposure to diseases that may affect pregnancy such as rubella or Fifth's disease (human parvovirus B-19).
D. Medications used since conception.
   1. Inquire about use of
       a. Over-the-counter medications.
       b. Home remedies and herbal preparations.
       c. Prescribed medications.
       d. Progesterone in infertility patients.
       e. Vitamins, folic acid, or mineral supplements; particularly calcium and iron.
   2. Drugs are rated as classes A, B, C, D, and X (Box 7.1).
   3. Medications should be checked in a drug reference if the examiner is unsure of classification or effect on pregnancy.
E. Weight gain since onset of pregnancy and recalled or documented pregravid weight.
   1. Overweight and obesity may be related to pregnancy complications of hypertension, diabetes, fetal macrosomia and to delivery complications.

VIII. Medical history: Include diseases that could affect the woman's health or fetal well-being during pregnancy.
A. Diabetes: Correlates with an increased risk for multiple maternal and fetal complications, such as preterm labor, infectious illnesses, hydramnios and hypertension (maternal), and congenital anomalies, fetal macrosomia, intrauterine fetal death, delayed fetal pulmonary maturation, and metabolic abnormalities.
   1. Diabetes in pregnancy of any type necessitates close control and consultation.
   2. Screening recommended for all pregnant women between 24 and 28 weeks' gestation, with initial laboratory work for diabetes with 1 hour, 50-g glucola test. Testing should be done earlier if indicated by history of gestational diabetes or high risk factors such as morbid obesity.

| *Drugs During Pregnancy: Food and Drug Administration Risk Categories* | **BOX 7.1** |

- *Category A*
Controlled studies in women do not demonstrate a risk to the fetus in the first trimester (and there is no evidence of risk in later trimesters), and the possibility of fetal harm appears to be remote.
- *Category B*
Either animal reproduction studies have not shown a fetal risk and there are no controlled studies in pregnant women, or animal reproduction studies have shown an adverse effect (other than a decrease in fertility) that was not confirmed in controlled studies in women in the first trimester (and there is no evidence of a risk in later trimesters).
- *Category C*
Either studies in animals have revealed adverse effects on the fetus (teratogenic, embryocidal, or other effect) and there are no controlled studies in women, or studies in women and animals are not available. Drugs in this category should be given only if the potential benefit justifies the potential risk to the fetus.
- *Category D*
There is positive evidence of human fetal risk, but the benefits from use in pregnant women may be acceptable despite the risk. The drug may be needed in a life-threatening situation or for a serious disease when safer drugs cannot be used or are ineffective.
- *Category X*
Studies in animals or human beings have shown fetal abnormalities, there is evidence of fetal risk based on human experience, or both, and the risk of the use of the drug in pregnant women clearly outweighs any possible benefit. The drug is contraindicated in women who are or may become pregnant.

Based on information from Yaffe, S. J. (1990). Introduction. In Briggs, R. K., Freeman, & Yaffe, S. J. (Eds.). *Drugs in pregnancy and lactation* (p. xiii). Baltimore: Williams and Wilkins; and Food and Drug Administration labeling and prescription drug advertising. (1979). Content and format for labeling for human prescription drugs. Federal Register 44 (June 26), 37434-37467.

3. Three types of diabetes to be considered in pregnancy.
   a. Type I: Insulin dependent: Should assess age at onset and amount and type of insulin used; refer the patient for insulin management and nutritional counseling.
   b. Type II: Noninsulin dependent: Refer for plan for monitoring serum glucose levels and to nutritionist for dietary counseling, and possible use of oral hypoglycemics.
   c. Gestational diabetes: diabetes during pregnancy. Refer for dietary counseling and glucose monitoring
   B. Hypertension: Consult as needed.

1. Chronic: Assess for method of control or use of antihypertensive medication.
2. Pregnancy-related: Must monitor and refer due to increased risk to current pregnancy.

C. Cardiac disease.
   1. Assess need for prophylaxis in labor if patient has mitral valve prolapse.
   2. Consultation necessary for other cardiac diseases

D. Liver disease.
   1. Assess risk factors for hepatitis and screen with blood testing as needed. Infants may require treatment with immunoglobulins soon after delivery if hepatitis present.

E. Renal disease.

F. Gallbladder disease: can be exacerbated in pregnancy.

G. Stomach or bowel disease.
   1. If abdominal surgery was performed, note type of surgery and location of any scarring.
   2. Consult specialist because the condition could cause deleterious effects during the antepartum or intrapartum period.

H. Pulmonary disease.
   1. If asthma is present, assess which medications or inhalers the patient currently uses.
   2. Assess current and recent status of asthma (mild, intermittent, severe).
   3. If pulmonary disease is present, evaluate early with consultation because of the possibility of the need for anesthesia in labor.

I. Congenital anomalies and genetic diseases: Must screen for risk to patient and fetus during pregnancy and labor.

J. Cancer.
   1. If cancer of the cervix treated with cone biopsy, the patient is at increased risk for preterm labor.

K. Genitourinary tract disease.

L. Varicosities and phlebitis: may worsen during prenancy.

M.Anemia.
   1. Inquire about sickle cell disease and sickle cell trait as well as thalassemia.
   2. Screen with initial laboratory work if status is unclear.

N. Infectious diseases.
   1. Hepatitis: Assess for type and current status.
   2. Tuberculosis.
   3. Human immunodeficiency virus (HIV) infection.

      a. Inquire about history of high-risk sexual behavior or intravenous (IV) drug use.

      b. Rate of transmission of HIV with retrovirals is down 2%.

  O. Autoimmune disorders.

    1. Increased rate of miscarriage in women with systemic lupus erythematosus (SLE).

  P. Neurologic disorders or any neurologic defects.

  Q. Psychiatric disorders.

    1. Screen for risk factors for postpartum depression

  R. Multifetal gestation.

  S. Allergies: document reaction.

IX. Obstetric and gynecologic history.

  A. Gynecologic.

    1. Abnormal uterine bleeding.

    2. History of sexually transmitted infections in self and partner.

      a. Treatment of sexually transmitted diseases; include human papillomavirus (HPV), herpes simplex virus (HSV), HIV, chlamydia, gonorrhea, *Trichomonas*, bacterial vaginosis, and syphilis.

      b. Note test of cures, if done.

      c. Any long-term sequelae.

    3. Contraception.

      a. Types ever used.

      b. Most recently used method.

      c. When contraception was most recently used.

      d. If patient became pregnant while actively using contraception, the examiner may need to discuss effects of contraceptive type on pregnancy.

    4. Gynecologic surgery. List date and reason.

  B. Infertility treatments performed.

    1. Include current or continuing infertility treatments.

    2. Use of ovulation induction.

    3. Previous attempts at pregnancy.

      a. Intrauterine insemination (IUI).

      b. Assisted reproductive technologies (ART).

  C. Past pregnancy history.

    1. Written as

      a. Gravida: number of total pregnancies.

      b. Para: Number of specific type of deliveries a woman has had (Box 7.2).

    2. Include

Terminology of Pregnancy   **BOX 7.2**

Gravida: Refers to the number of times a woman has been pregnant, regardless of the outcome of the pregnancy or the number of babies born from the pregnancy.

Parity: Technically means the number of pregnancies that ended with the birth of a viable fetus. In practice, used as a system of digits describing the outcome of pregnancies.
   First digit: Number of term babies (36 weeks' gestation or 2,500 g) delivered.
   Second digit: Number of preterm babies delivered (28–36 weeks' gestation or 1,000 to 2,499 g).
   Third digit: Number of pregnancies ending in spontaneous or elective abortion.
   Fourth digit: Number of currently living children.
Example: If a woman is currently pregnant and has one living child born at term, she is listed as G2 P1001.

---

     a. Abortions.
     b. Miscarriages, ectopic, and molar pregnancies.
     c. Preterm deliveries.
     d. Number of living children and their current health.
     e. Multifetal gestations.
     f. Complications with pregnancy, labor, or delivery.
     g. Cesarean section deliveries.

X. Surgical history.
  A. Include past surgeries, types of anesthesia received, feelings about or physiologic reaction to any anesthesia received, and any complications.
    1. List all surgical procedures. Include
      a. Abdominal or pelvic surgeries that could affect pregnancy or delivery.
      b. Scarring.
      c. Complications.
  B. Other hospitalizations.
  C. Types of anesthesia ever received and any reactions.
  D. Blood transfusions.
  E. Accidents that caused injuries that may affect the woman's ability to labor or deliver.

XI. General health and nutrition.
  A. Exercise (Box 7.3 lists recommendations).

Recommendations Relating to
Exercise During Pregnancy

BOX 7.3

- Exercise of any kind should not be fatiguing and should be combined with periods of rest.
- Consult with provider about current or new exercise program.
- Avoid high-risk sports and activities.
- Decrease intensity of exercise as pregnancy progresses.
- Exercise at least three times per week for 30-minute intervals, with maximum pulse rate 140 to 150 beats/min.
- Wear supportive bra and shoes.
- Drink liquids before and after exercise to avoid dehydration.
- Avoid vigorous exercise in hot weather to prevent hyperthermia.
- Stretch and warm up before exercise (prepare joints and muscles for activity); cool down with mild activity (avoid pooling of blood).
- Stop activity and consult provider if symptoms occur (palpitations, shortness of breath, dizziness, abdominal pain, bleeding, numbness and tingling, no fetal movement).
- Avoid sitting or standing for long periods.

---

  1. Discuss amount and type currently practiced.
  2. Use opportunity to discuss and recommend moderate, regular exercise during pregnancy.
 B. Diet.
  1. Inquire about current special diet requirements.
   a. Lactose intolerance.
   b. Vegetarian.
   c. Food allergies.
  2. Check for calcium intake, and recommend supplementation as needed.
   a. Sources vary; however, 1,000- to 1,500-mg daily calcium intake is usually recommended.
   b. Adequate calcium can prevent calf cramps later in pregnancy.
  3. Encourage appropriate weight gain considering woman's age, prepregnancy weight, and health status.
   a. Evaluate prepregnancy weight using standardized measure (e.g., body mass index [BMI], ideal body weight [IBW]). Although opinions vary, normal-weight woman gain is 25 to 35 lb during the course of the pregnancy; less if overweight and more if underweight at the onset of pregnancy.

      b. The average additional caloric consumption to a normal diet is approximately 300 calories per day.

   4. Folate.

      a. The Centers for Disease Control and Prevention (CDC) recommends 0.4 mg of folic acid per day for prevention of neural tube defects.

      b. It is best to begin 1 month before conception and continue through the first 3 months of pregnancy.

   5. Iron: Evaluate hemoglobin and hematocrit levels. If iron-deficiency anemia present, woman should supplement with 30 to 120 g/day. (Not routinely recommended at onset of pregnancy.)

XII. Social history.

  A. Substance abuse: Note past use and current use, including amount and frequency.

   1. Use of any of the following substances is not recommended during pregnancy: cigarettes, alcohol, or illicit drugs.

   2. If patient is using cigarettes, alcohol, or illicit drugs, she should be informed of the potential effects on her fetus.

   3. She should be advised to stop her use of the substance or substances, and be encouraged to accept a referral to an appropriate treatment or counseling center.

   4. Some states have requirements regarding reporting to state agencies if there is a history of known substance abuse.

   5. Inquire about:

      a. Smoking: include amount smoked in a typical day.

         (1) Associated with low birth weight, stillbirth, and sudden infant death.

      b. Alcohol use: include type, amount, and pattern of use.

         (1) Safety level unknown, no use of alcohol is recommended during pregnancy.

         (2) Associated with low birth weight, stillbirth, and fetal alcohol syndrome.

         (3) Fetal alcohol syndrome is a leading cause of mental retardation.

      c. Illicit drugs: include type, amount, and pattern of use.

  B. Physical abuse (see chapter 19, The Sexual Assault Victim).

   1. Current or past.

   2. Counseling done in past.

   3. Encourage patient to assess her current safety, and refer her to counseling or local agencies as needed. Abuse may intensify during pregnancy.

C. Sexual abuse.
1. Current or past.
2. Counseling done in past.
3. Encourage patient to assess her current safety, and refer her to counseling or local agencies as needed. Abuse may intensify during pregnancy.

D. Financial stressors.
1. Does patient have insurance coverage or private means to pay for pregnancy. If not, refer to social worker, financial aid worker, Medicaid, or local funding organizations as needed.
2. Does she have housing and adequate food during and after pregnancy? If not, refer to Women, Infants and Children (WIC), social services, or local agencies as needed.

E. Social support system.
1. Family or friends whom the patient can rely on during her pregnancy and after delivery.

F. Patient's plans for pregnancy and postpartum recovery.
1. Does she plan to attend prenatal classes?
2. What contraception is she planning at the end of her pregnancy; if she plans sterilization, does she meet criteria within state or institution?
3. Does she plan to breastfeed or bottle feed her baby?

XIII. **Family history.**
A. Used for screening for potential physical and emotional complications of pregnancy and familial patterns of health or illness. Document relationship to patient and type of condition, if known.
1. Diabetes.
2. Hypertension or gestational hypertension.
3. Heart disease.
4. Renal disease.
5. Cancer, including primary site, if known.
6. Anemia.
7. Other blood disorders.
8. Infectious diseases: Screen for patient exposure or immunization.
9. Neurologic disorders.
10. Psychiatric disorders.
11. Congenital anomalies.
12. Genetic diseases.
13. Multifetal gestations or births.

XIV. Physical examination.
   A. A complete physical examination should be performed, including breast, abdominal, and pelvic examinations.
   B. Explain to the patient specifically what you will be doing and what she may expect to feel just before and during the examination.
   C. Baseline vital signs, blood pressure, height, and weight: These items will act as baseline measurements for the duration of the pregnancy.
   D. Breast examination (see chapter 6, Assessment of the Female Breast). In addition to routine observation and palpation, the examination should include a check of the nipples' ability to evert with a gentle squeeze of the areola, to predict eversion of nipples during breastfeeding.
   E. The abdominal examination should include
      1. Notation of any abdominal scarring.
      2. Fundal height in centimeters from the symphysis pubis to the top of the fundus, if the fundus is palpable (Figure 7.1).
      3. Estimation of size and position.
      4. Assessment of fetal heart tones can be auscultated using Doppler ultrasonography.
         a. It is possible to assess fetal heart tones by 10 weeks' gestation.
      5. Assess for gradual uterine and abdominal enlargement.
   F. Pelvic examination (see chapter 4, The Physical Examination). In addition to a routine pelvic examination, evaluate
      1. Chadwick's sign.
         a. A bluish color of the cervix caused by increased vascularity in pregnancy.
         b. May also be apparent in the vagina and vulva.
         c. Evident at approximately 6 to 8 weeks' gestation.
      2. Goodell's sign.
         a. Mild softening of the cervix from the nonpregnant state.
         b. May be evident at approximately 7 to 8 weeks' gestation.
      3. Hegar's sign.
         a. Softening and compressibility of the lower uterine segment.
      4. Cervical position, length, and any dilation. Dilatation or effacement (thinning of the cervical length) is abnormal until late in the third trimester.
      5. Uterine size should be estimated by use of bimanual examination, and congruence with LMP should be considered in estimating the current gestational age.

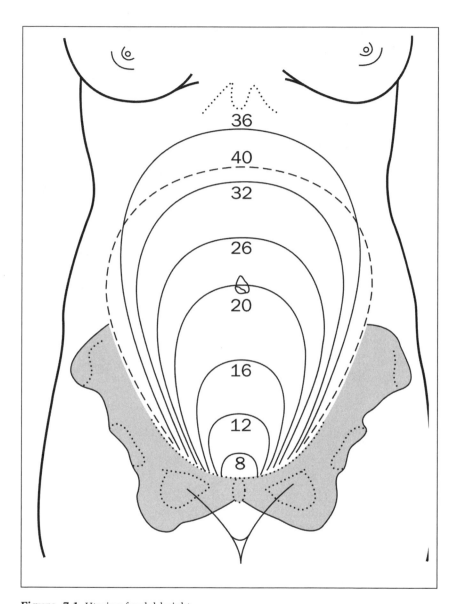

Figure 7.1 Uterine fundal height.

Risk Factors for Ectopic Pregnancy

BOX 7.4

1. Prior tubal pregnancy
2. Tubal surgery such as reversal of tubal ligation
3. Pelvic inflammatory disease, in which the tubes become scarred
4. Endometriosis
5. Intrauterine device

     a. If incongruence of size and dates is noted, ultrasonography should be considered to establish dating, fetal viability, and probable health status

  6. Adnexa should be palpated for pain or enlargement to screen for ectopic pregnancy.

     a. Ectopic pregnancy occurs when the fertilized ovum is implanted outside the uterus, usually in the fallopian tube.

     b. Symptoms initially are those of a normal pregnancy. Further symptoms may be vague or pronounced. They may include

       (1) Lower quadrant abdominal pain.

       (2) Spotting.

       (3) Syncopal symptoms (related to blood loss).

       (4) Adnexal tenderness.

       (5) Uterus may be normally enlarged.

       (6) Neck or shoulder pain with rupture.

     c. Obtain pelvic ultrasound and consider quantitative serum hCG to confirm diagnosis.

     d. Obtain consultation if ectopic pregnancy is suspected.

     e. Treatment is surgical.

     f. Risk factors are usually related to conditions that affect the lumen of the fallopian tubes or uterine cavity (Box 7.4).

  7. The bony pelvis should be evaluated during bimanual examination, including

     a. Diagonal conjugate.

     b. Sacral shape.

     c. Prominence of the ischial spines.

     d. Sacrosciatic notch.

     e. Coccyx mobility.

     f. Angle of the pubic arch.

     g. Diameter of the ischial tuberosities.

XV. Laboratory tests: Routine testing is performed to identify more

clearly pregnancies at risk and to provide an opportunity to prevent problems. It should include all of the following items:

A. Blood type and Rh factor.
   1. If patient is Rh negative and partner is Rh positive, Rh incompatibility may result. The patient should be advised that she will most likely receive RhoGAM during the pregnancy.
   2. If the patient's blood type is O and her partner's is A, B, or AB, there may be ABO incompatibility.
B. Antibody screen of serum.
   1. Antibodies are formed from major or minor blood group antigens.
   2. If the test yields positive results, the antibody should be identified and a titer should be performed.
   3. Screening should be repeated at 28 weeks' gestation in Rh-negative women.
C. Complete blood count (CBC) with differential smear.
   1. Hemoglobin and hematocrit.
      a. Blood volume increases 30 to 50% during pregnancy, with plasma volume increasing more than red blood cell (RBC) volume.
      b. A decrease in hemoglobin and hematocrit levels is normal during pregnancy.
      c. Mild anemia during pregnancy is defined as less than 11 g/dL hemoglobin; severe anemia is defined as less than 9g/dL.
      d. Anemia during pregnancy is usually iron-deficiency anemia; however, other types may coexist.
      e. Anemia should be treated using iron supplements, and severe anemia should be evaluated further, with referral made as needed.
   2. A platelet count should be performed to detect thrombocytopenia.
   3. Leukocytes: to screen for leukemia and infection. Pregnancy values may normally reach 17,000 leucocytes. RBCs and indices are used to diagnose various types of anemia.
   4. The differential is used to identify types of leukocytes, erythrocytes, cell abnormalities, and platelets.
D. Rubella titer to indicate immune status for rubella.
E. Serology.
   1. The venereal disease research laboratory (VDRL) test is usually used as a screening test for syphilis; if the test result is positive, a fluorescent treponemal antibody (FTA) test is performed to confirm diagnosis.

2. Current CDC guidelines state that parenteral penicillin is the only recommended treatment for syphilis during pregnancy

F. Hepatitis B surface antigen (HBsAg).
   1. If the test result is positive, the infant will need immunoprophylaxis at delivery.
   2. Vaccination is acceptable during pregnancy.

G. HIV screening.
   1. Recommended for all pregnant women as routine testing in prenatal care.
   2. Treatment for HIV can substantially lower transmission to infants of infected women from 15 to 20% to less than 2%. All pregnant women with HIV should be referred for treatment during pregnancy.

H. Urinalysis to screen for asymptomatic kidney or bladder disease (see chapter 11, Urinalysis).
   1. The presence of bacteria, leukocytes, and erythrocytes may indicate infection.
   2. The presence of casts or RBCs may indicate pyelonephritis.
   3. Glucose level may be normal in relation to increased glomerular filtration rate, or it may indicate carbohydrate intolerance. If the second test result is positive, testing for carbohydrate intolerance should be performed.
   4. Protein: Value greater than 1+ is abnormal and may be related to
      a. Urinary tract infection.
      b. Pregnancy-induced hypertension.
      c. Kidney disease.

I. Other screening to be considered for patients at risk.
   1. Sickle cell preparation or hemoglobin electrophoresis for sickle cell trait, thalassemia, or other hemoglobinopathy.
   2. Tay-Sachs screening for couples at risk.
   3. Toxoplasmosis screening should be performed if the woman is exposed to cat feces or undercooked meat.
      a. Women should be warned not to change cat litter or work in the garden without gloves during pregnancy.
   4. Cytomegalovirus screening with known exposure.
   5. Tuberculosis testing (purified protein derivative [PPD]).
   6. Thyroid screening if symptoms are present or as indicated.

J. Cervical or vaginal tests to consider.
   1. Papanicolaou (Pap) smear.
      a. All pregnant patients should receive a Pap smear within a year before the pregnancy ends.
         (1) Screens for cervical cancer and HPV.

(2) DNA testing should be ordered with Pap smear for high-risk HPV strains where available.

2. Chlamydia culture.
   a. Chlamydial infection necessitates treatment during pregnancy.
   b. Culture should be repeated after treatment for confirmation of cure.
   c. If the results are positive, treat per current CDC guidelines.
      (1) Current recommendation for treatment is: azithromycin 1 g orally in a single dose or amoxicillin 500 mg orally three times a day for 7 days.

3. Gonorrhea culture.
   a. Positive culture must be treated.
      (1) Current recommendation (April 2007) for treatment: ceftriaxone 125 mg intramuscularly in a single dose or cefixime 400 mg orally in a single dose or 400 mg by suspension (200 mg/5 ml).
      (2) plus treatment for chlamydia if chlamydial infection is not ruled out.
   b. The culture should be repeated 2 weeks after treatment for confirmation of cure.

4. Bacterial vaginosis: If there is a positive wet mount, treat the condition; treatment may lower incidence of preterm labor.

5. Herpes simplex virus.
   a. Women should be questioned regarding history of HSV, and if positive history, for prodromal symptoms and symptoms of outbreaks.
   b. Testing is necessary only to confirm the diagnosis of active herpes.
   c. Vaginal delivery is preferred if no lesions are visible at the onset of labor. If active lesions are present, cesarean section is the preferred mode of delivery.
   d. Risk to neonate varies by type of HSV and whether outbreak is initial infection or recurrence.
   e. Women should avoid any sexual contact with partners with known or suspected herpes during the third trimester. Efficacy and safety of retroviral medications has not been definitively established.

6. Group B streptococcus infection.
   a. Screening recommended for all pregnant women at 35 to 37 weeks' gestation.
   b. Treatment of choice is IV penicillin administered during la-

bor. Susceptibility testing should be done on specimens from patients with known penicillin allergy.

7. *Trichomonas.*
   a. Wet mount or culture.
   b. Usually treated after first trimester with metronidazole.
8. *Candida* infection.
   a. Infections tend to be more frequent during pregnancy.
   b. Seven-day course of topical azole is the only recommended treatment during pregnancy.

K. Other antenatal screening.
   1. Use of ultrasonography.
      a. May be performed for dating if unknown LMP or if there is a size/date discrepancy.
      b. Routine screening: frequently done at 19 weeks' gestation.
      c. To look for particular anomalies or complications of pregnancy.
         (1) Multiple gestations.
         (2) Molar pregnancy.
         (3) Fetal anomalies.
         (4) Maternal anomalies.
         (5) Placenta previa.
   2. Amniocentesis should be performed at approximately 17 weeks' gestation when indicated.
   3. Chorionic villus sampling at approximately 10 weeks' gestation is offered when indicated in women older than 35 years for screening for chromosomal abnormalities.
   4. The maternal serum alpha-fetoprotein (AFP) screen is offered at approximately 19 weeks' gestation as a screen to detect
      a. Neural tube defects.
      b. Down syndrome.
      c. Various other defects.

L. Table 7.4 summarizes common laboratory tests, indicating changes with pregnancy and timing of the test.

XVI. Planning at initial visit.
A. Most patients in the United States expect to be prescribed vitamins regardless of nutritional status. Prenatal vitamins are available over the counter or by prescription.
B. Laboratory tests should be ordered, and testing necessary in first or early second trimesters should be discussed and arranged.

Table 7.4 **Common Laboratory Values in Pregnancy**

Test	Normal Range (Nonpregnant)	Change in Pregnancy	Timing
Serum Chemistries			
Albumin	3.5–4.8 g/dL	↓ 1 g/dL	Most by 20 weeks', then gradual
Calcium (total)	9–10.3 mg/dL	↓ 10%	Gradual decrease
Chloride	95–105 mEq/L	No significant change	Gradual increase
Creatinine (female)	0.6–1.1 mg/dL	↓ 0.3 mg/dL	Most by 20 weeks'
Fibrinogen	1.5–3.6 g/L	↑ 1–2 g/L	Progressive
Glucose, fasting (plasma)	65–105 mg/dL	↓ 10%	Gradual decrease
Potassium (plasma)	3.5–4.5 mEq/L	↓ 0.2–0.3 mEq/L	By 20 weeks'
Protein (total)	6.5d > 8.5 g/dL	↓ g/dL	By 20 weeks', then stable
Sodium	135–145 mEq/L	↓ 2–4 mEq/L	By 20 weeks', then stable
Urea nitrogen	12–30 mg/dL	↓ 50%	First trimester
Uric acid	3.5–8 mg/dL	↓ 33%	First trimester, increase at term
Urinary Chemistries			
Creatinine	15–25 mg/kg per day (1–1.4 g/d)	No significant change	
Protein	Up to 150 mg/d	Up to 250–300 mg/d	By 20 weeks'
Creatinine clearance	90–130 ml/min per 1.73 m²	40–50%	By 16 weeks'
Serum Enzymatic Activities			
Amylase	23–84 IU/L	↑ 50–100%	Controversial
Transaminase	5–35 mU/dL	No significant change	Glutamic pyruvic (SGPT)
Glutamic oxaloacetic (SGOT)	5–40 mU/dL	No significant change	
Hematocrit (female)	36–46%	↓ 4–7%	Lowest values at 30–34 weeks'
Hemoglobin (female)	12–16 g/dL	↓ 1.5–2 g/dL	Lowest values at 30–34 weeks

(continued)

Table 7.4 *(continued)*

Leukocyte count	4.8–10.8 x 10³/mm³	↑ 3.5 x 10³/mm³	Gradual
Platelet count	150–400 x 103/mm³	Slight decrease	
Erythrocyte count	4.0–5.0 x 10⁶/mm³	↑ 25–30%	Begins 6–8 weeks
Serum Hormone Values			
Coritsol (plasma)	8–21 µg/dl	↑ 20 µg/dL	Peaks 28–32 weeks' then constant to term
Prolactin (female)	25 ng/dL	↑ 50–400 ng/dL	Gradual, peaks at term
Thyroxine, total (T₄)	5–11 g/dL	↑ 5 mg/dL	Early sustained
Triiodothyronine, total (T₃)	125–245 ng/dL	↑ 50%	Early sustained

C. Nutrition should be discussed with referral to a nutritional service, as needed.

D. Consultation should be arranged as needed for physical or emotional problems discovered during the visit, and the patient should be referred to social services or for medical consultation as needed.

E. The patient should be referred for consultation if she is not within normal limits in any aspect of her medical, gynecologic, or obstetrical status.

F. The patient should be given a short outline of Box 7.5 and instructed to return.

　1. 1 to 28 weeks' gestation: every 4 weeks.

　2. 28 to 37 weeks' gestation: every 2 weeks.

　3. 37 weeks' gestation to delivery: weekly.

　4. Centering, or group, prenatal care may be recommended if available

G. The patient should be asked whether there is any further information that she needs to share or questions she wishes to ask before her departure from the visit.

H. The patient should be instructed to call with any questions or problems (see Table 7.5 for warning signs).

I. Any prescription should be researched, and its benefits weighed against its potential hazards.

J. Inform the patient about prepared childbirth classes.

Questions to Ask at Each Subsequent Prenatal Visit

BOX 7.5

Since your last visit have you had problems with:

Physical symptoms, such as:

Headaches	Leaking urine
Eyes (blurred vision, blind spots, flashing lights or lines)	Not being able to wait to use the toilet
Swelling of face	Bleeding or spotting from vagina
Swelling of hands	Leaking fluid from your vagina (watery)
Swelling of legs or feet	Vaginal discharge or change in discharge
Pain in your chest	Vaginal burning, itching, or bad smell
Pain in your back	Increase in sores or growths in genital area
Pain in your abdomen	Illnesses or fever
Urination (burning or pain)	Exposure to sick children or adults

Signs of labor, such as:

Contractions	Pelvic pressure
Cramping	Low back ache
Any changes in the way the baby moves	Any visits to another doctor, midwife, nurse, clinic or emergency room?

Any medicines or substances you have used, including:

Medicines (prescription, vitamins, or over the counter)	Plants or herbs/herbal teas used to help you feel better or treat an illness
"Street" or illegal drugs you have used (if any)	Kind and amount of alcohol you have used (if any)
Number of cigarettes you have smoked per day (if any)	Do you need any prenatal vitamins, iron or other medicines?

Since your last visit, have you had any accidents, falls, been hit, hurt, or threatened?

(continued)

BOX 7.5 *(continued)*

There are many common discomforts of pregnancy. If there is one particular thing that is bothering you or that you want information about, or help or suggestions on how to work with or relieve the discomfort, please mark below. If none of these worry or bother you, skip this section.

Nausea (feeling sick to your stomach)

Diarrhea

Hemorrhoids

Heartburn

Varicose veins

Shortness of breath

Numbness or tingling of hands or legs or feet

Tired all the time (fatigue)

Sciatica (sharp pains down your leg)

Heart jumping, skipping, or beating very fast

Changes in desire for sex or way sex feels

Angry or irritable

Vomiting (throwing up)

Constipation

Not feeling hungry

Breast tenderness

Trouble sleeping

Leg cramps

Backache

Sad or crying for "no reason"

Unusual or intense dreams

Any other concern not on this list

On a scale of 1 (*awful*) to 10 (*wonderful*), how are you doing right now? If things are not so good, what would help?

Please tell us about anything else that is worrying you or about any information you want.

1. These classes are readily available throughout the country.
2. Provide the patient with valuable knowledge about labor and delivery to decrease anxiety.
3. Exercise and toning in preparation for labor often makes labor easier for most women.
4. Classes are a good way to help partners or support people be involved with pregnancy.

K. Additional concerns.
   1. Sexual intercourse.
      a. May be unrestricted in normal pregnancy as long as the cervix is not significantly dilated.
      b. Avoid if vaginal bleeding, ruptured membranes, or premature labor is present.
   2. Travel.

Table 7.5 **Warning Signs During Pregnancy**

Danger Sign or Symptom	Potential Cause
Marked decrease in fetal movement	Fetal compromise, anoxia
Vaginal bleeding Abdominal pain or cramping	Impending miscarriage, spontaneous abortion, or ectopic pregnancy
Leakage of fluid from the vagina	Premature rupture of membranes (PROM)
Persistent headache Dizziness Spots before the eyes Swelling of the hands or face Elevated blood pressure	Preeclampsia or pregnancy-induced hypertension
Fever or chills	Infection
Recurrent vomiting	Hyperemesis gravidarum

    a. Travel in itself is not necessarily harmful.

    b. Avoid long periods of sitting, which may cause venous stasis.

    c. Patient should consider possibility that competent obstetrical care may not be immediately available in some areas.

    d. Pressurized aircraft poses no additional risk. Airlines may have restrictions on overseas flights related to gestational age.

L. Box 7.6 lists questions to review at subsequent prenatal visits.

Continuing Assessment During Uncomplicated Pregnancy

BOX
7.6

Schedule of Return Visits
Once monthly, 1 to 28 weeks' gestation
Every 2 weeks, 27 to 36 weeks' gestation
Once weekly, 37 to 40 weeks' gestation

Weeks' Gestation	Assessment	Rationale
Every visit	Weight	Evaluate fetal growth, screen for maternal edema, pregnancy-induced hypertension (PIH), under and overnourishment
	Blood pressure (BP)	Screen for PIH
	Fundal height (McDonald's Rule)	Evaluate fetal growth
	Leopold's maneuvers after 32 weeks' gestation	Determine fetal position
	Fetal heart rate (FHR) after 10 weeks' gestation	Evaluate fetal well-being with Doppler after 10 weeks' gestation, with fetoscope if desired after 20 weeks' gestation
	Edema	Screen for PIH, fluid retention
	Symptoms	Identify problems, discomforts
	Adjustment	Identify problems, provide support
	Nutrition	Determine adequacy of diet
	Urinalysis	Glucose screen for gestational diabetes, protein screen for PIH
6 to 12 weeks	Chorionic villus sampling*	Detect fetal chromosomal abnormalities
10 to 12 weeks	Ultrasound if indicated	Determine fetal age, development
	Hemoglobin (Hgb) electrophoresis*	Detect sickle cell, thalassemias, other hemoglobinopathies
15 to 20 weeks	α-Fetoprotein	Screen for fetal neural tube defects
	Amniocentesis*	Detect fetal genetic abnormalities
	Ultrasound if indicated	Determine fetal age, development, screen for anomalies
24 to 28 weeks	Glucose 50 mg	Detect gestational diabetes
28 to 34 weeks	Hematocrit/Hgb	Detect anemia
37 to 42 weeks	GBS screening	Identify cervical changes preceding labor onset
	Pelvic examination, with STD screening, if indicated	Screen for current changes in STD infection status

*For clients at risk.

Assessment and Clinical Evaluation of Obesity in Women

CHAPTER 8

Yolanda R. Hill

I. **Obesity explained.**
    A. Obesity is a women's health issue because obesity disproportionately affects women.
        1. Obesity is the result of a higher intake of calories and a lower output of physical exercise.
        2. Obesity can dramatically influence the risk for development of disease.
        3. With more Americans spending less time performing physical activity, along with an increase in the abundance of food and portion sizes, obesity is inevitable in the American population.
        4. Overweight, obesity, and healthy weight ranges are determined using weight and height to calculate a number called the body mass index (BMI) in adults (see section VB in this chapter).
        5. Reasons for gender differences are related to biologic and psychological issues (i.e., pregnancy and menopausal changes).

6. Female sex hormones, specifically progesterone, influences food intake and energy expenditure.
7. Menstruation and exogenous hormones for contraception or symptoms of menopause may affect weight.
8. Most women in developed countries live substantial portions of their lives in a postmenopausal state.
9. The American culture excessive drive for female slimness may promote restrictive eating patterns, which may trigger overeating binges.
10. Obesity affects quality of life and quantity of life.

II. **Prevalence/etiology.**
   A. United States: Overall.
      1. In the United States, more than 64% of Americans are defined as overweight or obese. According to the National Health and Nutrition Examination Survey (NHANES) IV, the prevalence of obesity is higher in women (34%) than in men (28%). This is an 8% increase from the NHANES III 1988-1994 results, which showed the prevalence of obesity in women was 26% and in men was 21%.
      2. For women ages 20 to 74 years, 62% are overweight with a BMI of 25 or more. Of the 62%, 31% have a BMI of 40 or more.
   B. Ethnicity.
      1. The rates of obesity are disproportionate in ethnic groups. There is a higher prevalence of obesity among African American and Hispanic women than among White women.
      2. African American women are 80% more obese than African American men.
      3. Minority women have a higher prevalence of obesity.
      4. Obesity rates are 40% for Mexican American women and 50% for African American women, compared with 30% for Non-Hispanic White women.
      5. Overweight prevalence increases as women age (Table 8.1).
   C. Genetic: usually associated with extreme obesity, the conditions necessitate special care, identified early in age, based on features such as retardation and abnormal physical findings. Appropriate referrals by primary care clinicians and weight management teams for further genetic assessment and counseling.
      1. Prader-Willi syndrome: short stature, hypogonadism, short extremities.
      2. Angleman's syndrome: normal stature, movement disorder, happy affect.

Table 8.1   **Prevalence of Obesity Among U.S. Women
According to Age**

Increase in Overweight Prevalence With Age Among U.S. Women (1999 to 2000)	
Age (y)	Prevalence (%)
20–39	54.3
40–59	66.1
≥ 60	68.1

Note: Women are more likely to become overweight (BMI ≥ 25) as they become older.

3. Down syndrome: short stature, typical facial features, cardiac malformation, hypotonia.
4. Bardet-Biedl syndrome: normal/short stature, rod-cone dystrophy, polydactyly, renal structural defects.
5. Alstrom syndrome: normal/short stature, deafness, cardiomyopathy, rod-cone dystrophy.
6. Albright's osteodystrophy: normal/short stature, bradydactyly [short fingers], subcutaneous ossification.
7. Cohen syndrome: normal/short stature, distinctive facial features, retinochondrial dystrophy, granulocytopenia.
8. Carpenter syndrome: short stature; acrocephaly, polydactyly, hypogonadism.

D. Hypothalamic obesity.
   1. Hypothalamic obesity is rare, with bilateral injury to the ventromedial hypothalamus, the paraventricular hypothalamus, or the amygdala.
   2. Symptoms consist of increased intracranial pressure (headache, vomiting, blurred vision), hypopituitarism, and neurologic problems (seizures, coma, somnolence, temperature dysregulation).
   3. Hypothalamic obesity is caused by an increase in the early phase of insulin secretion from insulin sensitivity.

E. Endocrine causes.
   1. Hypothyroidism is common in older women. It is associated with small weight gain; however, most of the weight gain is not fat.
   2. Adrenal syndrome: Cushing's syndrome is characterized by central obesity, hypertension, and plethoric facies. Common characteristics are central obesity and thin extremities with atrophic skin.

      3. Polycystic ovarian disease is a manifestation of insulin resistance.
- **F.** Eating disorders.
  1. Prevalence is twice as high in the nonobese population (21% vs. 9%)
  2. Usually associated with emotional distress.
  3. Psychiatric referral necessary to establish the treatment plan.
- **G.** Exogenous obesity.
  1. Metabolic syndrome: a cluster of coronary heart disease risk factors sharing insulin resistance in common.
     a. Insulin resistance is the hallmark.
     b. Central feature is increased visceral fat.
     c. The increased release of free fatty acids impairs insulin clearance by the liver and alters peripheral metabolism.
     d. The reduced production of the protein adiponectin by fat cells is another potential factor in the development of insulin resistance.
     e. If at least three of the five criteria are abnormal, the metabolic syndrome is present.
        (1) Waist circumference more than 88 cm (> 35 in.).
        (2) High-density lipoprotein (HDL) level less than 50 mg/dL.
        (3) Triglyceride level 150 mg/dL or more.
        (4) Fasting glucose level 110 mg/dL or more.
        (5) Blood pressure (BP) ≥130/≥85 mmHg.
- **H.** Critical key biological periods.
  1. Puberty: has been shown to be a vulnerable period for development of obesity. Studies have shown that the onset of menses may contribute to the development of obesity later in life. During menarche, the gonadal steroids exert strong influences on body composition related to adipose tissue growth. Early onset of puberty is associated with high adiposity in adults.
  2. Postpartum: Retention of weight after pregnancy may be a factor in obesity in young women. The weight gain may reflect the changes in the lifestyle of the woman rather than the physiologic changes associated with childbirth. After delivery, women have a higher intake of food, have more accessibility to food during the day, experience decreased physical activity, spend more time watching television, and experience decreased social support.
  3. Postmenopause: Weight changes in older women may be as-

sociated with aging rather than with menopause. The reduction of lean body mass causes increase in weight due to the reduction in the body's metabolism rate. During this time, it is easier for aging women to gain weight than to lose it.

4. Menopause.

   a. Studies have shown women at menopause had significant increases in total cholesterol, low-density lipoproteins, and insulin levels.

   b. Studies have suggested that abdominal fat distribution is strongly influenced by hormonal replacement therapy.

   c. Weight is increased in aging women because of a decrease in physical activity during leisure time and because of a decreased resting metabolic rate.

   d. Decreases in metabolic rate may be due to the loss of lean tissue mass and loss of the luteal-phase increase in energy expenditure.

   e. Estrogens promote lower body fat accumulation, whereas androgens have been associated with upper body fat distribution.

   f. The ratio of androgens to estrogens shifts, thereby increasing abdominal fat distribution.

III. **Risks associated with obesity or health consequences.**

A. Nonmodifiable risks.

   1. Hypertension: BP greater than 140/90 mmHg or the use of any antihypertension medications.

   2. High HDL cholesterol level: greater than 160 mg/dL.

   3. Low HDL cholesterol level: lower than 35 mg/dL.

   4. Impaired fasting glucose level: 110 to 125 mg/dL.

   5. Family history of premature coronary heart disease.

   6. Atherosclerotic disease.

   7. Sleep apnea.

   8. The metabolic syndrome.

   9. Age older than 55 years in women.

   10. History of polycystic ovarian syndrome.

B. Modifiable risks.

   1. Cigarette smoking.

   2. Lack of physical exercise.

C. Complications of obesity are summarized in Box 8.1.

IV. **Health history.**

A. Age.

   1. Age older than 65 years is a cardiac risk factor.

Medical Complications of Obesity

BOX
8.1

Diabetes mellitus (type 2)	Hypertension
High cholesterol levels	Coronary heart disease
Congestive heart failure	Angina pectoris
Stroke	Asthma
Osteoarthritis	Musculoskeletal disorders
Gallbladder disease	Sleep apnea
Respiratory problems	Gout
Bladder control problems	

B. History of weight gain.

    1. Weight gain greater than 10 kg (22 lb) at 18 to 20 years of age increases the health risk.

C. History of eating disorders: bulimia or anorexia nervosa; referral to specialist.

D. Breastfeeding or pregnancy: defer weight loss.

E. Sleep apnea: At a higher risk for obesity; necessitates a more intensive treatment regimen.

F. Coronary artery disease.

G. Arteriosclerotic vascular disease/dyslipidemia.

H. Diabetes.

I. Thyroid.

J. Polycystic ovarian syndrome

K. Physical activity.

L. Diet.

M. History of smoking.

N. Social history/socioeconomic status.

    1. Employment status and type of occupation.

    2. History of drug abuse.

    3. Living arrangements.

O. Family history of premature coronary artery disease, diabetes, eating disorders, gallbladder disease.

P. History of use of medications associated with weight gain (Box 8.2).

V. Focused physical assessment.

    A. Height, weight and BMI.

        1. Height.

        2. Weight.

        3. Body shape (Figure 8.1).

            a. Pear-shaped body.

Medications Associated With Weight Gain   BOX 8.2

1. Glucocorticoids
2. Megace
3. Cyproheptadine
4. Antidepressants (tricyclic, MAO inhibitors, selective serotonin reuptake inhibitors [SSRIs], mirtazapine)
5. Mood stabilizers (lithium)
6. Antipsychotics and phenothizianes (clozapine, olanzapine, risperidone)
7. Antiepileptic medications (valproate, gabapentin)
8. Hormones (contraceptives, corticosteroids, progestational steroids)
9. α-Adrenergic-blocking drugs
10. Antidiabetic agents (sulfonylureas, insulin, thiazolidinediones, and drugs that stimulate insulin release)

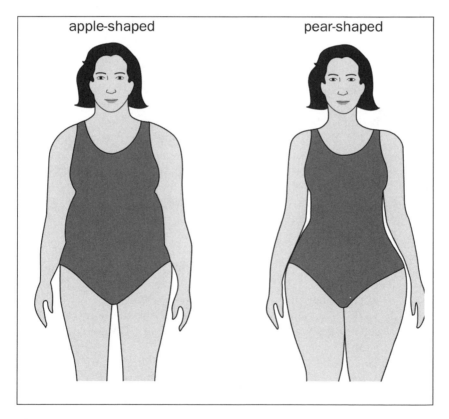

Figure 8.1 Apple-shaped and pear-shaped bodies.

	120	130	140	150	160	170	180	190	200	210	220	230	240	250
4'6	29	31	34	36	39	41	43	46	48	51	53	56	58	60
4'8	27	29	31	34	36	38	40	43	45	47	49	52	54	56
4'10	25	27	29	31	34	36	38	40	42	44	46	48	50	52
5'0	23	25	27	29	31	33	35	37	39	41	43	45	47	49
5'2	22	24	26	27	29	31	33	35	37	38	40	42	44	46
5'4	21	22	24	26	28	29	31	33	34	36	38	40	41	43
5'6	19	21	23	24	26	27	29	31	32	34	36	37	39	40
5'8	18	20	21	23	24	26	27	29	30	32	34	35	37	38
5'10	17	19	20	22	23	24	26	27	29	30	32	33	35	36
6'0	16	18	19	20	22	23	24	26	27	28	30	31	33	34
6'2	15	17	18	19	21	22	23	24	26	27	28	30	31	32
6'4	15	16	17	18	20	21	22	23	24	26	27	28	29	30
6'6	14	15	16	17	19	20	21	22	23	24	25	27	28	29
6'8	13	14	15	17	18	19	20	21	22	23	24	25	26	28

Figure 8.2 Body mass index measurements.

         (1) Hips wider than shoulders due to body stores of fat there; lower risk for diabetes and heart problems.
      b. Apple-shaped body.
         (1) Body fat is stored around middle; higher risk for heart problems.
         (2) Common in midlife and menopause due to decreasing levels of estrogen.
   B. BMI measurement (Figure 8.2).
   C. Weight in kilograms divided by height in meters squared.
      1. Determine correct height (cm) and weight (kg) of the patient.
      2. Convert height to meters by dividing the number of centimeters by 100:
         a. cm of height/100 (Do not round the value.)
      3. Take the square (obtained by multiplying the number by itself) of the resulting number and save it. (Do not round the value.)
      4. To calculate BMI: Divide the weight by the square of the height calculated in No. 3. (Do not round either of these values.)
      5. This answer, the BMI, should be rounded to the nearest tenth.

Sample Recording of BMI

BOX 8.3

1. Convert weight from pounds to kilograms.
   Weight: 130 lb = 59.09 kg (1 lb = 2.2 kg)

2. Convert height from inches to centimeters.
   Height: 5 ft 4 in. = 64 in. × 2.54 = 162.56 cm (1 in. = 2.54 cm)

3. Convert the height to meters by dividing the number of centimeters by 100:
   162.56 cm/100 = 1.6256 (Do **not** round the value.)

4. Take the square of the resulting number and save it. (Do **not** round the value.) To get the square, multiply the number by itself.
   1.6256 × 1.6256 = 2.6425753

5. To calculate the BMI: Divide the weight by the square of the height calculated in No. 4. (Do **not** round either the weight or the square of the height.)
   59.09 kg ÷ 2.6425753 = 22.36; BMI = 22.4

Definition of BMI: kg of body weight
$\overline{\qquad\qquad\qquad\qquad}$
M² of body height

---

      a. Example: 29.85 is expressed as 29.9.
      b. Example: 29.84 is expressed as 29.8.
  6. Example of calculation of BMI for a patient who weights 130 lb and is 5 ft 4 in. (Box 8.3).
  7. The advantage of using the BMI is that it is gender nonspecific.
  8. The BMI provides an approximation of mortality risk for obesity.
  9. The BMI is used because it correlates with the amount of body fat; however, it is not a measurement of body fatness. An adult who has a BMI between 25 and 29.9 is considered overweight. An adult who has a BMI of 30 or higher is considered obese.
D. Waist and hip circumference: provides an indication of trunk or visceral obesity, often associated with diabetes and heart disease. To determine the circumference:
  1. The patient should stand up straight in the upright position with feet together.
  2. Instruct patient to relax and stand with arms to the side.
  3. Expose the waist with the undergarments pulled below the waist.

| *Calculating Daily Caloric Requirements* | **BOX 8.4** |

Step 1
Estimate the recommended individual caloric requirement (kcal per day) by calculating the resting energy expenditure (REE).

For adult women:
REE = 10 x weight (in kg) + 6.25 x height (in cm) – 5 x age (in years) – 161

Example = 10 x 59.09 + 6.25 x 162.56 – 5 x 36 – 161 = 1587.9
590.9   +   1016   –   19   = 1587.9

Weight: 130 lbs = 59.09 kgs
Height: 5"4 = 64 inches × 2.54 = 162.56 cm

Step 2
Multiply REE by an activity factor (AF) of 1.5 for women for light activity to estimate daily caloric need or by 1.6 for women for higher activity.

Example = 1587.9 x 1.5 = 2381.85 kcal

REE x AF = estimated total caloric need (kcal per day) to maintain weight
REE = resting energy expenditure

4. Find the natural waist, which is the narrowest part of the torso. This area is midway between the inferior border of the rib cage and the superior aspect of the iliac crest.
5. Place the tape measure at the measuring point and locate the point on the tape where the zero aligns with the measuring point. Record to the nearest 0.1 cm. Hold tape horizontally.
6. If necessary, ask the obese patient to elevate any sagging abdominal wall.
7. Take measurement at the end of normal expiration.
E. Calculating daily caloric requirement (Box 8.4).
F. BP: elevation with plethora: consider Cushing's syndrome.
G. Ear, nose, throat (ENT): noisy breathing, sleep disturbance, daytime sleepiness.
H. Funduscopic examination: intracranial pressure increased?
I. Plethora and thin skin: consider Cushing's syndrome.
J. Respiratory: shortness of breath, coughing with exercise, cannot climb two flights of steps without cough/wheeze.
K. Cardiac: heart palpitations.
L. Gastrointestinal: regular patterns of diarrhea, constipation, vomiting (bulimia, secret eating or binge eating).

Table 8.2   **Metabolic Assessment of Obesity**

Parameter	Measurement	Critical Value
Obesity	Body mass index (BMI)	Up to 24.9 = normal 25–29.9 = overweight 30–34.9 = class I obesity 35–39.9 = class II obesity ≥ 40 = class III obesity
Body fat distribution	Waist circumference	Women > 35 in. (89 cm)
Fasting lipid profile	High-density lipoprotein (HDL)	Women < 50 mg/dL
	Triglycerides	Women > 150 mg/dL
	Low-density lipoprotein	Women > 100 mg/dL
Insulin resistance	Fasting blood glucose (mmol/L)	HOMA-IR ≥ 5mmol/L
	Fasting insulin	60 pmo/L
Hypertension	Blood pressure	Systolic > 130 mmHg Diastolic > 85 mmHg

M. Abdominal examination: aneurysm or atherosclerosis: high risk.

N. Polyuria (polycystic ovarian syndrome): irregular menses or absence of menses.

O. Hypogonadism: Consider genetic syndrome.

P. Orthopedics: hip pain, knee pain, or limp.

Q. Peripheral edema: consider sleep apnea, increased intraabdominal pressure, or heart failure.

R. Pedal pulses: atherosclerotic vascular disease is a risk factor for obesity.

S. Arrest of linear growth: consider childhood Cushing's syndrome or other endocrine cause for obesity.

T. Metabolic assessment summary (Table 8.2).

VI. **Laboratory testing.**

A. Fasting blood glucose level: diabetes is a high risk factor for obesity; impaired glucose tolerance is a risk factor.

B. High levels of triglycerides, low HDL cholesterol levels: risk factor.

C. High LDL cholesterol level: risk factor.

D. Electrocardiography: myocardial infection is a high risk factor

E. Dual-energy x-ray absorptiometry: accurate way to measure total body fat.

F. Computed tomography (CT): can quantify the amount of visceral fat in the abdomen.

VII. Interventions.

A. Behavioral.

B. Pharmacologic.

  1. Many state boards of nursing prohibit the prescription of antiobesity medication by an advanced practice registered nurse (APRN). Check with your state board of nursing for guidance on antiobesity medications.

VIII. Development of a weight management plan: An effective weight management plan is designed to help an overweight or obese person reach and stay at a healthy body weight. There are several options for weight control in practice today.

A. The NHLBI (National Heart, Lung, and Blood Institute) panel recommends treatment for obesity for patients with a BMI of 25 to 29 kg/m^2 and with two or more risk factors and for patients with a BMI of 30 or more with no risk factors.

B. The overall goals of weight management are to reduce body weight and maintain a lower body weight long-term, prevent further weight gain, and control potential risk factors.

C. Nurse practitioners should counsel their patients about dietary interventions, increasing the amount of physical activity, behavior therapy, pharmacotherapy, and a combination of all techniques.

D. The ability to prescribe obesity drugs varies by state. Check with your state board of nursing regarding the rules and regulations for prescribing antiobesity medication.

E. The most effective therapy for weight loss and maintenance is a combination of a low-calorie diet, an increase in physical activity, and lifestyle modifications. Table 8.3 shows recommendations for the average daily allowance.

F. Using this therapy for at least 6 months and setting a goal for a 10% reduction in weight should be the initial goal for the patient. Patient continued participation is the most important outcome in weight management.

G. Results of recent clinical trials suggested that weight management plans should be created according to a woman's current phase of life. The critical phases that should be targeted include puberty, postpartum, and during menopause. There are key weight management interventions during these critical periods that produce weight loss.

H. Women should see the Internet sources listed in Box 8.5 for further information.

Table 8.3   **Recommended Average Daily Energy Allowances for Women**

Population Group	Age (y)	Kcal/kg	Kcal/day
Women:	11–14	47	2,200
nonpregnant,	15–18	40	2,200
nonlactating	19–24	38	2,200
	25–50	36	2,200
	> 51	30	1,900

Note: This is based on women engaged in light to moderate physical activity, with no underlying medical condition.

Selected Internet Resources for Patients   **BOX 8.5**

www.eatright.org
The American Dietetic Association offers information on nutrition, healthy lifestyle, and how to find a registered dietician.

www.nal.usda.gov/about/oei/index.htm
The National Heart, Lung, and Blood Institute Obesity Education Initiative offers information on selecting a weight loss program, menu planning, food label reading, and BMI calculation and interpretation.

www.niddk.nih.gov/health/nutrit/win.htm
Weight Control Information Network has weight loss articles from the National Institutes of Health.

www.fitday.com
FitDay.com gives nutrition analysis of calories, fat, protein, carbohydrates, and fiber in table and graph form as well as offering journals, and goal-setting and activity-tracking tools.

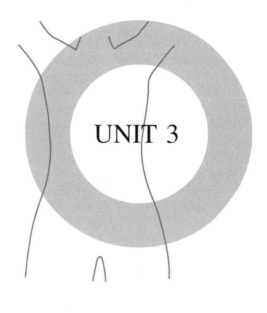

UNIT 3

Investigative Procedures

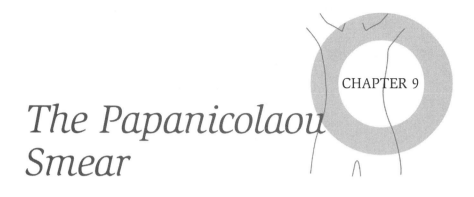

CHAPTER 9

The Papanicolaou Smear

Rebecca Koeniger-Donohue

I. **The Papanicolaou (Pap) smear explained: The Pap smear, or test, named for Dr. George Papanicolaou in the 1940s, is a periodic screening test based on cytologic examination of cervical cells. The Bethesda system terminology is used for cytologic classification. Please refer to the algorithms detailing the different management recommendations for cytologic and histologic management, available at the American Society for Colposcopy and Cervical Pathology (ASCCP) www.ascccp.org.**

A. Conventional or liquid based Pap smear is the standard method of screening for cervical cancer. It is used to detect changes in the cervix that may be related to cancer, precancerous conditions, infection, inflammation, or hormonal changes.

B. The test is relatively inexpensive and extremely valuable as a screening tool because laboratory evaluation of the cells can detect precancerous conditions long before they become cancerous.

C. The test is a screening test; it is not a diagnostic test. However, it is the most effective screen ever developed.

D. The Pap screening test suggests potential appropriate next steps in the diagnostic process. Colposcopy is diagnostic.

E. Some statistics.

  1. Since the introduction of the Pap smear, there has been a dramatic decrease in the number of deaths from cancer of the cervix.

2. It is estimated that 11,070 women will be diagnosed with cervical cancer, and 3,870 women will die of cancer of the cervix uteri in 2008 in the United States.

3. The incidence of cervical cancer in young women is low: incidence rate of invasive cervical cancer: 0/100,000/year for ages 10 to 19 years, 1.3/100,000/year for ages 20 to 24 years.

4. Many lesions will regress spontaneously: Research indicates that 91% of human papillomavirus (HPV) infections in college-aged women resolve within 2 years[1]; 61% of low-grade squamous intraepithelial lesions (LSILs) in young women regress at 12 months and 91% regress at 36 months; 3% of LSILs progress to high-grade SILs (HSILs).

5. More Black and Hispanic women get cervical cancer and are diagnosed at later stages of the disease than women of other races, possibly due to decreased access to Pap testing or follow-up treatment. Cancers missed by laboratories represent only a tiny fraction of cervical cancers. Of women who develop cervical cancer, 22% do not regularly undergo Pap testing in the first place.

F. Assess risk factors for cervical cancer (Box 9.1).

G. Provide preventive education and counseling. Box 9.1 lists measures that can be used to reduce the risk for cervical cancer.

H. Limitations of the Pap smear.

1. Errors in Pap smear testing can be broadly categorized as errors in sampling and preparation, screening, or interpretation.

a. Sampling and preparation represent the greatest limitation because the sample must contain a representative smear.

II. Cervical cancer.

A. Infection of the cervix with high-risk HPV is a requirement for diagnoses for virtually all cervical carcinomas (squamous cell and adenocarcinoma).

---

[1]Author note: Visit the ASCCP Web site for information on the first HPV genotyping assay, which was approved in March 2009. Based on this approval, ASCCP released the Management Algorithm for Using HPV Genotyping to Manage HPV High-risk Positive/Cytology Negative Women 30 Years and Older. This also includes the descriptions of the new FDA-approved P HPV DNA designed to identify 14 high-risk types of HPV. This test will be marketed under the name Cervista HPV HR for use with ThinPrep samples. Available at: http://www.asccp.org/pdfs/consensus/hpv_genotyping_20090320.pdf. Click on 2009 Algorithm: Use of HPV Genotyping to Manage HPV HR Positive/Cytology Negative Women 30 Years and Older.

Risk Factors for Cervical Cancer	BOX 9.1

Unprotected sex, particularly if with multiple partners
Early coitarche (age of first intercourse < 18 years)
A sexual partner with more than one sexual partner or a history of multiple sexual partners
A personal history of
    Exposure to other sexually transmitted diseases
    HPV, particularly if a smoker
    DES exposure
    Previous abnormal Pap smear
    HIV
    Malnutrition

DES = diethylstilbestrol; HIV = human immunodeficiency virus; HPV = human papillomavirus.

B. The addition of cofactors may trigger malignant transformation. These include
    1. Other sexually transmitted diseases.
    2. Infection with human immunodeficiency virus (HIV).
    3. Smoking.
    4. Nutritional deficiencies.
C. Of the more than 100 known HPV types that may infect humans, only approximately 40 infect the female genital tract, 14 of which are considered oncogenic or high-risk carcinogenic types for cervical carcinoma.
D. Two types—HPV 16 and HPV 18—account for nearly 70% of cervical carcinomas.
E. HPV testing should target only high-risk carcinogenic cancer–associated types.
F. Types of cancer detected.
    1. Squamous cell carcinomas: 90%.
    2. Adenacarcinomas: 10%.
G. Clinical description: HPV depends on the differentiation of the epithelium to regulate its replication and complete its life cycle.
    1. Low-grade lesions are characterized by abnormal proliferation up to the lower third of the epithelium.
    2. Cervical intraepithelial neoplasia (CIN) lesions are graded based on the extent of abnormal proliferation of the basal layer of the cervical epithelium. In mild dysplasia (CIN-I), proliferation occurs up to the lower third of the epithelium. CIN-I includes mild dysplasia and condyloma (anogenital warts).

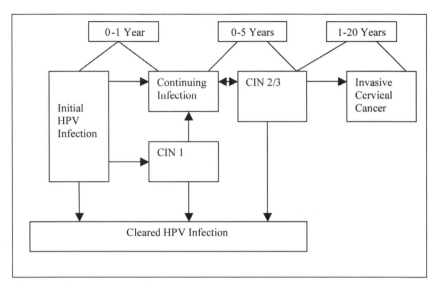

Figure 9.1 Progression of invasive carcinoma.

3. Enlarged keratinocytes, termed koilocytes, are present in the upper layers of the epithelium. These cells serve as a typical marker of HPV infection.
   a. The shedding of dead keratinocytes releases HPV virions to infect other cells or transmit the virus to another individual.
H. Cervical cancer may arise either in situ (undifferentiated malignant cells) or as invasive disease.
   1. The peak incidence of carcinoma in situ occurs between the ages of 35 and 45 years.
   2. Cervical cancer is rare in adolescents.
   3. Cervical malignancy usually occurs after years of dormancy, which may last as long as 10 to 20 years.
   4. Rapid development of invasive carcinoma is rare (Figure 9.1).
I. Symptoms.
   1. Abnormal uterine bleeding is the most significant finding, and it is usually associated with friability of the diseased cervix, occurring as postcoital or midcycle spotting.
   2. The condition may go undetected for years if a Pap smear is not performed during the invasive stage.
J. Women should be taught measures to reduce the risk for cervical cancer (Box 9.2).

Measures to Reduce the Risk of Cervical Cancer	**BOX 9.2**

Avoid early coitarche (age of first intercourse).
Practice bilateral sexual monogamy.
Use condoms 100% consistently and correctly.
Pap test screening per clinician recommendation.
Avoid smoking cigarettes.
Consume a diet rich in vitamins A and C and folate.

III. Screening.

    A. Start at age 21 or 3 years after first intercourse (whichever comes first) (ACS, 2002; USPTF, 2003; ACOG, 2003).

    B. Start annually, and then extend to every 2 to 3 years.

    C. Most organizations recommend two to three normal Pap smears at the annual visits before extending the interval (United States Preventive Services Task Force [USPSTF], 2003).

    D. Extend the interval to every 2 to 3 years when the woman is older than 30 years of age and has had 3 prior normal Pap smears (American Cancer Society [ACS], 2002; American College of Obstetrics and Gynecology [ACOG], 2003).

    E. Continue annual screening in women who are HIV positive or immunocompromised or have a history of diethylstilbestrol (DES) exposure.

    F. Discontinue screening at age 65 to 70 years if the woman has had regular screening and zero abnormal Pap smears in the previous 10 years (USPSTF, 2003; (age 65); ACS, 2002 (age 70); ACOG does not set an upper age limit).

    G. HPV DNA Screening.

        1. Women 30 years of age and older who have a negative test result for high-risk HPV DNA and for whom cytology is negative should be rescreened after 3 years and not before.

        2. Dual screening with HPV DNA testing and cervical-type cytology, either conventional or liquid based, is recommended by the American Cancer Society for primary screening of women 30 years of age and older.

            a. Types 6 and 11 are low risk and are responsible for genital warts.

            b. Types 16 and 18 are high risk and cause approximately 70% of cervical cancer worldwide.

            c. HPV types classified as high risk or as carcinogenic:

Types 16, 18, 31, 33, 35, 39, 45, 41, 52, 56, 58, 59 are considered precursors of cervical cancer.

   d. HPV types classified as probable high risk: 26, 53, 66, 73, and 82.

   e. HPV types classified as low risk: 6, 11, 40, 42, 43, 44, 54, 61, 70, 72, 81, and 89

3. A woman who is scheduled to have a Pap smear every 2 to 3 years may change her sexual partner and fall into a high-risk category.

H. Women who underwent hysterectomy.

1. Elicit reasons why hysterectomy was performed.

   a. Benign: ACS and USPSTF guidelines recommend ceasing routine Pap screening for women who have undergone total hysterectomy for benign disease (such as fibroids or uterine prolapse).

   b. Malignancy: If hysterectomy was performed because of cervical dysplasia, Pap smear testing should be performed every 3 months for 2 years, every 6 months for 3 years, then yearly.

I. DES offspring.

1. Use of DES was discontinued by the U. S. Food and Drug Administration (FDA) in 1971; therefore, treatment of DES offspring now includes those women who are age 37 years of age and older.

2. Women whose mothers took DES while pregnant may have a very large area of columnar tissue on the outside of the cervix. The cervix often appears to have a collar. This tissue is more fragile and subject to infection.

   a. Recommended testing.

   (1) Baseline colposcopy.

   (2) Vaginal and cervical Pap smears every 6 to 12 months until 30 years old.

   (3) Yearly cervical and vaginal Pap smears.

IV. Obtaining the Pap smear.

A. Patient instructions: When the patient schedules her appointment for a Pap smear, she should be instructed in the following:

1. Do not schedule Pap smear during menses because the presence of blood may obscure results. If the patient is ovulatory or if other excessive mucus is present, remove with a swab.

2. Avoid intercourse for 48 hours before the test.

3. Abstain from vaginal douches, creams, or medications for 48

hours before the Pap test. Douching and medications may remove or contaminate those cells necessary for diagnosis.
Pap smears can be obtained under these conditions if abso-
lutely necessary, but the woman must understand that the results may be altered.

    4. If the woman is in postpartum recovery, schedule the smear
for 6 to 8 weeks after delivery, by which time the cervix will
have undergone reparative changes.

B. Equipment: The following equipment should be assembled:

    1. Nonsterile gloves.

    2. Speculum (metal or plastic).

    3. A good light source (a speculum with a light is ideal).

    4. One frosted glass slide (some facilities use the two-glass
slide system) or liquid-based container.

    5. A pencil for labeling the frosted portion with the woman's
name or a marker for the liquid-based container.

    6. A single or double cardboard slide cover.

    7. A cytobrush, broom, or cotton swab.

    8. An Ayer wooden or plastic spatula—"notched."

    9. Aerosol fixative if conventional smear.

C. Preparation of the conventional slide.

    1. The cells on the slide must be clearly visible to be accurately
interpreted. Characteristics of an adequate smear include

        a. An adequate number of squamous epithelial cells.

        b. Lack of excessive amounts of blood, inflammatory exu-
date, or ovulatory discharge.

        c. Good fixation of smear, with minimal air-drying artifact.

        d. Spreading of cells sufficiently thin in monolayer, properly
distributed on the slide.

        e. Adequate labeling of slide. The name should be printed in
pencil on the frosted portion of the slide.

D. The technique: The conventional Pap smear is obtained during
the routine speculum examination. Careful sampling techniques
are vital to ensure an adequate sample for accurate interpretation by the pathologist.

    1. Insert a lightly lubricated speculum into the vaginal canal.

    2. Gently open the speculum to clearly visualize the cervical
os.

    3. With a large swab, carefully clear any excessive cervical mu-
cus from the cervix. If the discharge is colored or has an
odor, obtain a pH test of the secretions, taken from the lateral wall of the vagina, and perform a wet mount before

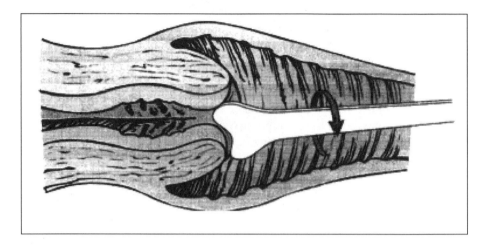

Figure 9.2 Cervical scrape.

sending the Pap smear to the laboratory. If an inflammatory condition is present, the condition should be treated; the woman asked to return for the Pap smear in 1 or 2 months.

4. Any areas that look suspicious should be scraped and sampled.

5. The sample should include squamous epithelial cells from the ectocervix and columnar cells from within the transformation zone within the endocervix. Cells from the squamo-columnar junction are reported as "endocervical" cells.

6. Cells that are undergoing change and within the transformation zone are called metaplastic, which is a normal finding.

7. Obtaining the ectocervical sample using the Ayer spatula (Figure 9.2).

    a. Firmly place the longer projection of the notched end of the Ayre spatula into the os and rotate 360°. A small sample of cells will be collected on the spatula. The objective is to scrape the exfoliated cells or those cells held loosely on the surface of the cervix.

    b. Use firm pressure; be careful to avoid excessive abrasion that may cause bleeding.

    c. Hold the horizontal surface with the sample on it in the upright position as the spatula is withdrawn from the cervix.

    d. Place the flat side of the paddle against the labeled glass

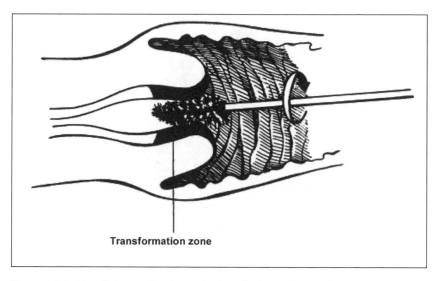

Figure 9.3 Use of the cytobrush to obtain cells from the transformation zone.

slide and smear uniformly to create a monolayer across two thirds of the side, using one firm motion. A counterclockwise circular or zigzag pattern may be used. Be careful not to use too much pressure because it may alter or destroy the cell structure.

8. Obtaining the endocervical sample using the cytobrush.
   a. Insert the cytobrush into the cervical os and rotate, gathering a sample of cells and taking care to sample the squamocolumnar junction (transformation zone; Figure 9.3).
   b. Unroll the specimen on the slide in the opposite direction of that taken when collecting the specimen.
   c. Add to the remaining third of the slide, being careful not to overlap the ectocervical sample.
   d. Some providers prefer to obtain the endocervical component first. However, because the os tends to bleed with use of the cytobrush, it is best to obtain the ectocervical sample first before it becomes obscured with blood resulting from obtaining the endocervical sample.
   e. Use in pregnancy: It is controversial whether the cytobrush should be used in a pregnant woman because trauma from the brush may cause the cervix to bleed. It is becoming the standard of care to use the cytobrush

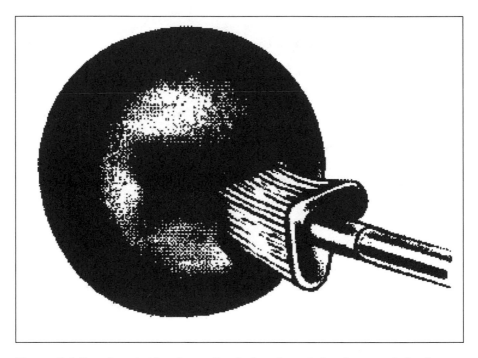

Figure 9.4 Use of cervical brush to collect both endocervical and extocervical cells.

gently in pregnant women. However, the manufacturer of the cytobrush still cautions against its use in pregnant women.

9. Obtaining a combined endocervical and ectocervical sample.
   a. Recent studies suggest that use of the "broom" results in the best yield of endocervical cells (Figure 9.4)
   b. A paintbrush-type (broom) instrument may be used instead of the cytobrush or the spatula. It is used for collecting both the ectocervical and the endocervical samples. It uses flexible plastic bristles, which reportedly cause less blood spotting.
   c. The brush is introduced into the vagina, with the central long bristles inserted into the os or until the lateral bristles bend fully against the ectocervix.
   d. Maintain gentle pressure, and rotate the brush by rolling the handle between the thumb and the forefinger three to five times to the left and right, simultaneously collecting

Comparison of Cytobrush and Broom   BOX 9.3

Advantages and Disadvantages of Using the Cytobrush for Endocervical Samples
Advantages
   High efficiency for collection of endocervical cells
   Can insert into a narrow os more easily
Disadvantages
   May cause more discomfort and bleeding
   Controversy regarding whether safe for use during pregnancy

Advantages and Disadvantages of Using the Broom for Endocervical Samples
Advantages
   Causes less spotting
   Highly effective for endocervical cell collection
   Simultaneously collects both the endocervical and ectocervical sample
Disadvantages
   Cannot be used during pregnancy
   More expensive
   May not be as effective in obtaining endocervical cells in a tight
   cervical os with the transformation zone high in the canal

cell specimens from both endocervical and ectocervical cells.

   e. Withdraw the brush.
   f. Transfer the sample to the slide with two single paint strokes, applying first the one side of the bristle, then the other side, painting the slide again in exactly the same area. Apply fixative as before.
   g. The brush should only be used on nonpregnant patients. Box 9.3 compares different applicators.
10. Vaginal specimens. Some clinicians also like to use a vaginal swab to capture exfoliated cells from the uterus and tubes that may be present in the vaginal pool. Others believe it is not necessary and may only serve to decrease the quality of the sample by adding degenerating cells. It is not reliable for screening for cervical cancer.
   a. Women with a cervix.
      (1) Moisten cotton-tipped applicator with saline or use the handled end of the spatula.
      (2) Insert the applicator into the vagina, and rotate it against the vaginal wall, just under and lateral to the cervix (Figure 9.5).

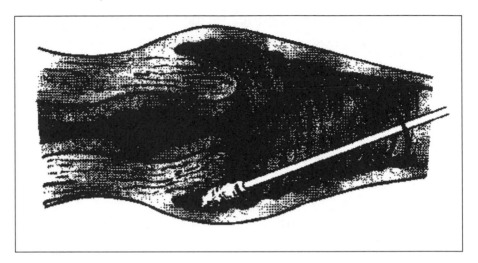

Figure 9.5 Vaginal pool.

           (3) Wipe the applicator gently across a glass slide, uniformly spreading secretions.

           (4) Spray with fixative.

           (5) Transport: The slide is placed in a cardboard container and sent to the cytologist for evaluation.

        b. Women without a cervix (those who have undergone hysterectomy).

           (1) Using the handle of the spatula, gently scrape the walls of the vagina in all four quadrants.

           (2) Wipe the applicator across the slide, uniformly spreading the secretions.

    E. Special considerations.

        1. If the examiner is obtaining additional cultures, remember that the likelihood of bleeding increases with each sample obtained. Therefore, the Pap smear should probably be obtained first, the chlamydia smear second, and the gonorrhea smear last.

    F. Fixation.

        1. The sample should be fixed immediately to avoid air drying. Spray the slide with fixative (97% ethyl alcohol) as soon as possible; however, patient comfort should not be compromised.

           a. The woman should not be left with the speculum in place while the clinician is fixing the slide. The speculum should be removed; the woman, gently assisted to a sitting position.

2. The fixative should be held 12 in. from the slide.

G. Liquid-based Pap.

1. The FDA approved a test in May 1996 as a replacement for the conventional Pap smear (ThinPrep Pap Test, Hologic Corporation).

a. This represented the first such advance in 50 years.

b. Liquid-based testing reduces the chance that the Pap test will need to be repeated, but it does not seem to find more precancers than a regular Pap test.

c. The liquid helps remove some of the mucus, bacteria, yeast, and pus cells in a sample. It also allows the cervical cells to be spread more evenly on the slide and keeps them from drying out and distorting.

d. A key point is that the cells kept in the liquid can also be tested for HPV.

2. The technique.

a. Liquid based: Instead of smearing the cells over the slide, cells are immersed in a vial of preservative solution.

b. The whole sample is captured, rather than whatever portion can be transferred from the collecting device to the slide.

c. Addresses sampling preparation, screening, and interpretation errors.

d. Cells are collected in the standard manner.

(1) Liquid-based cytology: Place the sample of cells from the endocervix and ectocervix into a special preservative liquid (instead of placing them on a slide directly), using the same techniques described previously for conventional collection.

(2) Some laboratories require that the tip of the collection brush or spatula be sent to the laboratory in the preservative container.

(3) Technicians use special laboratory instruments that spread the cells in the liquid onto glass slides to evaluate under a microscope.

e. The fluid medium is used to preserve cells, and a uniform, thin layer of cells is transferred to the slide.

f. In the laboratory, clumps of cells are gently disaggregated by a spinning cylinder that is lowered into a special specimen vial.

g. Next, the sample is homogenized and filtered.

      h. A thin, even layer of cells is then applied to the slide.

      i. The final sample is fixed, stained, and evaluated microscopically.

      j. This method, also known by brand names ThinPrep or AutoCyte, is more expensive than a conventional Pap test.

H. Liquid-based versus conventional Pap smears.

  1. Pros and cons.

    a. Liquid-based pros.

      (1) Less risk of air-drying artifact

      (2) More sensitive

      (3) May have lower risk of "partially obscuring inflammation"

      (4) HPV testing can be performed from the same specimen.

    b. Liquid based cons.

      (1) May be more false-positives

      (2) More cytopathology resources.

  2. Liquid-based cytology has increased sensitivity for high-grade lesions. It is unclear whether specificity differs.

    a. There have been no random controlled clinical trials comparing liquid-based and conventional smears.

    b. Either method is acceptable.

  3. Computerized Pap instruments are another method used to improve the Pap tests.

    a. Computerized instruments that can detect abnormal cells in Pap tests.

    b. The AutoPap instrument was approved by the FDA to read Pap tests first (instead of a technologist).

    c. AutoPap is also approved by the FDA for rechecking Pap test results that were read as normal by technologists.

    d. Any smear identified as abnormal by AutoPap would then be reviewed by a physician or a technologist.

    e. Computerized instruments can find abnormal cells that technologists may miss.

    f. Most of the abnormal cells are in early stages, such as atypical squamous cells (ASCs), but high-grade abnormalities may be missed by human testing.

    g. It is not known whether the instrument can find enough high-grade abnormalities missed by human testing to have a significant effect on preventing invasive cervical cancers.

    h. Automated testing also increases the cost of cervical cytology testing.

4. The best way to detect cervical cancer early is to make certain that all women are tested according to American Cancer Society (ACS) guidelines.
5. Follow-up: Communication of Pap smear results to women varies by clinic and facility.
    a. The woman is told that the results may take a week to 10 days.
    b. A good practice is to send a normal Pap letter, having a standardized template to simplify the approach.
    c. Abnormal results should be clearly and verbally communicated because the woman may easily misinterpret information owing to her fear of cervical cancer. She may panic when you first contact her. If she hears that the results are abnormal, she may automatically conclude that she has cancer.
    d. Other clinicians simply tell the woman that she will be contacted only if the results are abnormal. Because this is a common practice, it is accepted by the woman. If the woman still seems concerned, make it a point to contact her with the results.

V. **Management of abnormal Pap results using the Bethesda classification system. (Please refer to the end of the chapter for the Management of Pap smear results in algorithmic form by the American Society for Colposcopy and Cervical Pathology [ASCCP]).**
    A. The Bethesda Classification System is the most widely used protocol for classifying Pap smears. It is named for the town in Maryland where the National Cancer Institute developed the classification.
    B. Indications of a negative smear.
        1. A negative smear indicates a prediction that there are no premalignant or malignant cells in the cervix.
        2. A lack of endometrial cells is not considered a negative result; however, it indicates a lack of proper sampling from the squamocolumnar junction.
        3. A normal result indicates the presence of normal exocervical squamous epithelial cells with benign nuclear characteristics consistent with the clinical hormonal state of the woman.
        4. Squamous metaplasia is considered a normal, benign process in which there is the changing of columnar cells into squamous epithelial cells.
        5. Unsatisfactory for evaluation (Box 9.4).
    C. Inadequate sample due to absence of endocervical cells.
        1. The squamocolumnar junction.

Unsatisfactory Conventional Pap Test Finding	BOX 9.4

Problem	Description
Scant cellular material	Not enough epithelial cells present to obtain a representative sample
Smear too thick	Many epithelial cells piled on top of each other, making it difficult to view the characteristics of an individual cell
Artifact present	Characteristics obscured by menstrual debris or inflammatory exudate (leukocytes)
Sample poorly fixed	Slide not sprayed in a timely manner Air drying artifact present (sides of the epithelial cells curl, resembling corn flakes)

Note: Repeat pap smear in 3 to 6 months, as indicated by risk factors.

  a. The cervix is the lower part of the uterus, the knoblike cylinder projecting into the vagina. It surrounds a tiny canal leading out from the uterus. There are two types of cervical cells.
   (1) Columnar epithelial cells: The interior of the canal is lined with columnar tissue that contains mucus-secreting glands.
   (2) Squamous epithelial cells: The knob of the cervix is covered with a different type of flat tissue, called squamous epithelial tissue. This tissue is pink and shiny.
   (3) These two types of tissues meet at the squamocolumnar junction, or the transformation zone. The endocervical cells are found in this area.
 2. Metaplasia.
  a. This is an area of normally changing tissue. However, precancerous and cancerous cells are most likely to proliferate in this area; therefore, it is the area of greatest importance to sample by a Pap test.
  b. This area is referred to on a Pap smear as endocervical cells.
 3. Cellular damage causes the columnar cells to proliferate. This is the probable point of susceptibility to oncogenes.
 4. Significance of the transformation zone.

Table 9.1 Transformation Zone (Squamocolumnar Junction) Shifts in Response to Age and Hormonal Alterations

Developmental Period	Pathophysiologic Process	Location of Transformation Zone
Puberty	Squamous tissue slowly replaces the glandular tissue on the ectocervix under the influence of estrogen	Junction on the surface of the cervix
Early to middle years	Remains relatively stable	Junction at the cervical os
Menopause	Lack of estrogen causes the squamous cells to migrate up the endocervical canal	Junction recedes inside the os

a. A majority of malignant and premalignant diseases arise in the transformation zone. This is an area of rapidly changing metaplastic cells that varies with hormonal status (Table 9.1).

b. The presence of endocervical components indicates that the transformation zone has been adequately sampled.

c. There is question whether the presence of endocervical cells is always necessary. Some recent studies indicate that the presence of the cells is not necessary. The reason is that it is possible to find dysplastic and malignant cells in the cervical smear without endocervical cell elements because the endocervical cells often exfoliate into the cervical mucus. However, most clinicians consider the presence of these cells vital.

d. These cells are absent in 10% of Pap smears in premenopausal women and in 50% in postmenopausal women (because the transformation zone has receded up the endocervical canal).

D. Unsatisfactory for evaluation (see Box 9.4).

E. Infection.

　　1. Etiology.

　　　　a. Inflammation usually indicates the presence of neutrophils (usually in the form of polymorphonuclear cells).

　　　　　　(1) This is generally associated with vaginal conditions such as *Candida* or *Trichomonas* infection.

(2) Severe inflammation is often due to the cervicitis associated with a chlamydial infection. It is not always clinically apparent.

b. Nonspecific inflammation: If severe inflammation is present, the woman should return for a wet mount examination and possible cultures, particularly if she is at risk for chlamydial infection. Risk factors for chlamydial infection include

(1) Multiple partners.

(2) Lack of condom use.

(3) History of other sexually transmitted disease or pelvic inflammation.

c. Moderate inflammation: The woman may return for wet mount sampling, or, if the patient does not have symptoms, the provider may elect to repeat the Pap smear in a year. Three months after the organism has been treated, the Pap smear should be repeated.

d. Noninfectious causes of inflammation may exist, such as allergy, vaginal atrophy, or trauma. Oral contraceptive pills, which cause the transformation zone to fall on the ectocervix, may cause inflammation.

e. If the organism is identified on a Pap smear, the condition should be treated and the Pap smear should be repeated in 3 months.

F. Koilocytosis: a cellular change that may represent the presence of a viral infection such as HPV. This finding is often associated with the presence of venereal warts (condyloma). The cells have a large cytoplasmic vacuole, irregularity of the nucleus, and hyperchromatism.

G. Predominance of coccobacilli consistent with a shift in vaginal flora.

1. Return to evaluate for and treat bacterial vaginosis (the Pap smear is not diagnostic).

2. The clinician may or may not repeat the smear.

H. *Actinomyces*.

1. Usually associated with *Actinomyces* colonization in women using an intrauterine device (IUD).

2. Examine the patient to exclude pelvic actinomycosis (presents like pelvic inflammatory disease [PID]).

a. If there is no pelvic tenderness, remove the IUD and repeat the Pap smear in 1 to 2 months. If the Pap smear is negative, the woman can insert a new IUD.

  b. If tenderness is present, refer to the Centers for Disease Control and Prevention (CDC) guidelines for treatment with an antibiotic.

I. Herpes simplex virus (HSV) infection.

  1. The Pap smear provides poor sensitivity but good specificity for HSV.

  2. A positive smear usually is associated with asymptomatic shedding of virus.

  3. HSV culture is usually negative by the time the results of the Pap smear are available.

  4. It is not a cost-effective strategy to perform the culture in the absence of a lesion.

J. Reactive or repair-related changes.

  1. These changes may be seen with infection or a recent cervical procedure, such as a biopsy, or even vaginal atrophy.

  2. An IUD may cause reactive changes on the cervix as a result of slight irritation from the IUD string. A diaphragm may also cause cervical irritation.

  3. Generally, no further evaluation is needed if one of the aforementioned conditions is determined. If the cause is not known, a subsequent examination may be suggested.

K. Atrophy with inflammation.

  1. Common in states of estrogen deficiency.

  2. If associated with atypical squamous cells of undetermined significance (ASCUS) or LSILs, treat with vaginal estrogen for 4 to 6 weeks, and then repeat the smear. Basilar cells are found in both conditions.

L. ASCUS: Abnormal squamous epithelial cells are present, but the exact cause of the abnormality is not clear.

  1. The report often suggests that the cause is more likely to be either inflammation or a precancerous lesion.

  2. The Pap smear should be repeated in 3 to 6 months.

M. Endometrial cells: These are cells shed from the lining of the uterus.

  1. Normal finding: If the Pap smear was taken during the time of menstruation, this finding is normal.

  2. Abnormal: This finding is abnormal in nonmenstruating women and in postmenopausal women. Endometrial biopsy is necessary to rule out endometrial cancer.

N. Atypical glandular cells (AGCs). These glandular cells are abnormal in appearance without any apparent cause. Cancer of the glandular tissue usually starts deep in the tissue and may not shed until it is well established.
   1. The cells may possibly represent the presence of infection, HPV, or adenocarcinoma.
   2. Diagnosis necessitates aggressive diagnostic efforts and colposcopy.

O. ASCUS: This term simply means that the cytologist was unable to classify the abnormality of the cells on the surface of the cervix. It is unknown whether they are significant or not.
   1. Managed with HPV testing with liquid-based Pap smears; colposcopy is necessary if HPV is high risk.
   2. Routine follow-up if results of liquid-based Pap smear are negative for HPV.

P. LSIL and CIN-I.
   1. Refer for colposcopy.
      a. In adolescents, colposcopy is deemphasized and cytology follow-up is recommended for 2 years in the absence of HSIL. Adolescents are defined as individuals 20 years of age or younger.
      b. Treatment of CIN-I in adolescents is particularly discouraged.
      c. CIN-I management: Follow-up as the primary approach to managing all groups of women.

Q. HSIL: Cells appear to be moderately or severely precancerous. The cells almost always contain high risk viral types. The full thickness of the lining is involved (carcinoma in situ). There is a 50 to 75% likelihood that cells will become cancerous.
   1. Colposcopy with biopsy.

R. Dysplasia.
   1. Etiology: The term *dysplasia* is derived from *dys*, meaning bad, and *plassein*, meaning to form; consequently the term means a bad, abnormal formation of tissue.
   2. Normal stratified squamous epithelium of the cervix: Composed of four layers that mature from the basal layer to the superficial layer under the influence of estrogen.
      a. A one- to two-cell layer of basal cells.
      b. A three- to four-cell layer of parabasal cells.
      c. A wider zone of intermediate cells.
      d. A superficial outer layer of cells.
   3. Dysplasia results when there is a delay in the maturation of

Table 9.2   **Classification of Dysplasia**

Dysplasia	Mild	Moderate	Severe	Carcinoma in situ
Cervical intraepithelial neoplasia	I	II	III	in
Squamous intraepithelial lesion	Low grade	High grade	High grade	High grade

the basal cells as they attempt to move toward the surface. The cells with abnormally large nuclei and minimal cytoplasm will appear to be closer to the surface of the epithelium.

4. Classification of dysplasia by biopsy study (Table 9.2).
   a. Mild dysplasia (CIN-I): the presence of the larger nucleated cells present in the lower third of the stratified squamous epithelium. Mild dysplasia may regress to normal in some cases.
      (1) Follow-up: Evaluate every 3 to 6 months by either Pap smear or colposcopy.
   b. Moderate dysplasia (CIN-II): the presence of the larger nucleated cells in the lower half of the epithelium.
   c. Severe dysplasia (CIN-III).
   d. Carcinoma in situ: if the abnormal cells extend from the basal cell layer all the way to the surface, with no maturation of the cells.

S. The maturation index: assesses the level of estrogen in relation to the maturation of the epithelial cells. Screens for the presence of basal or parabasal cells, which may indicate estrogen deficiency. The mucus is thin and dries rapidly.
   1. Estrogen effect is sampled by scraping the inner third of the lateral vaginal wall.
   2. Estrogen therapy will restore the natural epithelial cell layers in postmenopausal women.

VI. **Special situations.**
   A. Referral.
      1. In some situations, it may not be possible to sample the transformation zone adequately. Cervical scarring may occur

after laser, cryotherapy, or cone biopsy surgery, making the os difficult to penetrate with the cytobrush. The risk factors and any special patient circumstances should be considered. If it is determined that the transformation zone must be sampled, refer the patient to a specialist for cervical dilation.

B. Special indications for older women.

    1. Inadequate sample from the transformation zone.

        a. In postmenopausal women, inadequate sampling of the squamocolumnar junction can occur. This often happens because

            (1) The transformation zone travels inward, up the columnar area of the cervical canal as estrogen levels decrease, moving the transformation zone out of reach of the cytobrush or broom.

            (2) The os atrophies and becomes stenotic, making the penetration of the os nearly impossible.

            (3) If the woman is at low risk for cervical cancer, and if she has had a history of normal Pap smears and a monogamous relationship, further attempts are not recommended.

            (4) The clinician may repeat the Pap smear using a cytobrush.

    2. The presence of endometrial cells in postmenopausal women is cause for concern. It indicates microscopic shedding of the endometrium, which suggests that the uterus is still active and bleeding. This type of bleeding should be treated as any postmenopausal bleeding. An endometrial biopsy should be performed.

C. Accuracy of the Pap smear: The accuracy of the Pap smear is 80 to 90%.

    1. False-negative results (test does not identify a cell abnormality that is present).

        a. Range of 5 to 20%: Some studies indicate it may be as high as 70%.

        b. One half are due to sampling errors.

        c. One half are due to laboratory errors.

    2. The false-negative rate of adequate Pap technique interpreted by a reliable laboratory is less than 10%. The rate is dependent on

        a. The technique of the provider.

        b. Characteristics of the instrument used (cytobrush vs. swab).

        c. Skill of the cytopathologist.

3. False-positive results rarely occur (abnormal cells were reported when the cells were normal).
4. The rate of false-positive results is one reason why women at risk should have yearly Pap smears because the likelihood of a false-positive test for two consecutive years is very low.

D. Recommended follow-up.

1. No endocervical cells: If previous Pap smears have been normal and the woman is at low risk for an abnormal Pap smear, then the Pap smear can be delayed until the next annual examination. If either of the aforementioned conditions exists, or if there was a "no endocervical" finding on the last Pap smear, a more aggressive approach is necessary. The Pap smear should be repeated in 3 months, with special attention to the cytobrush technique.
2. Table 9.3 summarizes the follow-up for a Pap smear.

E. Patient education handouts: Free to download from the CDC

1. http://www.cdc.gov/std/HPV/pap/HPV_Patient_English_ booklet.pdf

F. Strategies for increasing use of Pap smears.

1. Increasing the knowledge base so that women understand that they are at risk for cervical cancer and must be screened.
2. Reducing the costs associated with the procedure.
3. Providing easy access to screening.

VII. The Pap smear and beyond: Several new technologies have received clearance from the FDA.

A. HPV vaccine Gardasil (Merck): Licensed June 2006.

B. Quadrivalent HPV 6/11/16/18 L1 viruslike particle (VLP) vaccine.

1. Each 0.5-ml dose contains HPV types 6, 11, 16, and 18 (20, 40, 40, and 20 ìg L1 protein, respectively).

C. Quadrivalent HPV vaccine.

1. Dose and Administration.

   a. Three intramuscular injections over a 6-month period, 0.5-ml dose.

      (1) Can be administered at same visit as other age-appropriate vaccines (e.g., tetanus, diphtheria, and pertussis [Tdap]; adult diphtheria and tetanus [TD]; meningococcal conjugate [MCV4] and hepatitis B).

      (2) Costs approximately $140.00 per dose (~ $420 for full series).

Table 9.3   **Summary of Pap Smear Follow-Up Measures**

Findings	Implications of Descriptions of Findings	Implications/ Follow-Up
Normal	Normal finding	Repeat Pap smear every 1 to 3 years, as indicated by risk factors
Metaplasia	Normal finding	Repeat Pap smear every 1 to 3 years, as indicated by risk factors
ASCUS	May be caused by inflammation, infection Can be found with cervical cancer	Screen for inflammation secondary to vaginitis or cervicitis, such as *Candida*, bacterial vaginosis, or *Trichomonas* If negative HPV, follow per protocol.
ASCUS favor mild dysplasia	Consistent with HPV, koilocytosis, parakytosis	Recommend colposcopy
ASCUS favor inflammation	Caused by inflammation or infection	Screen for infection
CIN-I or LSIL	Includes mild dysplasia (CIN-I) and changes linked to HPV	Colposcopy for diagnosis Observation, topical therapy/cryotherapy LEEP/LLETZ/CO_2 laser
HSIL (potentially precursor lesions of carcinoma)	Includes CIN-II, CIN-III, and CIN-IV	Includes moderate and severe dysplasia (CIN-II and III) and CIS. CIS is not a true invasive form of cancer; is a precancer that must be treated
Colposcopy and biopsy for diagnosis	LEEP-LLETZ/CO_2 laser/ cone biopsy for CIS or high-grade Pap smear and normal biopsy	
Cancer	Cells have progressed beyond dysplasia (CIN) and have become invasive	Colposcopy and biopsy Gynecology-oncology consults for staging and definitive therapy

Note: Follow-up varies considerably from provider to provider.
ASCUS = Atypical squamous cells of undetermined significance; CIN = cervical intraepithelial neoplasia; CIS = carcinoma in situ; HSIL = high-grade squamous intraepithelial lesion; HPV = human papillomavirus; LEEP = loop electrocautery excision procedure; LLETZ = large loop excision of the transformation zone; LSIL = low-grade squamous intraepithelial lesion.

  (3) Pregnancy category B: Not recommended for use in pregnancy
  (4) Can be given to lactating women.
  (5) Available in single-dose vial or a refillable syringe.
  (6) Store at 2°C to 8°C (36°F to 46°F) and not frozen.
D. HPV vaccination schedule.
  1. Routine schedule is 0, 2, and 6 months.
  2. Minimum intervals.
     a. 4 weeks between doses 1 and 2.
     b. 12 weeks between doses 2 and 3.
     c. Do not restart the series if the schedule is interrupted.
     d. Administer at the same visit as other age-appropriate vaccines (e.g., hepatitis B).
E. HPV vaccine and cervical cancer screening.
  1. Cervical cancer screening: no change.
     a. 30% of cervical cancers caused by HPV types are not prevented by the quadrivalent vaccine.
     b. Vaccinated women could be subsequently infected by non-vaccine HPV types.
     c. Sexually active women may have been infected before vaccination.
     d. Educate women who received the HPV vaccine regarding the importance of cervical cancer screening.
F. Contraindications.
  1. Moderate or severe acute illnesses: Defer until after illness improves.
  2. Acceptable to administer during minor acute illnesses (e.g., diarrhea or mild upper respiratory infection with or without fever).
  3. History of immediate hypersensitivity or severe allergic reaction to yeast or to any vaccine component.
G. Management of Pap smear results in algorithmic form by the American Society for Colposcopy and Cervical Pathology (ASCCP) available at: http://www.asccp.org/pdfs/consensus/algorithms_cyto_07.pdf

CHAPTER 10

Vaginal Microscopy

Helen A. Carcio and Mimi Clarke Secor

I. **Vaginal microscopy explained.**
   A. The value.
   1. Vaginal microscopy is an important laboratory tool for the differential diagnosis of vaginitis. It is also used to assess normal vaginal flora. Five common conditions cause the majority of discharge or infection (Box 10.1).
   2. Vaginal microscopy allows observation of living vaginal organisms to study the ecology of the lower genital tract in women.
   3. It is a direct, rapid, inexpensive test with high sensitivity and specificity for most conditions.
   4. It acts as an accessory tool to patient history, inspection of the vulvar and vaginal mucosa, and pH determination to arrive at a presumptive etiologic diagnosis.
   5. The two components involved are saline wet mount and potassium hydroxide (KOH) wet mount.
   B. The wet mount.
   1. Nomenclature: Microscopy involves use of the wet mount.
      a. Other similar terms include *wet smear, wet prep, vaginal smear, vaginalysis,* or *hanging drop.*
   2. Basic principles.
      a. A 5-minute microscopic search is necessary before stating that a slide is negative for a certain condition.

---

*The Five Conditions Causing the Majority
of Vaginal Discharge or Infection (in Order)*   **BOX 10.1**

1. Bacterial vaginosis
2. *Candida* vulvovaginitis
3. Cervicitis (usually caused by *Chlamydia*)
4. Excessive but normal secretions
5. *Trichomonas* vaginitis

---

    b. Examination under oil immersion is rarely needed.
    c. The sample should be taken from the vaginal side walls.
    d. The sensitivity rate depends on the expertise of the clinician and the adequacy of sample.
    e. Remember to consider cervical factors when working up studies of a patient reporting vaginal discharge; if you are in the differential diagnosis phase, also perform a cervical wet mount.
  C. Indications: Vaginal micrsopcopy should be performed
    1. On every patient presenting with vaginal symptoms or with clinical features suggestive of a cervical or vaginal condition.
    2. Even if the diagnosis is clinically obvious (such as with a curdlike discharge associated with candidiasis) because many conditions can mimic other conditions.
    3. In a patient with urine sediment that contains white cells and many squamous epithelial cells to determine the exact source of infection (vagina or urinary tract).
    4. To determine the reason a routine Papanicolaou (Pap) smear shows an inflammatory response.
    5. As a follow-up test in a woman after treatment for a vaginal or cervical infection.
    6. During the routine health maintenance visit to assess for normal flora or asymptomatic vaginal infection.
    7. As a complement: A thorough and comprehensive health history is necessary to establish a differential diagnosis (Box 10.2). Table 10.1 presents the differential diagnoses.

II. Comments on the vaginal ecology.
  A. The vagina has minimal nerve endings; therefore, the symptoms of vaginal disorders may become evident only when the vaginal discharge irritates the sensitive vulvar skin.
  B. Normally, the vagina cleanses itself by the discharge of acidotic secretions.

Key History-Taking Questions and Considerations

BOX
10.2

History and chronology
Onset of symptoms
Duration of current episode
Date, diagnosis, treatment, and
    response of previous infection
Self-diagnosis and treatment
Monthly or seasonal variation
Affect on lifestyle
Evolution of chronicity
Sentinel events
History of IV drug use
Blood transfusion

Symptoms
Description (use patient's own words)
Location (use patient-guided drawing)
Radiation
Severity (use a rating scale of 0 to
    3+)
Full review of systems

Aggravating factors
Allergies
Activities
Positions
Dietary
Self-treatments
Prescription and OTC medications
Clothing
Sexual activities

Relieving factors
Vulvar care measures
Prescription and OTC medications
Alternative or home remedies
Stress reduction measures
Vitamins, supplements, and
    diet

Sexual history
Age of first sexual experience
Lifelong number of partners, gender,
    ages
STD exposure
Current sexual partner, duration of
    relationship, other partners
Partner history of STD, GU
    symptoms, circumcision
Sexual practices (i.e., anal
    intercourse, oral sex, order of
    activities, hygiene)
Condom use
Sexual devices or toys
Lubricants (specify brand)
Date of last coitus or genital contact
Dyspareunia (superficial, deep;
    before, during, or after penetration)

Obstetric and gynecologic factors
Last menstrual period
Duration of menses
Tampons versus pads
Dysmenorrhea or dysfunctional
    uterine bleeding
Pregnancy, birth, episiotomy,
    lacerations
Pain in pregnancy
Infertility
Pelvic or genital surgeries
Pap smear history
Vulvar care

GU = genitourinary; IV = intravenous; OTC = over the counter; STD = sexually transmitted disease.

Table 10.1 Differential Diagnosis of Vaginal Conditions

Condition	Vulvovaginal Symptoms	Vaginal Discharge	Lactobacilli	pH	Microscopy
Candida albicans	Mild to severe itching Cyclic Marked vulvovaginal erythema	Increased amount White, curdy, cottage cheese–like	Moderate	< 5	KOH Hyphae, pseudohyphae and spores "Spaghetti and meatballs"
C. glabrata	Mild to moderate burning/itching Chronic, cyclic Mild vulvovaginal erythema	Increased Unchanged to white	Moderate	< 4.5	KOH Spores only Vary in size and shape
Bacterial vaginosis	Mild to moderate itching Absent to mild inflammation Mild vulvovaginal erythema	Adherent, homogenous discharge Appearance of milk poured into vagina Fish odor, particularly after intercourse	Rare	> 4.5	Saline Clue cells, few to many WBCs KOH + Whiff test
Cytolytic vaginosis	Mild to moderate burning/itching Premenstrual, relieved with menses	Unchanged to increased white	Excessive	< 3.5-4	Saline Overabundance of lactobacilli Fragments of epithelial cells Rare WBCs
Lactobacillosis	Vaginal itching/ burning Chronic, cyclic	Thick White to creamy	Elongated Rare, short rods	4-5	Saline Very long rods Few short rods Rare WBCs
Trichomonas	Severe vulvar itching Petechiae of cervix and vagina Vulvar erythema	Copious Yellow-green May be frothy Malodorous	Plus or minus	> 5	Saline Unicellar trichomonads Many WBCs
Atrophic vaginitis	Pruritus, irritation Vaginal dryness and dyspareunia Smooth vaginal walls	Red, tender vestibule and vagina Scant discharge Lack of rugae	Rare	> 5-6	Saline Parabasal cells Few to many WBCs
Desquamative inflammatory vaginitis	Erythema of vulva, vagina, and cervix Dyspareunia Pruritus or irritation	Thick, profuse No odor	Rare	> 4.5	Saline Basal/ parabasal cells Many WBCs

KOH = Potassium hydroxide; WBC = white blood cell.

C. The pH is acidotic, approximatily 3.8 to 4.2.
　　1. Organisms live symbiotically in an acid environment.
　　　　a. Factors that increase the glycogen content (high levels of estrogen in pregnancy or medication) increase the acidity of the vaginal secretions.
　　　　b. Glycogen present in the epithelial cells is used by the peroxide-producing lactobacilli to produce lactic acid, which maintains an acid environment.
　　　　c. Acidity allows for the overgrowth of the yeast organisms.
　　2. This level of acidotic secretions is antagonistic to harmful bacteria.
D. Factors affecting normal vaginal flora.
　　1. Role of hormones.
　　　　a. Estrogen.
　　　　　　(1) Affects vaginal epithelium.
　　　　　　(2) Causes glycogen to be deposited in the vagina, mainly in the intermediate cells.
　　　　　　(3) Glycogen is metabolized to become lactic acid.
　　　　b. Progesterone causes shedding of these glycogen-rich cells into the vaginal pool. (This may be the reason symptoms of candidiasis increase premenstrually and are somewhat relieved after the menstrual flow.)
　　2. Effect of medications on the vaginal ecology.
　　　　a. Antibiotics may increase the incidence of *Candida* infection. There are many theories:
　　　　　　(1) *Candida* reproduce rapidly because they no longer have the competition from other bacteria, which were destroyed by the antibiotic.
　　　　　　(2) Secretion of an antifungal substance by bacteria stops when the bacteria are killed (more recent theory).
　　　　　　(3) Possible direct stimulation of growth of *Candida* by the antibiotic.
　　　　　　(4) Other theories describe reduction of host defenses, as in human immunodeficiency virus (HIV).
　　　　b. Certain medications can affect the growth of lactobacilli and thus affect the vaginal milieu.
　　　　　　(1) Some drugs, such as oral and vaginal metronidazole and ampicillin (modest), increase the number of lactobacilli.
　　　　　　(2) Intravaginal clindamycin decreases the number of lactobacilli (very temporary, only lasts 1 week).
　　　　　　(3) Drugs such as doxycycline, azithromycin, clotrimazole, and fluconazole have little or no effect.

(4) Antifungal agents can reduce the number of lactobacilli, possibly contributing to the problem of
recurrence.
  c. Corticosteroids.
    (1) Reduce inflammatory response of host.
    (2) Topical steroids do not aggravate candidiasis, as pre-
viously thought.
  3. Douching: decreases normal flora, and increases the risk for
bacterial vaginosis.
  4. Tampon use may also alter normal flora and increase the
risk for vulvovaginal infection.

III. **The microscope: The clinician must be familiar with all parts of
the microscope and know how to care for it properly.**
  A. Selection of magnification.
    1. Low-power objective (10x magnification, eye piece 10x =
100x magnification)
    2. High-power objective (40x magnification, eye piece 10x =
400x magnification)
  B. Light source: Helps increase the examiner's ability to visualize
details by controlling the illumination. The examiner must increase or decrease the light transmitted through the preparation.
The light source is controlled by the following features:
    1. Intensity setting of the light source.
    2. The light shutter.
    3. The position of the condenser.
      a. For the low-power objective, drop the condenser for a
lower intensity setting.
      b. For the high-power objective, increase the condenser for a
higher intensity setting.
  C. Mechanics of observing the saline smear. (Always wear gloves.)
    1. Position the slide on the stage of the microscope with saline
preparation under the objective and secure with stage clips.
    2. Turn light on under stage.
    3. Click low objective into place over the specimen (obtains a
larger view of the slide area, although the images are small).
    4. Turn the condenser to the lowest position; subdued light is
best to accentuate fine details. (Try increasing the light by
raising the condenser while viewing the specimen to see
how the cells and bacteria disappear from view.)
    5. Move objective and slide as close together as possible, until
just barely touching.

6. Adjust the eyepiece until a single round field is seen (interpupillary diameter).
7. While looking through the eyepiece, turn the coarse adjustment knob in the opposite direction until the microscopic field comes into focus. Use both eyes.
8. Turn fine-adjust knob back and forth to adjust to the different planes and bring image into sharper focus.
9. Adjust each eyepiece separately by closing one eye at a time.
10. Turn knob slowly to focus (some microscopes are very sensitive; turning too rapidly may result in missing the proper plane of visualization).
11. Move the saline specimen under the objective and scan the slide at low magnification to locate representative sections.
    a. Scan all fields because characteristic findings may be clumped in one section of the slide.
    b. When the side of the coverslip is reached, move the slide over one field's width, and then start scanning in the opposite direction.
12. Switch to high-power objective (40x × 10x = 400x) magnification.
    a. Facilitates identification of microbes by further magnifying the specimen.
    b. It may be necessary to increase the light source slightly.
    c. Watch stage when switching to make sure that the objective does not break the slide. This should not happen if low power is properly adjusted.
13. Turn fine adjustment back and forth; coarse adjustment should not require readjustment.
14. Using the stage adjustment knobs, move the slide laterally up and down and back and forth to view all fields because pathogens may not be distributed evenly throughout the slide and may be found in a limited number of fields.
15. Scan the slide systematically to evaluate the specimen fully.
16. Move the slide until you have a general impression of the number of squamous cells and any other findings.
17. Evaluate at least 12 fields.
18. Hint: If you immediately see one of the organisms that causes vaginitis you still must continue to examine the specimen to prevent missing a concomitant infection.

D. Mechanics of observing the KOH preparation. Observe same principles of microscopy described previously.

1. Move the KOH slide into position on stage.
2. Switch back to low-power objective to scan fields for yeast forms.
3. If yeast forms are noted, switch to high power to confirm their presence and type.

E. Concluding comments.
1. Thorough observation of both preparations should take at least 3 to 5 minutes.
2. Remember to turn off the light source and dispose of the slide in a special biohazard container.
3. Clean the microscope stage if it is soiled, and clean the lenses with special paper.
   a. KOH can damage the objective; must clean thoroughly.
4. Record findings, and review the findings with the patient.

IV. **Preparation for the wet mount procedure.**
A. Patient preparation: Any substance in the vagina can alter the accuracy of the microscopic findings. Instruct the woman in the following preparations:
1. Explain that the examination is similar to a Pap smear and should not cause any discomfort.
2. Menses cannot be avoided if a woman has symptoms during that time. However, it does make evaluation more difficult because of the presence of red blood cells in the smear.
3. Avoid coitus or douching for 24 hours before the examination.
4. Do not use over-the-counter preparations before the examination (avoid for as long as possible).

B. Perform clinical evaluation. (Box 10.3 shows the sequence of the examination.)
C. Observe characteristic of vaginal discharge (Table 10.2).
D. Equipment.
1. Gloves.
2. Speculum (metal or plastic).
3. Wooden handled cotton-tipped applicators or a wooden spatula, or both.
4. Glass slide (1 or 2).
5. Coverslips.
6. Bottle of normal saline (slightly warmed if possible).
7. Bottle of 10% to 20% KOH.
8. Vaginal pH test paper (Nitrazine; Squibb & Sons).
9. Microscope with 10x and 40x objectives.

*Sequence of Examination During an
Infection Check*

**BOX
10.3**

Perform a careful history.

Review procedure and expected outcomes with patient.

Insert speculum.

Inspect genitalia, noting signs of infection.

Determine vaginal pH.

pH should be collected first because cervical specimens may cause cervical bleeding, which might increase the pH level.

Procure sample of discharge.

Collect cervical culture or vaginal culture if indicated.

Remove speculum.

Label any specimens.

Perform wet mount evaluation.

Document results.

Review results with patient.

Treat any infection.

　　　10. Small test tubes (3 to 4 in. long) with 1 ml (or half inch) of saline if saline immersion method is used.
　　E. Perform pelvic examination as outlined in chapter 4, The Physical Examination.
V. **Saline wet mount.**
　　A. Obtaining and preparing the sample.
　　　　1. Obtain copious sample from the posterior and lateral vaginal walls using a wooden spatula or a cotton-tipped applicator.
　　　　　a. The collection technique may vary with the suspected diagnosis.
　　　　2. Place two separate samples of vaginal discharge on the same unfrosted glass slide. It takes practice to use only one slide, but it is time and cost effective; therefore, it is probably worthwhile to develop the skill. (Saline sample should be thin.)
　　　　　a. Alternate procedure: double-slide method.
　　　　　　(1) May use two separate slides.

Table 10.2   Analysis of Vaginal Discharge

Characteristic	Possible Findings

Magnitude (quantitate amount)	Stains on undergarment
	  dime size
	  quarter size

Color	Off white Creamy Whitish-grey Yellow Greenish Pink-red
Character	Watery Thick Curdlike Homogenous
Odor	Fishy Foul
Relation to menses	Premenstrual Midcycle After menses

Note: A yellow color indicates sloughing of leukocytes that have undergone a partial lytic breakdown. Mostly seen with endocervicitis.

    (2) Place smear of sample on one slide and a sample on the second slide. Add coverslip.

    (3) Blot with paper towel.

    (4) This method has the advantage of eliminating the possibility of the two solutions contaminating each other.

  3. Add one drop of normal saline to thinner sample.

    a. Be careful not to mix the solutions.

      (1) If the solutions are mixed, the sample must be collected again because the KOH will dissolve the cellular material on the saline portion of the slide.

    b. Mix each specimen, thoroughly stirring until smooth, to create a turbid suspension. (Use separate utensils.)

      (1) May use a wooden spatula or the opposite wooden end of a cotton-tipped applicator.

      (2) The saline specimen should be fairly diluted to separate the epithelial cells from each other.

      (3) If the cells are clumped on top of each other, the char-

acteristic of the individual form is difficult to determine and sensitivity is reduced.
  c. Alternate method: saline immersion.
    (1) Some believe that an undiluted smear is often too
        thick to interpret accurately and dries too quickly.
    (2) Place 7 to 10 drops (0.5 ml) of physiologic saline in a
        small test tube. (Saline must be room temperature or
        warmer.)
    (3) Roll a cotton-tipped applicator along the posterolat-
        eral vaginal walls.
    (4) Immediately immerse applicator into the saline-filled
        tube.
    (5) Place a drop of the suspension on the slide using ei-
        ther method described previously.
  d. Some comments.
    (1) Whether the diluted effect of this method affects the
        sensitivity of this test is controversial.
    (2) It may prevent drying of the specimen; therefore, the
        examiner may have more time—15 minutes—to read
        slide.
    (3) This procedure may best be reserved for those exami-
        nations when trichomoniasis is suspected to ensure
        the motility of the organism or when the examination
        does not allow the clinician to leave the room
        immediately.
    (4) Because the KOH cannot be prepared in similar fash-
        ion, it is more time consuming to prepare the slides
        two different ways.
4. Immediately place separate coverslips over each specimen
   just before viewing to prevent drying.
  a. Hold one edge of the coverslip against the slide, and
     slowly drop (like a hinged door) over the liquid specimen
     to reduce the number of air bubbles.
5. Place a paper towel over the entire slide and lightly blot up
   any excess fluid.
  a. Helps keep the microscope clean.
  b. The pressure of the blotting stabilizes the mixture under
     the coverslip.
6. Interpret findings immediately, viewing saline slide first
   (allowing KOH time to lyse).
7. At least 12 fields should be analyzed for a total of 3 to 5
   minutes.

B. Findings on saline wet mount.
  1. Vaginal epithelial cells.
    a. Slightly grainy cytoplasm-containing vacuoles.
    b. Distinct cell walls.
    c. Evaluate cells for the following features:
      (1) Quantity of mature cells present.
      (2) Presence of immature cells and their relative frequency. May indicate
        • Decreased estrogen.
        • Significant inflammatory reaction of chronic inflammation.
        • Presence of many immature cells indicates a severe inflammatory process of significant duration.
    d. Epithelial cells change as they mature in the presence of estrogen (Table 10.3). See chapter 23, Atrophic Vaginitis.
  2. Presence of significant bacterial adherence to cell surfaces.
    a. Often indicative of a virulent organism.
    b. Dynamic process involving bacterial fimbriae and epithelial surface characteristic.
    c. Attachment depends on pH, hydrophobic properties, and surface secretion.
  3. Lactobacilli
    a. Easily visualized in saline preparation (Figure 10.1).
    b. Pleomorphic, gram-positive, aerobic or facultative anaerobic, non–spore-forming organism.
    c. Elongated rod-shaped bacilli that appear as straight rods, which may be slightly motile if smear is made properly and not excessively dried out.
    d. Lactobacilli vary in length between 5 and 15 μm.
      (1) Super long bacilli may be a normal finding (previously termed *Leptothrix);* they may be longer than the diameter of an epithelial cell.
      (2) May indicate lactobacillosis.
    e. Lactobacilli usually dominate the flora of the normal estrogenized vagina (96%).
    f. Predominance in vagina of acidophilic *Lactobacillus* species.
      (1) Eighty species have been identified.
    g. Maintains a low pH of vaginal discharge by making lactic acid, which inhibits adherence of bacteria to epithelial cells.
    h. Known to inhibit growth of organisms that may normally be found in the vagina, such as

Table 10.3   Characteristics of Epithelial Cells in Relation to Menstrual Cycle

Early proliferative phase. Few cells found in smear because desquamation is slight	Precornified Polygonal shape Little tendency toward folding of the edges Transparent cytoplasm Nucleus with granular chromatin PMNs present
Late proliferative phase	Under estrogenic stimulation Small deeply pigmented, homogeneous nuclei Polygonal shape May appear flat or folded Rare PMN cells
Midsecretory phase	Progestational phase Increase in number of desquamated superficial cells Predominately precornified More angular with folded edges Nuclei are vesicular and elongated or oval Cytoplasm contains occasional granules Marked tendency toward folding and clumping Background clear Few PMN cells
Late secretory (premenstrual) phase	Clusters of desquamated, precornified cells Fragments of cytoplasm, mucus, and PMN cells Peak shedding

PMN = polymorphonuclear.

      (1) *Gardnerella vaginalis.*
      (2) *Mycoplasma hominis.*
      (3) Certain anaerobes.
    i. Little effect on candidiasis (may even increase) or trichomoniasis.
    j. Numbers increase after menarche and markedly decrease after menopause.
  4. White blood cells (WBCs or leukocytes).
    a. Present as dark and granular cells with clearly segmented nuclei.

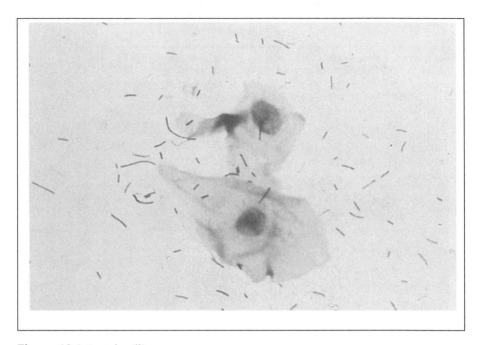

Figure 10.1 Lactobacilli.

(1) Termed polymorphonuclear (PMN).

(2) This lobulated nucleus is often fairly easy to distinguish.

a. May also appear as cytoplasmic granules with an indistinct nucleus (often with chronic infection).

b. Slightly larger than the nucleus of a mature epithelial cell.

c. Immobile trichomonal organisms are more similar to a teardrop in shape and slightly larger than mobile organisms; however, they may be difficult to distinguish from PMN cells.

d. The number of WBCs helps determine extent of inflammation (Table 10.4).

e. Increased in many conditions (Box 10.4).

5. Motile trichomonads.

6. Clue cells.

7. False clue cells.

8. Immature squamous epithelial cells (see chapter 22, Assessment of Menopausal Status).

Table 10.4 **Significance of White Blood Cells**

	Number in hpf	Ratio of WBC to Epithelial Cell
Normal	0–4	< 1:1
Mild	5–10	> 1:1 to 5:1
Moderate	10–20	5:1 to 10:1
Severe	> 20 WBCs/hpf	> 10:1 to TNTC

Note: May be influenced by the concentration of the smear. If inflammation is present, observe for the presence or absence of parabasal cells.
hpf = high-power field; TNTC = too numerous to count.

Causes of the Presence of Leukocytes (White Blood Cells) on Wet Mount

BOX 10.4

Moderate increase of leukocytes found with

· IUD use
· Postpartum reparative process
· Atrophic vaginitis
· Allergic reaction to spermicides and douches (may also see eosinophils)
· Depo-Provera users with low estrogen levels

Marked increase of leukocytes found with

· Trichomoniasis
· Candidiasis
· Chlamydia or gonorrhea
· Atrophic vaginitis with bacterial superinfection

Note: If many leukocytes are seen but neither *Candida* nor *Trichomonas* are present, consider a cervical culture for infections such as chlamydia or gonorrhea. Also consider dysplasia or metaplasia as a possible cause.
IUD = intrauterine device.

---

9. The presence of eosinophils may indicate an allergic response.
10. Mobiluncus.
    a. Easily visualized; be careful not to confuse with the rod-shaped lactobacilli.
    b. Comma-shaped, highly motile bacteria.
    c. Seen at one point as black dots that bounce off the coverslip and elongate in an eyelash shape.
    d. Gram stain is negative.
11. Red blood cells: visible as small concave spheres.
C. Normal findings include

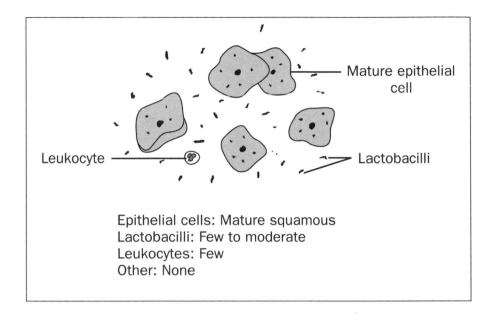

Epithelial cells: Mature squamous
Lactobacilli: Few to moderate
Leukocytes: Few
Other: None

Figure 10.2 Normal flora.

1. Absence of or less than 5 WBCs/high-power field (hpf).
2. pH less than 4.5.
3. Presence of moderate amounts of lactobacilli.
4. Absence of demonstrable pathogens such as *Trichomonas* or cocci.
5. Figure 10.2 shows the characteristics of a normal smear.
D. Hints on how to interpret a saline smear.
  1. Evaluate systematically (as with an electrocardiogram—each part is looked at; for example, the QRS complex rather than the whole rhythm strip).
  2. Picture the smear as an ocean (fluid medium) dotted with islands (vaginal epithelial cells) and boats or rafts that may be in the ocean or dotting the shores of the island.
    a. The boats can come in many sizes and shapes, and they may represent WBCs or trichomoniasis; smaller rafts represent cocci and rods.
  3. Ask yourself the following questions:
    a. Are there any islands? How many in each field? What do they look like? Are the edges clear or obscured? If they are obscured, are they obscured by dots or rods?

    b. What is in the ocean surrounding the islands? Are there rods or cocci, or a mixture of both? Adequate numbers? Too few? Too many?

    c. Is there anything swimming in the ocean (extracellular spaces)? Are there any motile trichomonads or mobiluncus?

    d. Are there any WBCs? How many?

VI. KOH.
  A. Some comments.
    1. Dissolves leukocytes, *Trichomonas,* and background debris, making identification of fungal structures easier.
    2. Effects on epithelial cells.
      a. KOH breaks down cell wall, changing the wall from cuboid and translucent to ovoid and transparent.
      b. Epithelial cells become enlarged and faint; called "ghost" cells, a mere shadow of their former selves.
    3. Branching and budding hyphae are alkali resistant and stand out in sharp contrast.
    4. Higher sensitivity for *Candida* using KOH than with saline preparations.
      a. Some sources believe that KOH is rarely necessary if the observer is skilled in the evaluation of saline preparations.
  B. Obtaining and preparing the sample.
    1. Use cotton-tipped applicator or wooden spatula to collect specimen from vaginal walls.
      a. Cotton may contaminate the sample with fiber artifact.
      b. If vulvar sample, use wooden spatula to scrape erythematous border.
    2. Dot onto slide.
      a. Material should be fairly thick with epithelial cells clustered to concentrate the yeast forms.
      b. This is in contrast to saline, in which the sample should be relatively thin.
    3. Add a drop of KOH (10%).
      a. Be careful not to mix with saline solution if a single slide is used for both preparations.
      b. Use solution mixed by the laboratory's own pharmacy or order a premixed bottle.
    4. Mix with the wooden end of a cotton swab or spatula to create a turbid mixture.
    5. Perform the whiff test.
      a. Volatile amines are released into the air when anaerobic

bacterial overgrowth comes in contact with an alkaline solution such as KOH.

b. Amines are produced by converting lysine to cadaverine, arginine to putrescine, and trimethylamin oxide to trimethylamine.

c. Immediately after mixing sample with KOH, smell the applicator (no need to bring entire slide to nose).

d. Note the presence of a foul or fishy odor.

e. If odor is present, it is recorded as a positive result. A positive result indicates an imbalance of the vaginal flora in which anaerobes dominate.

f. Usually indicates the presence of bacterial vaginoses but may also indicate the presence of trichomoniasis.

g. May not be positive in the presence of concomitant candidiasis.

6. Blot any excess fluid with paper towel.

a. KOH can damage the objective.

7. If a vulvar sample is obtained, must heat it slightly by passing it under a lighted match to dissolve the keratin.

C. Findings on KOH wet mount.

1. Wait 2 to 3 minutes, allowing time for the KOH to dissolve the cellular structures.

a. Examine the saline mixture during this time.

2. Scan slide.

a. Low power (10x): Locate sections of yeast forms, which may appear as thin sticks.

b. High power (40x): Focus on buds and pseudohyphae for further confirmation of morphologic characteristics.

3. Artifact may interfere with interpretation of the wet mount (Box 10.5).

4. Note the presence of any yeast forms.

D. For summary flow sheet instructions, see Tables 10.5A and 10.5B.

VII. pH.

A. Some comments about pH.

1. pH is representative of the acidity or alkalinity of the vagina, as determined by the presence of lactobacilli and other organisms.

2. Exacerbation or amelioration of clinical disease in relation to the menstrual cycle is a function pH.

3. Correlate pH findings with microscopic examination and clinical assessment.

Artifacts That May Interfere With the Interpretation of Candida *Species on Wet Mount*

BOX 10.5

In identification of spores

White blood cells

Nuclei of epithelial cells (particularly if clumped together)

Powder granules from gloves (resemble umbilicated marshmallows)

Tiny bubbles of emulsified vaginal creams (must elicit possibility of presence by history)

Dust on microscope lenses

In identification of filaments

Cotton fiber from cotton-tipped swab, undergarments, or tampons

Edges of epithelial cells rolled under the coverslip

4. Evaluation of pH of the vaginal secretions is a valuable diagnostic tool.
5. It is easy to perform and is inexpensive, with a high predictive value.
6. Women must avoid intravaginal medication and sexual activity 2 to 3 days before the visit.
7. pH of the vagina varies with the amount of vaginal estrogen during the various reproductive cycles of women (Table 10.6).

B. pH paper.
   1. Scale must begin at 4.0 at minimum.
   2. Record range of pH, as determined by the color of the tape, compared with the manufacturer's chart.
C. Collection: Cut off strip before inserting speculum.
   1. Use 1-in. strip of pH paper.
   2. Collect the sample from the upper lateral wall because it is less likely to be mixed with cervical mucus.
   3. Obtain sample directly from tape applied to vaginal wall or to discharge from the collecting spatula, or dip tape into discharge pooled on the upper blade of the vaginal speculum.
      a. Keep the speculum in the sink in the event that additional samples are needed.
         (1) Avoids woman having to undergo subsequent pelvic examination.
D. Interpretation of results.

Table 10.5A **Vaginal Microscopy: Secor Flow Sheet Instructions***

Date	
History	Brief history of symptoms, including self-care, medications
LMP, last coitus	LMP, last coitus, dyspareunia
Vulva, vagina, cervix	Erythema, lesions, tenderness
Vaginal mucus	Amount and characteristics pH (4.0–7.5)
Cervical mucus	Color, quality, and amount
(4 = normal)	Use 1-in. strip of nitrazine or ColorpHast (Merck) paper; dip pH paper into vaginal mucus collected on wooden spatula or from speculum.
Amine test (KOH)	Using spatula containing sample, stir x10 into 20% KOH on glass slide.
Wet mount saline (dilute w/scattered ECs)	Using spatula containing sample, stir x3 into saline solution on glass slide.
Low power (quality) magnification	Note general appearance and quality of sample, for example, proper concentration, too dilute, too concentrated.
High power (detail) magnification	Identify organisms and morphology.
Lactobacilli (0–5 +) appear as rods	1–2 + = few 3–4 + = dominant 5 + = false clue cells
Bacteria: anaerobes (0–5 +) appear as tiny dots	1–2 + = few 3–4 + = dominant background 5 + = clue cells
WBCs (0–3 +): lobulated nucleus	1 + = 1:1 ratio to ECs 2 + = 5:1 ratio to ECs 3 + = 10:1 or greater ratio to ECs
Other	ECs (true clue cells, false clue cells, grainy, furry) yeast, *Trichomonas*, *mobiluncus*, sperm, red blood cells, medications, artifact
Wet mount (KOH) (very concentrated)	ECs look like round, faint balloons, called ghost cells
Low power	Hyphae forms (cobwebs) visible but not buds
High power	Hyphae look like elongated circus balloons Buds look like spherical glass beads
Assessment	Specify, including rule-outs, list in order of most likely to least likely
Plan	Diagnostic tests, including yeast cultures, medications, education, and follow-up

EC = epithelial cell; KOH = potassium hydroxide; LMP = last menstrual period; WBC = white blood cell.
*Adapted from Secor Scale. Used with permission.

Table 10.5B   **Vaginal Microscopy: Secor Flow Sheet**

Date			
HPI			
LMP, last coitus			
Vulva, vagina, cervix			
Vaginal mucus			
Cervical mucus			
pH (4.0–7.5) 4 = normal			
Amine test (KOH)			
Wet mount (saline)			
Low power (quality)			
High power (detail)			
LB (0–5 +)			
Bacteria (0–5 +)			
WBCs (0–3 +)			
Other			
Wet mount (KOH)			
Low power			
High power			
Assessment			
Plan			

KOH = potassium hydroxide; HPI = history of present illness; LB = lactobacilli; LMP = last menstrual period; WBC = white blood cell.

Table 10.6   **pH in Relation to Lifecycle Changes Affected by the Presence or Absence of Lactobacilli**

Phase of Reproductive Lifecycle	pH
Preadolescence	7.0
Reproductive years	3.8–4.2
Postmenopausal years	6.6–7.0

Table 10.7   **Measurement of Vaginal pH**

pH	Condition	Color Change
4.0–4.7	Normal flora Cytolytic vaginosis Small number of immotile trichomonads may be present (not clinically significant)	Light yellow
4.0–4.7	Vulvovaginal candidiasis (not as diagnostic) Group A or B beta-hemolytic streptococcus	Medium to dark yellow
4.7–6.0	Bacterial vaginosis	Light to dark olive green
> 6.0	Trichomoniaisis Significant inflammation (i.e., chlamydia)	Bluish

1. Acidic finding (< 4.5) indicates the presence of vaginal lacto-bacilli in the vaginal flora.
2. A pH less than 4.5 effectively excludes
   a. *Neisseria gonorrhoeae.*
   b. *Gardnerella vaginalis.*
   c. *Haemophilus influenzae.*
   d. *Trichomonas vaginalis.*
3. *T. vaginalis* thrives on an alkaline milieu; *Candida* is inhibited.
4. Factors that interfere with the determination of pH, which, if present, eliminate use of pH as a diagnostic tool.
   a. Menses: 7.2.
   b. Semen: more than 7.
   c. Mucus: alkaline (cervical and vaginal).
   d. Lubricant from speculum.
   e. Intravaginal medications.
   f. Lubricating jelly.
   g. Tap water.
   E. Summary of findings (Table 10.7).

VIII. Candidiasis explained.
   A. The *Candida* species.
   1. More than 200 different strains of *Candida* species.
   2. Fungi share characteristics of both plants and animals but are classified into their own kingdom.
   3. They reproduce sexually by producing spores and asexually by budding.

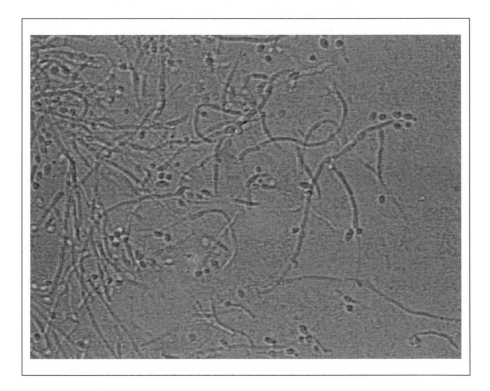

Figure 10.3 *Candida albicans.*

   4. Their growth is best supported in an environment that is
   warm, moist, and dark.
   5. They rely on sugar as their major source of energy (glycogen
   in the female vagina).
   6. Differentiation of terms: Yeast, fungus, mycoses, monilia,
   Candida are used interchangeably.
   7. Candidiasis is not considered a sexually transmitted disease.
B. Six genera most typically inhabit the vagina (in order of
   occurrence).
   1. *Candida albicans* (in 65% of cases, this is the cause of vulvovaginal candidiasis).
      a. They are dimorphic. They form both blastospores and my-
      celia (filaments, hyphae, and pseudohyphae) (Figure
      10.3).
      b. Sometimes referred to as "spaghetti and meatballs."

2. *Candida tropicalis* (23%): dimorphic.
3. *Candida glabrata* (previously called *Candida torulopsis)* (5–10%): monomorphic. Forms only spores (buds).
4. *Candida krusei.*
5. *Candida parapsilosis.*
6. *Candida pseudotropicalis.*

C. Relationship to estrogen.
   1. There is some evidence that there are estrogen receptors on *C. albicans* and that any condition that increases estrogen may increase risk for development of candidiasis, such as
      a. Pregnancy.
      b. Estrogen replacement therapy, either systemic or vaginal.
      c. Birth control pills. (New, lower dose pills do not seem to be as much of a problem.)

D. Relationship to pH.
   1. Presence does not usually change the acidity of the vaginal secretions.

E. Predisposing factors for the development of candidiasis.
   1. Resistance altered by immune status of the body.
      a. HIV.
      b. Pregnancy, corticosteroids, and stress may lead to depressed immunity.
   2. Vaginal allergens cause a chemical vaginitis (Box 10.6).
   3. Increased vaginal glycogen from sugar sources such as artificial sweeteners, wine, fruit juices, and processed sugar.

F. Clinical features of *C. albicans.*
   1. Subjective findings.
      a. Inflammatory response on the walls of the vagina.
      b. Produce erythema, edema, intense pruritus, pain, and dyspareunia.
         (1) Reactive increase in the production of PMN leukocytes.
      c. Clumplike cottage cheese on undergarments.
      d. Adherence to cells is necessary for symptomatic disease.
         (1) *C. albicans* adheres more than other species.
         (2) This characteristic may explain why this species is more frequently found.
   2. Objective findings.
      a. Invasion of *C. albicans* causes increased shedding, which leads ultimately to the thick curdlike discharge (sample for wet mount is best if taken from that discharge).
         (1) Variable: present 20 to 50% of the time.

Substances That May Cause Chemical Vaginitis

BOX
10.6

Substances associated with laundering

Chlorine bleach

Laundry detergent

Fabric softeners

Intravaginal preparations

Propylene glycol found in spermicides, lubricants, and vaginal medications

Feminine hygiene products

Deodorant tampons, liners, and sanitary napkins

Douches and vaginal sprays

Body secretions

Semen

Saliva

Vulvar or vaginal medications

Antifungals

Lidocaine

Crotamiton

Estrogen creams and suppositories

Antibiotic preparations

Clothing

Fabric dyes, especially in colored underwear

Nylon (can give off formaldehyde vapors)

Fiberglass particles on underwear (residual in washing machine after washing fiberglass)

---

(2) Loosely adherent to the vagina or vestibule.
(3) White or yellow.
(4) May coat entire vagina or stick like patches of a rolled-up piece of tissue paper.
(5) Will scrape off with a spatula.
　b. External dysuria (burning when the urine touches the vulva).

    c. Excoriation from scratching of affected tissues.

    d. Minimal odor.

G. Diagnosis.

  1. Use of vaginal microscopy in the diagnosis of candidiasis is about 60% sensitive.

  2. Yeast forms seen more easily with KOH preparation than with saline.

  3. Wooden spatula best to obtain sample because use of a cotton swab may create a fiber artifact, leading to an incorrect diagnosis.

  4. Observations using saline.

    a. Presence of varying numbers of leukocytes (PMN).

      (1) Helps determine the extent of inflammation.

      (2) Number increases with inflammation.

    b. Lactobacilli are present in moderate numbers.

    c. Negative whiff test.

    d. Possible concomitant infection.

      (1) Rare.

      (2) Determine if pH is increased.

    e. Presence of yeast forms.

      (1) Tinea cruris may have only hyphae.

    f. Abundance of epithelial cells (increase in exfoliation).

      (1) Many clumps are only sheets of sloughed squamous epithelium.

      (2) Carefully examine edges of these sheets for protruding Candida pseudohyphae.

  5. Observations using KOH

    a. Blanches cell wall transparent, making yeast forms more apparent.

    b. Note the presence of yeast forms (other yeast forms are described in Table 10.8).

H. pH less than 4.5 unless concomitant bacterial vaginosis is present.

I. Fungal cultures.

  1. Usually unnecessary because wet mount is often diagnostic.

  2. Expensive and may cause a delay in treatment.

  3. Indicated if the diagnosis is suspected but no yeast forms are seen on wet mount.

  4. More sensitive than wet mount but may confuse diagnosis.

    a. *Candida* may be part of normal vaginal flora.

    b. A positive culture does not indicate the presence of infection.

Table 10.8   **Candidal Forms in Relation to Species**

Yeast Form	Description	Species Name
Pseodohyphae	Long segmented sausages	*Candida albicans* or
Hyphae	Long continuous filaments	*C. tropicalis*
Chlamydiaspores	Clusters of glass beads at terminal ends of the hyphae Uniform in size, associated with hyphae forms	*C. albicans*
Blastospores	Budding ovoid spores of variable size 2–10 microns	*C. glabrata*
	Round to ovoid; no filaments	
	May be budding or grouped in clusters interspersed with filaments	*C. tropicalis*
	Smaller than red blood cells	
	Located at the proximal branches, appearing much like a fern	
	Tiny glass beads	

      c. The culture may be positive in up to 20% of women not infected with *Candida.*
    5. Nickerson culture.
      a. Standard medium for *Candida* growth.
      b. Most sensitive.
  J. Gram stain may be positive when wet mount is negative because of excessive cellular debris.
  K. Pap smear.
    1. Sensitivity is 50%.
    2. Not routinely used as a diagnostic tool.
    3. Asymptomatic *Candida* infection may be picked up on a routine smear.
    4. A Pap smear should not be performed when *Candida* infection is suspected because presence of an inflammatory process will alter results.

IX. Bacterial vaginosis explained.
  A. Description of terms.
    1. "*–osis*" means in excess of; "*–itis*" means inflammation of.

    2. Previously referred to over the years as haemophilus vagini-
tis, cornybacterium vaginitis, *Gardnerella,* nonspecific vaginitis, anaerobic vaginosis, bacterial vaginosis—now, vaginal
bacteriosis is being used more frequently.

    3. The term is defined as vaginal excess of bacteria, with little
or no inflammation.

B. Some comments.

    1. It is the most common cause of vaginal complaints, oc-
curring twice as frequently as candidiasis.

    2. It is a surface bacteria and does not usually invade vaginal
tissues or cause an inflammatory reaction.

    3. It is the most symptomatically benign of the common
infections.

        a. It may have serious implications, such as premature la-
bor, for pregnant women.

        b. Many infected women do not have symptoms.

    4. The condition can coexist with trichomoniasis.

C. Risk factors.

    1. Sexual activity, particularly multiple partners (may also be
found in women never sexually active).

    2. Often coined as a "sexually associated disease."

        a. Can be cultured from the prepuce of sexual partners.

    3. Douching, which may alter the vaginal environment.

    4. Presence of an intrauterine device (IUD).

D. Pathogenesis.

    1. Decrease in lactobacilli, particularly hydrogen peroxide
producing.

    2. Increase in various anaerobic bacterial pathogens (often by a
factor of 100–1,000 fold).

    3. Lack of inflammation.

        a. *Mobiluncus* and *Bacteroides* produce succinic acid, which
may inhibit leukocyte formation, producing infection without inflammation: in mild bacterial vaginosis, there is less
inhibition of leukocytes; therefore, inflammation may be
visible.

E. Clinical features.

    1. Subjective findings.

        a. Increase in vaginal discharge.

        b. Fishy odor, particularly after intercourse, due to presence
of alkaline secretions that release amines.

            (1) Semen has a high pH (7–9).

            (2) Lubrication secreted by the vaginal epithelial cells dur-
ing sexual stimulation also has a high pH.

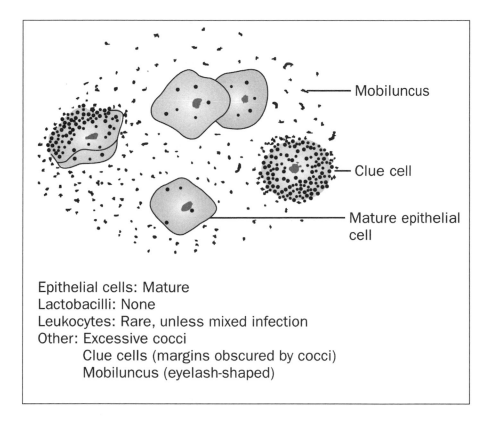

Mobiluncus

Clue cell

Mature epithelial cell

Epithelial cells: Mature
Lactobacilli: None
Leukocytes: Rare, unless mixed infection
Other: Excessive cocci
      Clue cells (margins obscured by cocci)
      Mobiluncus (eyelash-shaped)

Figure 10.4 Bacterial vaginosis.

    2. Objective findings.
       a. Uniform discharge that adheres to the vaginal walls like "spilled milk."
       b. Mild erythema or absence of inflammation of vulvar or vaginal tissues.
  F. Diagnosis: Requires three of the following four criteria (Amsel's criteria).
    1. pH 4.5 or higher.
       a. Highest sensitivity.
       b. Lowest specificity because it can be elevated in concomitant infections, semen, medications, douching, and blood.
    2. KOH: positive whiff test—amine volatilized when the pH is increased.
    3. Uniform, homogenous vaginal discharge.
    4. Presence of "clue cells" in saline preparation (Figure 10.4).

      a. Stippled or granular mature epithelial cells that appear speckled rather than translucent, resembling fried eggs sprinkled with pepper.

      b. The nucleus remains distinct, thus aiding identification of the cell.

      c. Small, pleomorphic, gram-negative coccobacilli adhering to surface of epithelial cells so that the cell wall becomes indistinct (75% of cell margin obscured).

         (1) May be confused with vacuolated squamous cells, which also contain small, dark spots.

         (2) Focus up and down to distinguish between coccobacilli stuck on the surface of the cell with bacterial vaginosis, and vacuoles found within the cell itself.

      d. Often comprise between 10 and 50% of epithelial cells.

      e. High sensitivity (91.2%) and specificity (94.3%).

   5. Additional findings.

      a. Absence or relative scarcity of lactobacilli.

      b. Possible presence of *Mobiluncus* species such as *Mobiluncus curtisii* or *Mobiluncus mulieris.*

         (1) Highly motile, anaerobic, gram-negative.

         (2) Short-curved, "comma" cells.

         (3) Present in 50 to 100% of patients.

      c. Few leukocytes (unless a concomitant infection is present, such as trichomoniasis).

         (1) Ratio of PMN cells to epithelial cells is less than or equal to 1.

      d. Floating background bacteria between epithelial cells, which usually outnumber lactobacilli.

G. Gram stain.

   1. Not usually necessary because wet mount study is often diagnostic.

   2. The diagnosis is based on the stippled appearance of epithelial cells due to uniformly spaced coccobacilli, a reduction of *Lactobacillus* morphotypes, and an increase in small gram-negative rods and gram-positive cocci.

H. Cultures.

   1. Not helpful.

   2. Anaerobes can be recovered from healthy women.

I. Pap smear.

   1. Unreliable for diagnosis of BV. Correlate with Amsel's criteria but do not use as solo criteria for diagnosis.

X. Trichomoniasis explained.

A. Some comments.

1. Causes about 10% of all cases of vaginitis; however, prevalence seems to be decreasing.
2. Almost exclusively sexually transmitted; present in 30 to 40% of sexual partners of infected women.
3. Can cause nongonococcal urethritis.
4. Chronic trichomoniasis can reduce the glycogen content of the cells, causing vaginal lining to become thinner and more prone to ulceration.
5. Primarily affects the vagina but can affect the cervix, Bartholin's glands, urethra, and bladder, including the Skene's ducts.
6. Many infections are asymptomatic.

B. Identification of trichomoniasis.
1. Trichomonads are unicellular, anaerobic protozoans.
2. Actively motile by virtue of four filaments of equal length.
   a. One to two times the length of the organism itself.
   b. Protrude from the forward end of the trichomonad.
3. Teardrop shape of various sizes.
   a. A little larger than PMN leukocytes.
   b. Smaller than a mature epithelial cell but larger than its nucleus.

C. Replication.
1. Binary division.
2. Transfer from one host to another only in the presence of moisture.

D. Effects of pH.
1. If less than 4.5, the organism is rounded. It is difficult to distinguish.
2. Usually pH is 5.0 (pH less than 5.0 virtually eliminates the possibility of trichomoniasis).

E. Predisposing factors.
1. Hypoacidity of vaginal secretions due to an increase in cervical mucus production (cervical mucorrhea; estrogen effect) or menstruation.
2. Exogenous estrogen, including estrogen replacement therapy, estrogen creams, and oral contraceptives (possibly).

F. Clinical features.
1. Subjective findings.
   a. Profuse, often malodorous discharge.
      (1) Variable appearance.
      (2) Classic appearance: frothy, yellow to green.
   b. Pruritus, vaginal burning.
2. Objective findings.

    a. Vulvar edema and erythema.

    b. Strawberry cervix (ecchymotic petechiae) occasionally present (30% of the time).

G. Diagnosis.

  1. Observations using saline.

    a. Patience and diligence at the microscope is often necessary.

    b. Trichomonads visible only in saline. Lysed in KOH.

    c. Time is a critical factor.

      (1) Susceptible to oxygen, cool temperature, and drying. (This may be another reason to examine the saline slide first.)

      (2) If wet mount cannot be performed immediately, place cotton-tipped applicator with vaginal secretions in a test tube with 0.5 inch normal saline, as described on p. 199.

      (3) The organisms will remain motile for at least a half hour unless they dry out or the saline is old (must change saline every 3 months or else it becomes hypertonic).

    d. May warm slide slightly by passing a match under it to increase motility. Microscope light may warm.

    e. Squamous epithelial cells present.

      (1) Immature parabasal and intermediate cells may be present with marked or chronic infection.

    f. Polymorphonuclear leukocytes are increased due to the inflammation (may be dramatic).

    g. Lactobacilli may be present.

    h. *Candida* may be noted concomitantly (rare).

  2. Characteristics of trichomonads in saline.

    a. Flagella never visible under low power and sometimes visible under high power.

    b. Healthy trichomonads undulate, jerk, or twitch or actively move in the direction of the flagellae.

    c. Unhealthy trichomonads assume a rounded shape, are more difficult to identify, are sluggish, and usually are visible only under high power.

    d. Mobility is reduced when cold.

      (1) Keep the saline warm, and view immediately.

      (2) Motility may be hampered by large numbers of PMN leukocytes.

    e. Trichomonads assume a rounder shape when they are dry or drying.

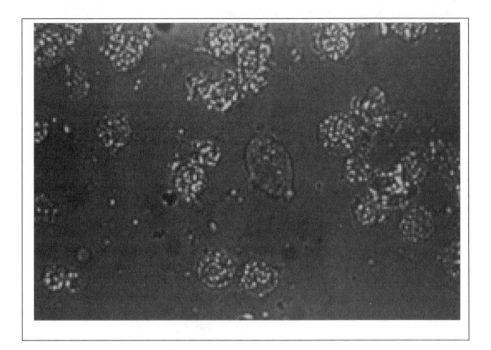

Figure 10.5 Characteristics of trichomoniasis.

    f. Trichomonads can provoke a strong WBC response. Carefully examine clumps of WBCs that may surround and attach to a trichomonad.

    g. Figure 10.5 demonstrates characteristics of trichomoniasis.

3. Observations using KOH preparation (Figure 10.6).

    a. Trichomonads are lysed.

    b. Possible presence of amine odor (50%).

4. Pap smear.

    a. Usually does not reveal trichomonads because they are immotile by the time they are evaluated.

    b. Positive predictive value only 40%.

5. Gram stain.

    a. Trichomonads can be identified by Gram stain but offers no real advantage over a careful wet mount.

    b. More difficult to distinguish from PMNs by this method.

6. Culture: *Trichomonas.*

    a. Most sensitive (95%).

      b. Easy to perform.

      c. Not readily available.

      d. Limit use to those in whom diagnosis is suspected but not seen on wet mount.

    7. Gonorrhea culture.

      a. Perform on all women with trichomoniasis because up to 60% of woman with trichomoniasis may also have gonorrhea.

    8. Urinalysis. Organism may be clearly visualized due to lack of other cellular debris.

XI. Cytolytic vaginitis explained.

  A. Some comments.

    1. Caused by destruction of vaginal epithelial cells by the acid environment caused by the overgrowth of lactobacilli.

    2. Previously termed *Döderlein's cytolysis* after the Döderlein species of lactobacilli.

      a. Over 100 different species of lactobacilli have been discovered.

    3. This infection is often confused with candidiasis because symptoms are similar, especially if premenstrual and chronic. However, microscopic findings are much different.

  B. Clinical features.

    1. Subjective findings.

      a. Pasty discharge.

      b. Pruritus, vulvar dysuria.

      c. Symptoms worsen during the luteal phase.

      d. Low-grade burning or discomfort; increased with sexual activity.

      e. Lack of odor.

    2. Objective findings.

      a. Vulvar tissues may be erythematous and edematous.

      b. Discharge may be thick or flocculent (clumpy).

  C. Diagnosis.

    1. Observations of saline preparation (Figure 10.6).

      a. Large number of epithelial cells.

      b. False clue cells.

        (1) Long rods (lactobacilli of varying lengths).

        (2) May be adherent to epithelial cells (intermediate)

        (3) May be confused with the clue cell of bacterial vaginosis.

      c. Contains cytoplasmic debris from fragments of epithelial cells destroyed by acid environment.

      d. Stippled nuclei.

      e. Negative for *Candida,* trichomonads, and clue cells.

      f. Rare leukocytes.

    2. Observations of KOH preparation.

      a. Bacteria lysed.

      b. Negative odor.

    3. pH is low (3.5–4.0).

    4. Culture recommended to rule out Candida infection.

    5. Pap smear.

      a. Shows cytolysis on routine smears.

      b. Should not be used as a diagnostic tool because wet mount is reliable and readily available.

D. Treatment consists of increasing the pH of the vagina by means of sodium bicarbonate douches or baths. Self-correcting with menses.

    1. Recommend 30 to 60 g per 1 L of warm water two to three times per week, then once weekly as needed.

XII. Lactobacillosis explained.

A. Some comments.

    1. Condition characterized by an increase in vaginal discharge and discomfort.

    2. May occur after antimycotic treatment after treatment of a *Candida* infection.

    3. The incidence is unknown because of scant research; condition is poorly understood.

    4. Bacteria elongates, particularly anaerobic lactobacilli.

B. Clinical features.

    1. Features resemble those of candidiasis.

      a. Thick, white, creamy, or curdy discharge.

      b. Associated with vaginal itching, burning, and irritation.

    2. Symptoms tend to occur 7 to 10 days before menses (second half of menstrual cycle), reaching a peak shortly before menstruation, after which it disappears after menses, only to recur before the next menses.

C. Diagnosis.

    1. Saline.

      a. Many long (40–75 μm) serpiginous rodlike lactobacilli, previously termed *Leptothrix.* Normal rods are between 5 and 15 μm.

      b. May be confused with filaments of candidiasis (thinner strands).

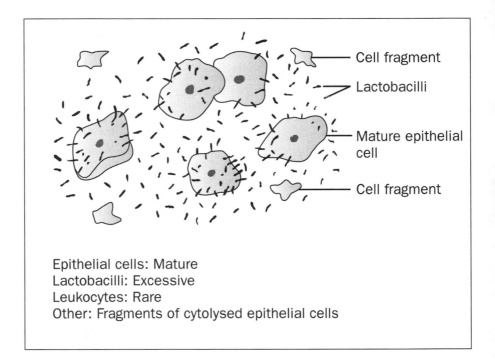

Epithelial cells: Mature
Lactobacilli: Excessive
Leukocytes: Rare
Other: Fragments of cytolysed epithelial cells

Figure 10.6 Cytolysis.

        c. Mature epithelial cells are present with few PMN cells.
     2. Differs from cytolytic vaginitis in that rods are longer and less abundant.
   D. Treatment with amoxicillin and clavulanate is clinically successful in 100% of patients. Baking soda douche is not as effective as it is with cytolysis.

XIII. Desquamative inflammatory vaginitis (DIV) explained.
   A. Some comments.
     1. Associated with overstimulation of vaginal mucosa from unknown causes.
        a. May be associated with lichen planus of the mouth and genitals.
        b. Overabundance of squamous cells, which act as a substitute for bacteria.
        c. Commonly misdiagnosed as *Trichomonas* infection; must rule out cervical cancer.

      2. Incidence may be underestimated.
- **B.** Clinical features: may resemble trichomoniasis or atrophic vaginitis with bacterial infection.
  - **1.** Subjective findings.
    - **a.** Thick, profuse discharge accompanied by dyspareunia and pruritus.
    - **b.** No odor.
  - **2.** Objective findings include ecchymotic and petechial lesions on the vulva, vagina, and cervix.
- **C.** Diagnosis.
  - **1.** Wet mount.
    - **a.** Many PM cells.
    - **b.** Many basal and parabasal cells (hallmark of the disease).
    - **c.** Few mature epithelial cells.
    - **d.** Naked nuclei.
    - **e.** Negative clue cells, yeast forms, or trichomoniasis.
    - **f.** Absent lactobacilli with few microorganisms.
    - **g.** Red blood cells may be present.
  - **2.** KOH.
    - **a.** Negative whiff test.
  - **3.** pH: more than 4.5.
  - **4.** Culture and Gram stain.
    - **a.** Gram-positive cocci (mainly group B streptococci).
- **D.** Treatment options include intravaginal Clindamycin or steroid creams. Relapses are more common with Clindamycin. Local estrogen may also be effective.

XIV. Atrophic vaginitis explained (see chapter 23).
- **A.** Some comments.
  - **1.** Inflammation of the vaginal epithelium occurs due wholly and in part to a lack of estrogen.
  - **2.** Found in breastfeeding women and those who underwent natural or surgical menopause, or in patients taking antiestrogen medications.
  - **3.** Epithelium is thin and lacks glycogen because of a decrease in endogenous estrogen.
- **B.** Clinical features.
  - **1.** Subjective findings.
    - **a.** Vaginal dryness.
    - **b.** Dyspareunia.
    - **c.** Vulvar and vaginal irritation and burning.
    - **d.** Possible spotting.

Table 10.9   **Microscopic Structures That May Be Identified in a Wet Mount Preparation (in Order)**

Saline	KOH
Lactobacilli	Yeast forms
Cocci	Hyphae
White blood cells (polymorphonuclear cells)	Pseudohyphae Mycelia
Squamous epithelial cells (varying degrees of maturity)	Spores Chlamydiaspores
Clue cells	Blastospores
False clue cells	
Trichomoniasis	
Red blood cells	

      e. Vulvodynia (see chapter 5).
   2. Objective findings.
      a. Thin and smooth vaginal walls; lack of rugae.
      b. Inflammation or exudate may be present.
      c. Smooth, shiny vulva with adherence of labia.
      d. Urethral caruncle or prolapse.
      e. Microscopy finding (Figure 10.7)
 C. Assessment of the Maturation Index in the diagnosis of atrophic vaginitis (see chapter 23).

XV. Vaginal cultures.
 A. Procedure: An adjunct to the wet mount; is needed only if the wet mount is inconclusive. Often performed too frequently.
   1. Wipe cervix free of discharge (particularly if copious, slippery estrogenic mucus may make collection of columnar cells difficult).
   2. Observe any special instructions or precautions from the laboratory.
   3. If a cervical culture is needed, sample columnal cells from the endocervical area.
      a. Insert the swab from the cervical sample into the cervical os.
      b. Rotate several times (some cultures indicate 30–60 seconds).

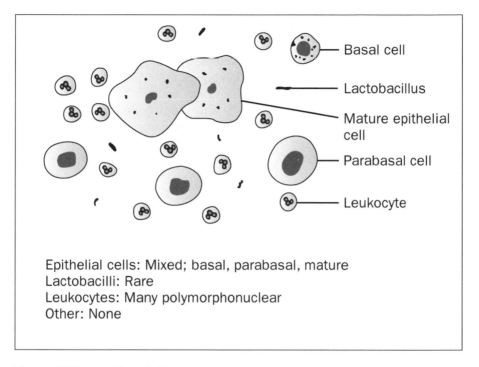

Epithelial cells: Mixed; basal, parabasal, mature
Lactobacilli: Rare
Leukocytes: Many polymorphonuclear
Other: None

Figure 10.7 Atrophic vaginitis.

     c. Withdraw sample and place in specified tube or
       container.
     d. Label with name and presumptive diagnosis.
   4. Vaginal culture: Take sample from vaginal pool. Label.

XVI. Gram stain of vaginal secretions.
   A. The procedure.
     1. Briefly heat-fix the slide that contains the smear of vaginal
       secretions.
     2. Flood the slide with gentian violet stain solutions for 10
       seconds.
     3. Wash the slide in water.
     4. Flood it with Gram's iodine solution for 10 seconds.
     5. Rinse it again with water.
     6. Decolorize it with acetone and alcohol solutions for 10
       seconds.
     7. Flood it with safranin stain for 10 seconds.

8. Wash it in water a third time.
9. Cover with a glass coverslip, and view it under a microscope.
10. Add a drop of saline on top of the coverslip to use the oil immersion lens (without having to add oil).

B. Stain of various organisms.
1. Gonorrhea: intracellular gram-negative diplococci.
2. Bacterial vaginosis: small pleomorphic gram-negative coccobacilli.
3. Trichomoniasis.
   a. Pale staining.
   b. Pear-shaped parasites.

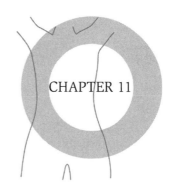

CHAPTER 11

Urinalysis

Helen A. Carcio

I. **Some comments related to urinary tract infection (UTI).**
   A. UTI is 50 times more common in women than in men.
   B. Ten percent to 20% of women develop a UTI at least once in their lives; 80% of these women develop a second infection.
   C. Definitions.
      1. Urethritis: Inflammation of the urethra. Cystitis: Inflammation of the bladder. Pyelonephritis: Inflammation of the kidney.
   D. Many factors may predispose a woman to the occurrence of a UTI (Table 11.1).
   E. Symptoms of cystitis include abrupt onset of
      1. Dysuria.
      2. Urinary frequency: voiding small amounts, particularly common in pregnancy.
      3. Urinary urgency.
      4. Suprapubic pain.
      5. Hematuria.
      6. Pyuria.

II. **Urinary evaluation.**
   A. Assessment of urine in women in a primary care setting is often performed to identify or rule out UTI in the evaluation of dysuria, frequency, and suprapubic pain. Other conditions that relate specifically to the vulvovaginal area, such as those caused by *Candida, Chlamydia, Neisseria gonorrhoeae,* or *Trichomonas* may also present with similar symptoms and must be explored.

Table 11.1   **Factors That Contribute to Infection of the Urinary Tract**

Factor	Result
Sexual activity	Results in introduction of bacteria into the urethra
Poor hygiene habits	Bacteria multiply in area of the urethra
Not bathing or showering routinely	Infrequent changing of underwear or peripads
Wiping from back to front	Introduces bacteria from the rectum into the urethra
Excessive use of caffeine	Causes urinary irritation and diuresis
Excessive stress	Reduces immune response
Contraception: Diaphragm use	Use of diaphragm may press on bladder, causing stasis of urine Spermicides inhibit growth of lactobacilli

Voiding habits
  Waiting long periods of time
  between urinating
	Results in stasis of urine
	Decreases flushing of bacteria from bladder

    B. A urine culture does not need to be ordered in young women with a history of previous uncomplicated UTIs who present with the usual symptoms. A dipstick test is sufficient.

    C. Urinary assessment may include a comprehensive health history, physical examination, a urine dipstick test, microscopy, or culture.

    D. A thorough evaluation should be performed
        1. For an initial episode.
        2. If diagnosis is uncertain.
        3. As an initial prenatal screen.
        4. In elderly women, particularly if a cystocele is present.
        5. In immunocompromised women.

    E. A physical examination should include the following:
        1. Vital signs, especially temperature.
        2. Abdominal examination to palpate the suprapubic area for tenderness.
        3. Percussion of costal vertebral angle (CVA) tenderness (present in pyelonephritis).
        4. Kidney palpation.

Solutes in Random Urine   BOX 11.1

Various solutes normally appear at different times of the day.

Glucosuria: more often after meals

Proteinuria: after activity or assumption of othostatic position from a recumbent position

Hemoglobinuria: After severe physical exertion, such as working out at a gym

     5. Pelvic examination and wet mount, if history indicates risk factors for sexually transmitted infection.
   F. The female anatomy predisposes a woman to bladder colonization with pathogens. This is related to
     1. Short urethra (2.5 cm).
     2. Proximity to the anal area.
     3. Pregnancy: bladder enlarged with decreased tone; unable to empty completely.
     4. Older age: Lack of estrogen may cause urethral atrophy.

III. Principles related to the procurement of urine.
   A. Freshly voided concentrated specimen provides more useful information than a diluted specimen.
     1. Use the first morning urine. However, a random specimen is more convenient (Box 11.1).
     2. Bacteria must have been in the bladder at least 4 hours for accuracy.
   B. Test within a few minutes of collection. (If this is not possible, cover tightly and refrigerate at 5°C [41°F].)
   C. Do not allow specimen to stand at room temperature. Urine that is allowed to stand at room temperature begins to grow bacteria within 30 minutes; if more than 2 hours elapses, it will be highly contaminated by bacteria.
   D. As urine sits, it becomes alkaline, decomposing important sediment.
   E. Red blood cells and casts lyse quickly in diluted or alkaline urine.

IV. The clean catch: In women, a clean catch is more difficult to obtain than in men, because external genitalia or vaginal discharge often cause contamination of the sample.
   A. Equipment.

1. Sterile urine container.
2. Three wipes saturated with soap.

B. The following steps should be explained.
   1. First, wash hands thoroughly to remove any potential sources of contamination.
   2. Remove the cover of a sterile specimen container, and put down with the lid side up. (Emphasize not to touch the inside of the lid or specimen container.)
   3. Spread the labia with the nondominant hand, and hold until after the specimen is collected.
   4. Using the dominant hand, wipe one side of the vaginal area with a cleansing towelette.
   5. Always use a single stroke, wiping the cleansing towelette from front to back.
   6. Cleanse the opposite side of the labia with the second towelette.
   7. Finally, cleanse the center area directly over the urethra, downward.
   8. Release a small amount of urine into the toilet to flush any bacteria from the distal portion of the urethra.
   9. Next, place the specimen container under the urethra (be careful not to touch the vulva), and urinate into the sterile cup while the labia remain separated.
   10. If there is heavy vaginal discharge, a tampon should be worn to absorb the vaginal secretions in an attempt to avoid contamination of the urine sample.
   11. Perform the urinalysis immediately, or refrigerate the urine sample.

V. **The chemical analysis: The complete analysis of urine is a simple, noninvasive, and inexpensive means of detecting abnormalities of the genitourinary tract. It is the single most important quantitative assessment of adequacy of renal function.**
   A. The dipstick: Analysis of the urine is performed with the dipstick, a chemically impregnated plastic strip. When the dipstick is placed in urine, the color changes in the various reagent strips provide an approximate quantification of the amount of substance present.
      1. Principles.
         a. Detects the presence of protein, occult blood, glucose, nitrites, and ketones in the urine.
         b. Determines the urinary pH.

   c. Color changes may be compared against a chart provided by the manufacturer.

   d. Store in a cool dry place and use before the expiration date.

 2. Technique: There are many rapid-agent tests for routine and special urinalyses. Most require dipping the stick into fresh, unspun urine and comparison of each reagent area with the corresponding colored area on the strip at varying suggested intervals (seconds to minutes).

B. Odor: Fresh urine is aromatic; stale urine smells ammonia-like. It may adopt the odor of certain ingested substances.

C. Turbidity.

 1. Description: Many normal urine samples appear cloudy.

 2. Normally, cloudy urine is often caused by the presence of phosphates and carbonates if the specimen is alkaline. It will clear as the urine cools.

 3. Significance: Abnormal turbidity may be caused by red blood cells (RBCs), white blood cells (WBCs), and bacteria, and may suggest UTI.

 4. Vaginal discharge may also cause cloudiness.

D. Color: Urine is often described as "straw colored" or yellow.

 1. Description: The amount of color depends on the density of urochromes (pigments formed by metabolism of bile). The intensity of the color is due to the concentration of the urine. Many substances may change the color of urine.

 2. Normal color ranges from almost colorless to deep yellow, depending on the concentration of urochrome pigment.

 3. Significance: May be a sign of disease or may indicate the presence of a pigmented drug, dye, or food (Table 11.2).

E. Specific gravity (SG): measures urine directly relative to the density of water.

 1. Description: SG is used as in indirect measure of the kidneys' ability to concentrate the urine.The normal range is 1.010 to 1.025, with urine isotonic to plasma.

   a. Diluted: under 1.010.

   b. Concentrated: over 1.025.

 2. Significance: If a first morning specimen is SG 1.025 or greater, it is generally taken as evidence of adequate concentrating ability and, therefore, adequate renal function.

F. pH.

 1. Description: The dipstick is impregnated with various dyes that respond with different color changes to a pH in the

Table 11.2   **Appearance of Urine in Relation to Products**

Urine Appearance	Association
Colorless	Dilute urine associated with water diuresis, or diabetes mellitus or insipidus
Red	RBCs or large amounts of free hemoglobin or myoglobin, bile pigments, food dyes, anthrocyanin (pigment in beets and blackberries)
Red-brown	Porphyria, urobilinogen, bilirubin
Orange	Fever and dehydration
Yellow	Normal due to the presence of a yellow pigment, urochrome
Yellow-red	Pyridium, vegetables, or phenolphthalein
Blue or green	Beets, methylene blue in IV
Brown or black	Porphyrins, melanin, acidification of hemoglobin content, rhubarb
Turbid	Frequently secondary to urates or phosphates (benign), RBCS, WBCs
Foamy	Protein, bile acids
Milky white	Heavy WBC content or precipitation of amorphous phosphate salts in alkaline urine
Cloudy	Pyuria

range of 5 to 11. Measurement of pH on random urine samples has little clinical value.

2. The normal range of urine pH is 4.5 to 8.5. The urine pH in a freshly voided urine sample from a woman on a healthy diet is about 6.0. Stale urine becomes alkaline:
   a. Diffusion of carbon dioxide into the air.
   b. Bacteria converts urea to ammonia.
3. Significance: If fresh urine is alkaline, a UTI urea-splitting organism (e.g., *Proteus, Klebsiella, Escherichia coli)* or bicarbonate excretion (e.g., renal tubular acidosis) must be considered.

G. Protein.
1. Description: The dipstick is sensitive to as little as 5 to 20 mg/dl of albumin (the prominent protein in renal disease). Normal: less than 50 mg/day.

2. Significance:
    a. Persistent proteinuria usually indicates renal disease.
    b. Transient proteinuria may be associated with orthostasis proteinuria, which results from prolonged standing after being in a recumbent position. Stress, cold, and contamination of the specimen with menstrual blood are other possible causes.
H. Nitrites.
    1. Description: Many practitioners use the dipstick as a screening test for occult bacteriuria. It is an insensitive screening test for women who do not have symptoms. It provides an indirect method of detecting bacteriuria because many organisms contain enzymes that reduce nitrate in the urine to nitrite.
    2. Significance: Any degree of pink should be considered positive for the nitrite test, suggesting the presence of 10^5 per ml. Negative nitrate tests do not always mean that no bacteria are present because some strains do not produce the necessary enzymes to convert to nitrites (*Streptococcus faecalis* and gonococci).
    3. Use of a random urine sample is not acceptable because sufficient time would not have passed for conversion of nitrate to nitrite.
I. Ketones: Ketosis is seen in starvation (fad diets) and with alcoholism, as well as in individuals with poorly controlled diabetes mellitus.
J. Blood: Normal: RBCs may normally be seen in extremely small numbers in normal urine, particularly after strenuous exercise.
    1. The normal level is two or fewer RBCs per high-powered field.
    2. Significance: Hematuria is virtually always significant (Table 11.3).
K. Sugar.
    1. Description: Can detect 100 mg/dl of glucose because the reaction relies on the enzyme glucose oxidase. However, results are qualitative.
    2. Normal: The absence of detectable glucose (negative dipstick) is considered a normal result.
    3. Significance: The dipstick method is extremely sensitive and specific for glucose. This test is the main method for the diagnosis of the common disease diabetes mellitus.

VI. **Microscopic examination (see chapter 10, Vaginal Microscopy).**

Table 11.3 Hematuria Differential Diagnosis: Red to Brown Discoloration

Symptom	Diagnosis
Without urinary tract pain	Renal or vesicle diseases
	Absence of RBC casts—tumor of bladder or kidney
	RBC casts—glomerulonephritis
	Stones, polycystic disease, renal cysts, sickle cell disease, hydronephrosis
Renal colic	Ureteral stone
Dysuria	Bladder infection or lithiasis

A. Description: Evaluation of sediment for cellular elements, casts, crystals and microorganisms.
B. Caution.
   1. Microscopic analysis is unreliable if more than 2 hours have elapsed between collection and evaluation.
   2. If SG is below 1.010, sample must be examined immediately after collection.
C. Principles.
   1. Turn condenser down to distance it further from the slide. Use varying light intensities to pick up subtle changes in various elements.
   2. Usc low power first, to identify elements in various fields.
   3. Examine near the four edges of the coverslip, where casts accumulate.
   4. Go to high power for cell counts and identification of casts and debris.
   5. If the urine specimen is purulent or bloody, remember to look at an unspun specimen first.
D. The technique.
   1. Pour 10 to 15 ml of freshly voided urine into a conical test tube.
   2. Check SG in remainder.
   3. Using dipstick, check for pH, protein, sugar, ketones, and heme in the remainder.
   4. If a UTI is suspected (leukocytes or nitrates present as seen by dipstick), check Gram stain of unspun specimen.
   5. Prepare spun specimen.

6. Spin at 1,000 to 2,000 rpm for 3 to 5 minutes.
7. Pour off top supernatant and discard, leaving one to two drops of urine at the bottom. A pellet is usually visible at the bottom.
8. Resuspend pellet immediately in the remaining urine (flick the bottom of the test tube several times with your fingers or tap it against a countertop).
9. Place two drops on a glass slide to dry for Gram stain.
10. While the Gram stain preparation dries, place two to three drops of sediment on another glass slide.
11. Cover the second slide immediately with a coverslip and examine under low power.
12. Use low power and scan entire slide to locate casts that may be present in only a few fields.
13. Examine under high dry power (never oil). Note presence of WBCs and vaginal cells.
14. Scan at least 10 to 15 high-power fields. Squamous epithelial cells are clearly visualized in urine without other vaginal contaminants.
15. Average the number of cells in the fields examined and record.

VII. **The sediment.**
   A. Common sediment in women (Table 11.4).
   B. Casts
      1. Description: Casts usually occur in the distal convoluted tubule of the nephron and are so called because they are casts of the nephron. They are distinguished from other debris by smooth, parallel sides (which may show the trapezoidal narrowing of the nephron collecting system).
      2. Rarely normal. Significance: They are often difficult to interpret. They may indicate renal disease.
         a. RBC casts indicate proliferative glomerular disease or vasculitis.
         b. Hyaline casts that indicate proteinuria can be normal in concentrated urine.
         c. WBC casts indicate interstitial nephritis or pyelonephritis.
         d. Broad casts indicate tubular atrophy, with waxy casts indicating nephron death. Both are the successive changes in degeneration of cellular casts seen in renal failure.
   C. Crystals.
      1. Description: Crystals occur because of precipitated chemicals

Table 11.4   **Common Urinary Sediment**

Sediment	Description	Clinical Significance

RBCs	Normal: presence of 0–3/hpf
	  Pale, biconcave discs
	  No nuclei
	  Can be crenated
	Menses can contaminate and give false-positive results
		Hematuria
		  Cystitis most common cause of hematuria
		  Can occur secondary to exertion, trauma, stress
		May be confused with yeast*

WBCs	Normal: presence of 0–5/hpf Polymorphonuclear leukocyte most common Segmented nuclei $1^1/2$ times as large as RBCs Cytoplasmic granules	Pyuria
Renal tubular epithelial cells	Round, single nucleus Slightly larger than WBCs	
Bladder epithelial cells	Varied shape: flat to cuboidal Larger than renal cells	
Squamous epithelial cells	Rectangular to round, flat cells Single small nuclei Usually from vaginal contamination	
Bacteria Gram stain	Normal urine does not contain bacteria Very small; difficult to identify microscopically Bacilli: short rods Cocci: tiny dots more difficult to identify	Significant bacteria may indicate a urinary tract infection Presence of WBCs may differentiate between an infection and contamination Almost always found but does not always indicate significant bacteriuria Presence in unspun specimen is significant and provides presumptive evidence of UTI Indicate presence of UTI or contamination Send for culture and sensitivity if suspicious If count is low and symptoms present, may be UTI

Table 11.4 *(continued)*

Yeast cells	May be seen in urine (diabetics) Ovoid, budding Variable size Similar in size to RBCs	*Candida* or contamination from vulvovaginal candidiasis If unable to differentiate from the RBC, drop acetic acid; RBCs will lyse, leaving the yeast intact.
Trichomonas	Most frequently seen parasite in urine Unicellular, ovoid with flagellate Undulates	Can be found in urine or urine contaminated from vaginal *trichomonas*
Spermatozoa	Ovoid to round, with long tails Forward trajectory, spinning, immobile	May be seen after contamination by vaginal intercourse
Artifact	Starch granules (powder) Cotton fibers	

hpf = high-powered field; RBC = red blood cell; UTI = urinary tract infection; WBC = white blood cell.

and cellular debris. Their interpretation depends on the clinical presentation involved and is beyond the scope of this chapter.

2. Crystals are formed in normal (alkaline) urine as the specimen cools.

3. Significance: Many different types of crystals are found in urine; however, a full discussion is beyond the scope of this chapter. Note: Normal urine contains no more than one or two RBCs, WBCs, and epithelial cells per high-powered field. An occasional hyaline cast may be seen.

VIII. Gram stain.

A. Description: The Gram stain technique can be used in the office setting. The preparation is more time consuming than microscopy; however, additional information can be obtained to help with diagnosis. The highlighting of cells and organisms during the staining process makes them easier to identify and facilitates making a diagnosis. The following are enhanced by the colors they become:

1. Gram-negative organisms appear pink.

2. Gram-positive organisms appear purple.

3. Cells stain purple.

4. Bacteria may be pink or purple.
5. WBCs: unstained at first, nuclei develop a red-blue stain with red cytoplasm.
6. Hyaline cast: bright blue.
7. Fine, granular casts: bright red.
8. *Trichomonas:* usually do stain but may appear bluish. Note: Some clinicians believe that the Gram stain is not necessary for diagnosis of most forms of vaginitis.

B. Technique.
1. Spread a thin smear of urine sediment on a glass slide.
2. Allow to air dry.
3. Fix by passing the underside of slide through a flame several times. Allow to cool.
4. Flood the slide with Gram crystal violet.
5. Wait 10 seconds, and rinse with tap water.
6. Repeat step 5, rinsing again.
7. Rinse the slide with decolorizer until all the violet has been rinsed away (fluid is colorless).
8. Immediately rinse again with tap water.
9. Flood the slide again with Gram safranin. Wait 10 seconds and rinse with tap water.
10. Dry or blot dry.
11. Place slide under microscope and put a small drop of oil on the stained specimen.
12. Using oil power objective with bright field illumination (diaphragm open), examine the slide.
13. View several fields.
14. Record findings.

C. Common errors leading to unsatisfactory urine sediment examination.
1. Contamination of collecting vessel with foreign material.
2. Inadequately resuspended sediment.
3. Failure to use both high- and low-power magnification.
4. Too much or too little light.
5. Dried specimen.
6. Artifacts such as cotton fibers from swabs or powder crystals.
7. Vaginal contamination.

IX. **Urine culture. (See Table 11.5 for the interpretation of WBC count in relation to symptoms.)**

X. **Management of positive findings. (See Table 11.6 for differential diagnoses.)**

Table 11.5   **Significance of WBCs in Urine Culture in Relation to Symptoms**

WBCs	WBC Count	Symptoms
100,000/ml	10^5	Symptoms Significant bacteriuria
10,000/ml	10^4	No symptoms Significant asymptomatic bacteriuria Symptoms Treat
1,000 to 10,000/ml	10^3–10^4	Contamination of external source Dilute urine Been in the bladder only a short period of time Early days of treatment with antibiotic No infection

WBC = white blood cell.

A. Uncomplicated UTI.
   1. Usually easy to cure because the infection is superficial and a high concentration of the antibiotic is readily achieved in the urine. Long courses of antibiotics are no longer necessary.
      a. Symptoms disappear 1 to 2 days after beginning treatment.
      b. Encourage the patient to continue medication even though symptoms are gone.
      c. Warn the patient that vulvovaginal candidiasis may develop secondary to antibiotic therapy. Tell her to call if she notices any vulvar itching or burning.
   2. Single-dose therapy.
      a. Amoxicillin, 3 g.
      b. Sulfamethoxazole/trimethoprim (Bactrim) two tablets
      c. Ofloxacin (Floxin), 100 to 250 mg.
   3. Three-day regimens (slightly increased efficacy).
      a. Bactrim DS bid.
      b. Nitrofurantoin macrocrystals (Macrobid) two times a day (somewhat decreased incidence of concurrent candidiasis).
      c. Amoxicillin, 500 mg three times a day.
      d. Ciprofloxacin (Cipro), 250 mg two times a day.

Table 11.6   Differential Diagnosis of Conditions That Affect the Urinary Tract

Condition/ Symptoms	Diagnosis	Description
Cystitis (most common)	10^5 Micro: 8–10 WBCs per hpf Red blood cells Bacteria	Infection of the superficial mucosa of the lower urinary tract Triad of symptoms Urinary urgency Frequency Dysuria
Upper urinary tract (pyelonephritis)	Involves renal parenchyma	Systemic manifestations of chills, fever, flank pain
Asymptomatic bacteriuria	10^3/ml of bacteria in the absence of symptoms	Negative symptoms
Acute urethral syndrome	Negative culture	Dysuria, frequency, urgency
Interstitial cystitis	Negative culture	Urgency and frequency associated with diminished bladder capacity

Note: If large numbers of vaginal epithelial cells are present, it may indicate contamination. A vaginal wet mount must be done to eliminate vaginal discharge as the primary source of the WBCs.
hpf = high-power field; WBC = white blood cell.

        e. Ofloxacin (Floxin), 400 mg two times a day.
    4. Box 11.2 summarizes those organisms found in urine cultures.
  B. Complicated cystitis.
    1. Use of the medications mentioned in Section III; increase use to 7 to 10 days.
    2. Needs further evaluation.
  C. If pylonephritis is suspected, continue the aforementioned regimens for 14 days.
  D. May prescribe phenazopyridine (Pyridium) 100 mg three times a day to relieve dysuria by preventing bladder spasm.

Most Common Organisms Identified in Urinary Tract Infection

BOX
11.2

Gram-negative organisms (found in large intestine)

Escherichia coli (70%)

Proteus mirabilis

Klebsiella spp.

Pseudomonas aeruginosa

Gram-positive organisms (less commonly identified)

Streptococcus faecalis

Staphylococcus epidermidis

Organisms commonly found in the absence of disease

Lactobacillus spp.

Cornebacterium

Micrococci

Neisseria spp.

Organisms that are not found in routine cultures but can cause UTI

Chlamydia trachomatis

Neisseria gonorrhoeae

Herpes simplex virus

Mycoplasma hominis—less common

Ureaplasma urealyticum—less common

Symptomatic bacteriuria—8–10 WBC/hpf is diagnostic

Culture and sensitivity—indicates the specific pathologic bacteria in the urine

Determines which antibiotics will be effective against it

hpf = high-powered field; UTI = urinary tract infection; WBC = white blood cell.

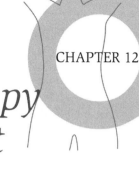

CHAPTER 12

Sonohysteroscopy (Fluid Contrast Ultrasound)

Helen A. Carcio

I. Sonohysteroscopy explained.

  A. Sonohysteroscopy is the infusion of sterile saline though the cervix and into the uterus, and the area is imaged by transvaginal ultrasound examination.

    1. The saline distends the normally collapsed uterus, allowing for a more accurate view of the inner surfaces.

      a. Reveals the presence of any abnormalities lining the uterus or in the cavity itself.

      b. Is an adaptation of standard pelvic ultrasonography.

    2. Provides a three-dimensional view of the uterine cavity and ovaries.

    3. Has the potential to replace the more invasive diagnostic methods, such as hysteroscopy and endometrial biopsy surgery.

    4. Is usually less costly and easier to perform than hysteroscopy, and is well tolerated by the patient.

    5. Findings are immediately viewed on a monitor, often making instant diagnosis possible.

    6. Can be done in an office setting without the use of anesthesia.

      7. Uses sound waves that are reflected from the tissue back to a receiver that records the different tissue densities.

B. Indications.

    1. To evaluate uterine bleeding in postmenopausal women.

    2. To investigate dysfunctional uterine bleeding in reproductive-age women if an area is unable to be visualized clearly with sonography.

    3. To monitor endometrial thickness in a patient undergoing tamoxifen therapy.

    4. To assess endometrial carcinoma.

    5. To investigate recurrent pregnancy loss in which uterine anomalies contribute to habitual abortion.

    6. To evaluate tubal infertility.

      a. Infusion contains albumin or lactose particles.

      b. Can actually view the proximal portion of the tube.

    7. Preoperative assessment of leiomyomata.

      a. Determines the exact size of uterine fibroids.

      b. Provides an excellent delineation of fibroid contour.

    8. Sonographic indications.

      a. Thickened or poorly defined endometrium in patients with abnormal uterine bleeding.

C. Uterine abnormalities detectable by saline infusion sonography.

    1. Endometrial cancer.

    2. Endometrial hyperplasia.

    3. Endometrial polyps.

      a. Sensitivity: 86%.

      b. Specificity: 81%.

    4. Dyssynchronous endometrium.

    5. Uterine fibroids: intraluminal, submucosal.

      a. Sensitivity: 87%.

      b. Specificity: 92%.

    6. Tamoxifen-induced changes.

    7. Intrauterine synechiae.

    8. Intrauterine fluid accumulation due to cervical stenosis.

D. Potential diagnostic and therapeutic applications.

    1. Directing endometrial biopsy.

    2. Identifying asymptomatic disease during routine examinations.

    3. Determining depth of invasions and sites of attachment of endometrial carcinomas.

    4. Retrieving "lost" intrauterine devices (IUDs).

E. Comparison with other diagnostic methods.

1. Hysterosalpingography.
   a. Necessitates use of radiation and iodinated contrast material.
   b. Provides only indirect information about the uterine cavity.
   c. Is more expensive.
2. Hysteroscopy.
   a. Provides an accurate topographic map of the cavity itself.
   b. Cannot determine the extent of submucosal myomas or the thickness of endometrial layers.
   c. Necessitates distention of the uterine cavity with liquid medium or gas.
   d. May necessitate anesthesia.
3. Magnetic resonance imaging (MRI).
   a. Provides excellent images of the uterus.
   b. Lesions within the uterus can be obscured.
   c. Expensive.

II. The procedure.

A. Patient preparation.
   1. Antibiotic prophylaxis in women with a history of mitral valve prolapse or regurgitation or joint replacement or other orthopedic hardware. Take 1 hour before saline-infusion sonography.
   2. The woman should take a nonsteroidal antiinflammatory agent 1 hour before the procedure to alleviate any discomfort.
   3. The woman should void immediately before the procedure.
   4. Determine that the woman is free of active pelvic inflammatory disease or vaginitis.
      a. Perform wet mount before scheduled procedure.
      b. Reschedule procedure if purulent discharge or cervical motion or adnexal tenderness is present.
B. Timing: It is essential to avoid encountering blood clots that can be interpreted as diseased (Box 12.1).
C. Equipment.
   1. Open-sided speculum: Advantages.
      a. User friendly.
      b. Does not dislocate the intrauterine catheter when it is removed.
D. Position.
   1. Place the patient in the dorsal lithotomy position.

| *Optimal Timing of Sonohysterography* | **BOX 12.1** |

Midfollicular phase of a spontaneous menstrual cycle

At least 4 days after a progestin-induced menstrual flow

After the progestin phase in women taking cyclic hormone replacement therapy

Anytime for women using combined continuous regimens

---

    2. If uterine retroversion is present, place the patient in the left lateral recumbent position.

  E. The technique.

    1. Must flush catheter to remove air bubbles because they can produce misleading images.

    2. Visualize the cervix through a vaginal speculum.

    3. Cleanse the cervical os with betadine solution.

    4. Insertion may be difficult because of adhesions or stenosis (common in postmenopausal women).

      a. Place tenaculum on cervix.

      b. Instruct woman to cough or perform the Valsalva maneuver while the catheter is placed on the anterior lip.

      c. Distraction technique seems to minimize the patient's pain.

      d. For marked stenosis, the clinician can use a dilator through the external and internal ora or a catheter that has been placed in freezer (becomes stiffer).

    5. Marked retroversion.

      a. Grasp the posterior lip of the cervix to straighten the uterine axis and to facilitate catheter placement.

    6. Withdraw speculum, and replace with the ultrasound probe.

      a. Anteverted uterus: Anterior to the catheter.

      b. Retroverted uterus: Posterior to the catheter.

  F. Instillation.

    1. Watch monitor closely during instillation because sonohysterography is a dynamic procedure that momentarily distends the uterus and thereby reveals any endometrial disease.

    2. Slowly inject 10 to 20 ml saline. The slow rate helps minimize discomfort.

      a. The saline causes the normally collapsed uterus to distend.

      b. It allows polyps and fibroids to be seen with greatly enhanced clarity.

      c. Optimal uterine distention is very important.

      d. Infusion rate depends on three factors.

          (1) The size of the uterus.

          (2) Amount of backflow into the vagina.

          (3) Patient discomfort.

   3. Place absorbent towels under the patient's buttocks.

G. The scan.

   1. Move slowly from cornu to cornu in the long axis to measure the endometrial echo.

   2. Rotate the probe 90°, and scan from the endocervix to the fundus.

   3. Note

      a. Echotexture and echogenicity of the endometrium.

      b. Symmetry of the myometrium.

   4. Visualize the adnexa in the semicoronal place, using one hand to gently palpate and push the adnexa toward the probe.

   5. If fallopian tubes are to be visualized, use Albunex (CSL Limited), a new ultrasound imaging agent that can enhance image clarity in fallopian tube studies when added to the saline.

   6. View the cervix and cul-de-sac as the probe is removed.

   7. Document the size, location, and characteristics of any masses.

   8. The study usually requires less than 10 minutes.

III. Conclusion.

   A. The advanced practice clinician is in an advantageous position to learn this new technique and offer it to patients.

   B. Although the advanced practice clinician can certainly learn the technique of inserting the catheter and instilling the solution, a physician certified in ultrasound interpretation is required for diagnosis.

CHAPTER 13

Bone Densitometry

Mimi Clarke Secor

I. **Some comments concerning osteoporosis.**
   A. Because most women with osteoporosis will not have symptoms, bone densitometry is an attempt to establish some means of recognizing those women who have the potential to develop fractures and those who will not.
   B. Bone mass measurements provide a quantitative value so that an osteoporosis diagnosis can encourage the patient to modify her lifestyle and diet, and help her decide on estrogen replacement therapy or use of other medications.
   C. Debates about bone mass measurement revolve around the techniques, frequency of measurements, site of measurement, and cost-effectiveness. No method can be endorsed at this point as part of the routine preventative care regimen of postmenopausal women.
   D. Bone mass densitometry (BMD) predicts the risk for fractures even more accurately than hypertension predicts risk for stroke.
   E. Many clinicians will be treating women with osteoporosis. It is imperative that they understand the indications for BMD and the implications of treatment.

II. **Osteoporosis explained.**
   A. Definition.
      1. Osteoporosis is defined as a skeletal disorder characterized

by compromised bone strength predisposing a person to increased risk for fracture.

2. It is a condition of porous bones that is underdiagnosed because it is a silent disease process.

3. Most serious fractures are those of the hip because they contribute substantially to morbidity rate, mortality rate, and health care costs.

4. There is an increased risk for osteoporosis with advancing age; it begins at the wrist and progresses to the vertebrae and last to the hip.

5. Osteoporosis is a generalized disease that affects all skeletal sites. Low bone density at any site is significantly associated with a risk for fracture.

B. Related statistics.

1. Osteoporosis causes approximately 2.3 million fractures annually at a cost of more than $23 billion in the United States and Europe.

2. One in three elderly women, or nearly 25 million postmenopausal American women are affected.

3. Seventy-five percent of women between the ages of 45 and 75 years have never talked to their doctor about osteoporosis.

4. A woman's relative risk for hip fracture is equal to her combined risk for breast, uterine, and ovarian cancers.

5. Numerous studies have shown that exogenous estrogen reduces the risk of hip fracture by 50% if treatment begins at the onset of menopause and continues for at least 7 years.

6. Vertebral fractures are the most common (700,000 annually), whereas the occurrence of hip fractures is 300,000 annually.

C. No method of bone density measurement can be endorsed at this point as part of the routine preventative care regimen of postmenopausal women. It is prudent to screen women at risk for osteoporosis (Box 13.1).

D. Some facts related to hip fractures.

1. Equal in number to wrist fractures.

2. More expensive than wrist fractures because of immobility and prolonged hospitalization.

3. The mortality rate associated with hip fractures is 12 to 20% during the year after injury.

4. Less than 50% of patients with a hip fracture ever return to their prefracture level of function.

Risk Factors for Osteoporosis

BOX 13.1

Dietary and weight-related factors

Slight build with loss of body fat

High caffeine intake

Excessive alcohol consumption

Lifetime low intake of dietary calcium (lactose intolerance)

Lack of weight gain since age 25

Eating disorder

Estrogen deficiency

Early menopause

Nulliparity

History of breastfeeding (eliminated from newer lists)

Family history of osteoporosis, particularly maternal hip fracture

Smoking

Lack of exercise

Inability to rise from a chair without using the armrest for support

Immobility

Less than 4 hours per day on feet

Tallness

Other conditions and medications may also increase risk

Hyperthyroidism or hyperparathyroidism

Long-term steroid therapy in those women with rheumatoid arthritis or chronic lung disease

Heparin treatment

Intestinal malabsorption

Cushing's disease

Type 1 diabetes

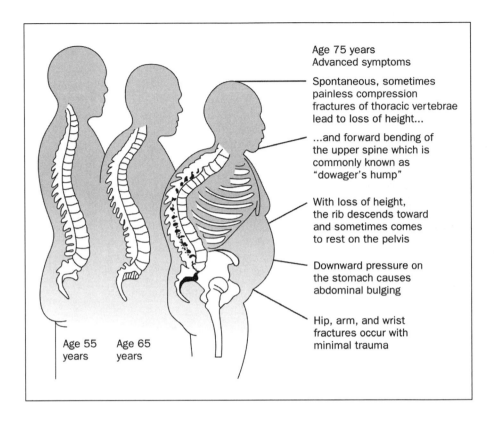

Age 75 years
Advanced symptoms

Spontaneous, sometimes painless compression fractures of thoracic vertebrae lead to loss of height...

...and forward bending of the upper spine which is commonly known as "dowager's hump"

With loss of height, the rib descends toward and sometimes comes to rest on the pelvis

Downward pressure on the stomach causes abdominal bulging

Hip, arm, and wrist fractures occur with minimal trauma

Age 55 years   Age 65 years

Figure 13.1 Silent vertebral fractures can lead to loss of height and related symptoms.

     5. One in seven women experiences osteoporosis-induced hip fractures.

  E. Some facts related to vertebral fractures.

     1. They are twice as common as hip fractures.

     2. They are less readily diagnosed.

     3. Up to 50% are asymptomatic.

     4. Successive fractures lead to a loss in height.

       a. A loss of 1 in. or more is highly indicative of osteoporotic spinal fractures.

       b. Figure 13.1 visually shows how fractures can lead to loss of height throughout the life span.

III. Measurement of bone density.

  A. Bone density is measured in grams per square centimeter.

1. Bone density varies throughout the body.
2. Used to define osteoporosis in terms of standard deviations from the average peak bone mass.
3. *Standard deviation* is a statistical term used to express the average amount by which an individual's bone density varies from the norm.
4. Values are matched against average bone density for women in their 30s, when bone mass generally is at its peak.

B. Parameters for diagnosis: Both the World Health Organization (WHO) and National Osteoporosis Foundation (NOF) categorize a patient's bone density using standard deviation (*SD*) but use a slightly different scale for diagnosis.

1. The WHO Scale.
   a. Low risk of osteoporotic fracture: Patients with an *SD* of 0 to 1.0 below peak bone density is normal.
   b. Greater risk of fracture: Patients with an *SD* between 1 and 2.5 are diagnosed with osteopenia (low bone mass).
   c. Have osteoporosis: Patients with an *SD* greater than 2.5 are diagnosed with osteoporosis, even though they have not had a bone fracture.
   d. The cutoff between osteopenia and osteoporosis is 2.5 *SD*s below peak bone mineral density.
   e. Using these criteria, the WHO classifies 30% of postmenopausal women in the United States as having osteoporosis.
   f. The WHO recommends that all individuals who are categorized with osteoporosis should be treated. (Many clinicians also treat the patient when osteopenia is present.)
2. NOF Scale.
   a. An *SD* 0 to 1.0 below peak bone density is normal, the same as that used by WHO.
   b. The cutoff between osteopenia and osteoporosis is 2.0 *SD*s below peak BMD (compared with the WHO scale of 2.5 *SD*s below peak).
   c. NOF criteria would classify 45% of postmenopausal women as osteoporotic.
3. Low BMD at spine, hip, or forearm is sufficient for a diagnosis of osteoporosis.
4. One *SD* at the spine or hip increases the risk of fracture approximately twofold.

C. Disadvantage of conventional radiography.
1. Insensitive and inaccurate if vertebral fracture is not present.

2. Subjective.
3. Influenced by radiographic exposure factors, patient size, and film-processing techniques.
4. Bone mineral content must decrease by as much as 35% before it can be detected.
5. Increased exposure to ionizing radiation.

IV. **The procedure.**
   A. Assess and monitor various disease states and conditions.
   1. Evaluate those women at risk for osteoporosis who are unsure whether to initiate estrogen replacement therapy.
   2. Detect osteopenia and assess its severity.
   3. Evaluate patients with metabolic bone disease that affects the skeleton.
   4. Identify those individuals at risk for traumatic fracture.
   5. Assess the effectiveness of prevention or treatment measures for osteoporosis.
   6. Monitor a patient undergoing long-term glucocorticoid therapy.
   7. Evaluate a patient with a hip, radial, or vertebral compression fracture.
   8. Assess women who have not taken estrogen in 3 years, in whom the results of the study will influence therapy.
   B. Contraindications to BMD evaluation.
   1. Pregnancy.
   2. Administration of radioisotopes.
   3. Spinal deformity.
   4. The presence of orthopedic hardware. Note: BMD results can be affected by the presence of metal objects such as a belt, button, or corset. It also can be affected by the patient's recent ingestion of calcium-containing tablets.
   C. Accuracy: generally good (90–95%).
   D. Many types vary in precision, accuracy, and discrimination and differing fundamental methods, in clinical and research usefulness, and in general availability. They include the following:
   1. Radiographic.
      a. Single X-ray absorb: Limited to measuring bone density in the arm or heel.
      b. Dual photon absorptiometry (DPA): Measures spine or hipbone density.
      c. Dual-energy X-ray absorptiometry (DXA): Most effective.
      d. Quantitative computed tomography (QCT): Measures bone density in the spine.

    e. Quantitative ultrasound.
    f. Quantitative MRI.
    g. Magnetic resonance microscopy.
E. The DXA. The most used technique at the present time.
    1. Has emerged as the most reliable and practical approach.
    2. Computes the density of bone with greater speed and less radiation than DPA (uses only a fraction of normal x-ray radiation).
    3. Measures the density of bone at two major sites.
      a. Hip.
      b. Spine.
    4. Accuracy: within 3–5%.
    5. Precision: within 0.5 to 2.0%.
    6. Best correlation to predict the risk of fractures at the hip.
    7. Process takes 10 to 15 minutes, with the woman lying on a table while an imager passes over her body.
    8. A computer calculates the density of the patient's bones and compares with normal bone at peak mass, as well as the average bone density for the patient's age.
    9. Results are expressed in grams per square centimeter in *SD* of peak value of matched controls.
    10. Bones with normal mineralization produce a higher reading in grams per centimeter than does osteoporotic bone.
    11. Disadvantages.
      a. Cost: between $100 and $250, depending on the geographic area.
        (1) Makes it prohibitive as a mass screening tool.
        (2) Medicare reimburses approximately $125.
      b. Only 2,200 machines in use nationwide.
F. Quantitative ultrasound.
    1. Advantages.
      a. May be indicated for mass screening.
      b. Lack of ionizing radiation.
      c. Relative portability.
      d. Low cost.
G. Quantitative ultrasound is similar to DXA in fracture-risk prediction.
H. Quantitative MR and computed tomography (CT) need further investigation.
I. Diagnosis at single or multiple bone sites. Controversial.
    1. Some studies have determined that there is not a great difference in bone density at different sites.

Table 13.1   **Daily Recommendations for Dietary Supplements**

Supplement	Age (years)	Daily requirements
Calcium	< 50	1,000 mg
	> 50	1,200 mg
Vitamin D	< 50	400–800 IU
	> 50	800–1,000 IU

　　2. Other studies reported that BMD at several sites increased the predictive accuracy.
　J. Biochemical tests: Blood and urine tests measure the rate of bone remodeling.
　　1. They indicate a high rate of bone turnover, which can be a sign of rapid bone loss.
　　2. At this point, they do not provide enough information on which to base treatment and management decisions.

V. Lifetime monitoring and recommendations
　A. The recommended follow-up interval for bone density testing.
　　1. Every 1 to 2 years to monitor women using estrogen therapy who have osteoporosis.
　　2. Every 1 to 2 years in woman at risk for osteoporosis after a bone densitometry with negative results.
　B. Dietary recommendations (Table 13.1).
　C. Fracture Risk Assessment Tool (FRAX) Risk Assessment Tool.
　　1. The FRAX tool was developed by the WHO to evaluate the fracture risk for patients.
　　2. It is based on individual patient models to integrate the risks associated with clinical risk factors and BMD at the femoral neck.
　　3. The algorithms give the 10-year probability of fracture.
　　4. Recommends that the patient be treated if the risk of fracture is more than 20% even if the BMD is normal.
　　5. The tool is found at www.shef.ac.uk/FRAX/

Acknowledgment

The authors thank Cathy Kessenich for her comments and suggestions regarding the material in this chapter.

CHAPTER 14

BRCA *Testing*

Helen A. Carcio and Paula Brooks

I. The *BRCA* (BReast CAncer) gene in breast and ovarian cancer. Advanced practice clinicians need to be aware of the indications for *BRCA* testing and the implications for the woman of any positive and negative results.

II. The relationship between breast cancer and ovarian cancer.
   A. In American women, breast cancer is the most common cancer and the second most common cause of cancer death, killing about 44,000 women each year.
   B. Ovarian cancer is the fourth most frequent malignancy affecting women.
   C. The risk of any woman developing breast cancer is 12.5% (1 in 8), and for developing ovarian cancer, is significantly less at 1 to 2%.
   D. According to the American Cancer Society, in 1997 approximately 180,200 new cases of invasive breast cancer were diagnosed among women in the United States, as well as 1,400 cases among men.
   E. The etiology of these diseases is thought to be multifactorial in the carcinogenesis.
      1. Genetics.
      2. Hormonal milieu.
      3. Environment.
   F. The frequency of breast and ovarian cancers occurring together suggests that genetic alterations causing these two malignancies are related. This relation, the so-called "breast–ovary" syn-

drome, refers to women who usually develop a breast cancer in the third or fourth decade of life followed by an ovarian cancer 5 to 10 years later.

G. This "breast–ovary" syndrome suggests that there may be a gene or group of genes involved with the establishment of both of these tumors.

III. **The history of *BRCA* gene identification.**

A. The *BRCA* gene.

1. The *BRCA* gene itself is classified as a tumor-suppressor gene because mutations in the gene increase the risk of breast and ovarian cancer. However, inherited mutations in several genes have been found to increase a woman's risk of developing breast cancer.

B. The *BRCA1* gene.

1. In 1989, researchers at the University of California at Berkeley analyzed several families with breast cancer and showed a linkage with the polymorphic locus (D17S74) on the long arm of chromosome 17. A similar association was made in families with breast–ovarian cancer by other researchers, and this common locus was named *BRCA1* for "BReast CAncer 1."

2. In 1990, a report was made linking a region containing *BRCA1* on chromosome 17 to the onset of familial breast cancer.

3. In 1994, the *BRCA1* gene was identified and cloned.

4. More than 340 distinct mutations capable of disrupting the *BRCA1* gene have been reported, but only a few, specifically 185delAG and 5382insC, have been shown to present themselves in multiple families.

5. The contribution of these inherited mutations to the overall risk of breast cancer, however, remains unclear, but it is thought that approximately half of all hereditary breast cancers can be attributed to mutations in *BRCA1*.

C. The *BRCA2* gene.

1. The second breast cancer gene *BRCA2* was localized to chromosome 13 in 1994, and more than 100 different mutations have been identified. As with *BRCA1*, only a few cases have been observed in multiple families.

a. As with the *BRCA1* gene, women with a mutation in *BRCA2* appear to have a lifetime risk of breast cancer similar to that seen in patients with *BRCA1*.

   b. Unlike *BRCA1*, however, *BRCA2* mutations also increase
      the risk of male breast cancer.
   2. *BRCA2* mutations have also been associated with cancers of
      the prostate, pancreas, and colon in families that carry the
      gene.

IV. The relationship of the *BRCA* gene to breast and ovarian cancer.
   A. More than 125 variations of the *BRCA1* gene have been identi-
      fied so far.
   B. Approximately 2/1000 have inherited a clinically significant alter-
      ation in a *BRCA1* gene.
   C. *BRCA1* variants, in and of themselves, do not cause cancer, and
      all women have two copies of the *BRCA1* gene.
   D. When it functions properly, this gene is thought to help suppress
      the growth of cancerous cells. If one copy of this tumor-suppres-
      sor gene becomes damaged, the other copy can act as a brake
      on uncontrolled cell growth.
   E. A woman born with one damaged version of the *BRCA1* gene
      has only one working set of brakes for uncontrolled cell growth.
      If her second *BRCA1* gene (her second set of brakes) becomes
      damaged by exposure to environmental carcinogens, the woman
      can develop cancer.
   F. Women afflicted with a germline mutation to *BRCA1* have a sig-
      nificantly elevated risk of both breast and ovarian cancers com-
      pared with the general population.
      1. In the presence of a germline *BRCA1* mutation, researchers
         have found that the risk skyrocketed to 85 and 50% for
         breast and ovarian cancer, respectively.
      2. In families with both ovarian and breast cancer, the associa-
         tion with the *BRCA1* locus may be close to 100%.
   G. A germline *BRCA1* mutation puts women at greater risk for de-
      veloping cancer at a young age.
      1. It has been estimated that up to one third of breast cancer
         cases diagnosed before the patient was age 30 may be in
         part caused by an inherited allele on chromosome 17q.
   H. Only some of these gene variants appear to be linked to an in-
      creased risk of breast and ovarian cancer.
      1. Mutations to this gene play a role only in the development
         of approximately one half of the cases of familial breast can-
         cer, which accounts for 2 to 19% of cases of all breast can-
         cer and about 10% of the cases of early-onset breast cancer.

  2. Inherited *BRCA1* mutations appear to play a role in only 5%
  of breast and ovarian cancer cases. The remaining 95% do
  not involve inherited mutations in the *BRCA1* gene.
  I. Nevertheless, researchers have established that women who in-
  herit certain *BRCA1* variants appear to be more susceptible to environmental carcinogens.

V. **Factors that are associated with an increased chance of having
an altered *BRCA* gene.**
  A. A blood relative who has been found to have an alteration in a
  BRCA gene.
  B. Women with both breast and ovarian cancer.
  C. An individual diagnosed with breast cancer or ovarian cancer,
  and one or more close relatives with breast or ovarian cancer.
    1. Especially breast cancer before age 50.
  D. Individuals with a strong family history of breast or ovarian can-
  cer in many relatives across two or more generations.
    1. Especially breast cancer before age 50.
  E. Personal history of breast cancer diagnosed before age 30.
  F. Women of Ashkenazi Jewish descent who have breast cancer before age 40 or who have ovarian cancer.
    1. The mutation has been found in approximately 1 to 1.5% of
    Ashkenazi individuals.
    2. This mutation may affect as many as 1 in 40 Ashkenazi
    individuals.
  G. A personal history of bilateral breast cancer or multiple primary
  tumors within the same breast.
    1. Especially before age 50.

VI. **Pretest education and counseling.**
  A. All women in whom the risk of hereditary cancer is questionable
  must be referred to a genetic counselor.
  B. Educate clients about the meaning, inheritance pattern, and car-
  cinogenic potential of *BRCA* mutations.
    1. Construct a detailed pedigree for patients who have a famil-
    ial risk for hereditary breast and ovarian cancer.
  C. Inform client about genetic testing, which should include:
    1. Benefits and limitations.
      a. Varying sensitivity of specific tests.
        (1) At present, more than 100 mutations have been identi-
        fied as occurring within the *BRCA1* gene over a broad
        distribution of the genome. Such heterogeneity of mu-
        tations makes it technically difficult to design a test
        with reasonable sensitivity and specificity.

      (2) A positive test for a cancer-associated variant of *BRCA1* will not determine that a woman will develop breast or ovarian cancer. It simply means that the woman has one of many possible factors that may increase the likelihood of developing cancer, and therefore, she may have a higher-than-average risk of developing this condition.

      (3) A negative test result for a specific *BRCA1* variant does not mean that a woman will not get breast or ovarian cancer. It means that her risk is approximately the "average" lifetime risk for breast cancer.

    b. Possibility that a new mutation of uncertain significance might be found.

    c. *BRCA* testing and counseling can cost almost $3,000.

    d. Takes 6 to 8 weeks to obtain results.

D. Counseling should be nondirective, allowing the patient full autonomy in deciding whether to be tested, and should include:

    1. Exploration of patient's expectations regarding testing.

    2. Discussion of the psychological implications of testing for her and other family members.

E. Discuss the potential risks of genetic testing.

    1. Loss of health.

    2. Loss of life.

    3. It is possible that mutations in the *BRCA1* gene will be found that may not cause an increased cancer risk (benign polymorphisms).

    4. The value of a positive test is questionable as well, because there is a lack of convincing data supporting the hypothesis that clinicians can prevent breast or ovarian cancer in women known to have the *BRCA1* gene mutated. Even measures such as prophylactic mastectomy and oophorectomy must be considered of uncertain therapeutic value in light of case reports detailing breast and ovarian cancer arising after such operations, and in the absence of clinical trials detailing their efficacy.

    5. A positive test result can have devastating psychological effects. This event can affect not only the individual being tested but her entire family, all of whom may share her genetic risk status.

      a. Positive test results can lead to discrimination.

      b. Healthy people who carry genes linked to risk of future disease may be at risk of losing health insurance.

      c. Survivor's guilt.

d. Loss of disability insurance.
(1) Several states have prohibited insurance companies from using genetic test results as a criterion on which to deny coverage. However, women whose health insurance is paid for by their employers are exempt from these laws.
6. Tests with limited predictive value may lead to women having unnecessary surgery, such as prophylactic mastectomies and oophorectomies.
7. The overemphasis on genetic factors in cancer, when environmental carcinogens are known to make major contributions, takes attention away from environmental clean-up measures that could, in fact, reduce the incidence of cancer.
8. The "geneticization" of cancer creates a blame-the-victim mind-set that obscures these social and environmental factors.

VII. Management of mutation-negative patients.
A. Interpret results with caution.
1. If a mutation has not previously been identified in the family:
a. Emphasize continued risk of unidentified familial mutation.
b. Provide an individual risk-management plan.
c. Refer for counseling as needed.
2. If a mutation has previously been identified in the family:
a. Emphasize continued risk of unidentified familial mutation.
b. Reassure the patient that she has not inherited the known familial mutation and that her cancer risk is the same as the average population risk for women her age.
c. Emphasize continued risk of sporadic cancer.
d. Refer for counseling as needed.

VIII. Management of mutation-positive patients.
A. Psychological support.
1. Assist the client in making informed decisions with regard to available options.
B. Genetic counseling:
1. The woman and her family members are in immediate need of counseling.
C. Management of cancer risk.
1. Surveillance (Table 14.1).
a. Begin monthly breast self-examination by age 18 to 21.

Table 14.1 **Surveillance of Mutation-Positive Patients**

Technique	Timing	Age
Breast self-examination	Monthly	18–21
Clinical breast exam	Annual or semiannual	25–35
Mammography	Annual	25–35
CA-125	Annual or semiannual	25–35
Transvaginal ultrasound	Annual or semiannual	25–35
Fecal occult blood and sigmoidoscopy	Every 3 to 5 years	50

    b. Annual or semiannual clinician examination beginning at age 25 to 35 years.

    c. Yearly mammogram beginning at age 25 to 35.

    d. Annual or semiannual serum CA-125 levels testing beginning between age 25 and age 35.

        (1) Benefits of CA-125.

           • Levels of CA-125 decrease postmenopausally; thus, the test becomes more valuable in women who have not undergone an oophorectomy before menopause.

        (2) Limitations of CA-125.

           • False-negative results.

             ◦ CA-125 is elevated in fewer than 50% of patients with stage I tumors and in only 21% of patients limited to diagnosis using microscopy.

             ◦ Oral contraceptives can suppress CA-125.

           • False-positive results.

             ◦ CA-125 levels can increase because of pregnancy, uterine fibroids, benign ovarian cysts, and endometriosis.

             ◦ CA-125 levels are relatively high during the follicular phase of the menstrual cycle.

    d. Transvaginal ultrasound annually or semiannually beginning at age 25 to 35.

        (1) Benefits of transvaginal ultrasound.

           • Distinguishes between benign and malignant pathologies.

        (2) Limitations of transvaginal ultrasound.

- Ovaries can be difficult to visualize.
- False-positive results can result in unnecessary surgery.
- Neoplasms detected are often further advanced than in stage I disease.

  e. Annual testing for fecal occult blood and sigmoidoscopy every 3 to 5 years beginning at age 50.

  (1) Research has shown that patients with *BRCA1* mutations also have an increased risk of colon cancer.

2. Box 14.1 lists those measures to be employed early on to reduce risk.

3. Prophylaxis.

   a. Chemoprophylaxis.

   (1) Tamoxifen has been shown to reduce rates of recurrent and contralateral disease in breast cancer patients.

   b. Oral contraceptives.

   (1) May provide risk reduction for ovarian cancer but may increase the risk of breast cancer.

   c. Prophylactic mastectomy.

   (1) Does not provide absolute protection against disease.

   (2) Cancer subsequent to mastectomy has been reported in 1 to 19% of high-risk patients.

   d. Prophylactic oophorectomy.

   (1) Does not provide absolute protection against disease.

   (2) Is likely to reduce breast cancer risk in *BRCA1* and *BRCA2* mutation carriers but increases the risk of osteoporosis and heart disease as a result of surgical menopause.

IX. **Figure 14.1 is an example of a pedigree for patients with a familial risk for hereditary breast and ovarian cancer.**

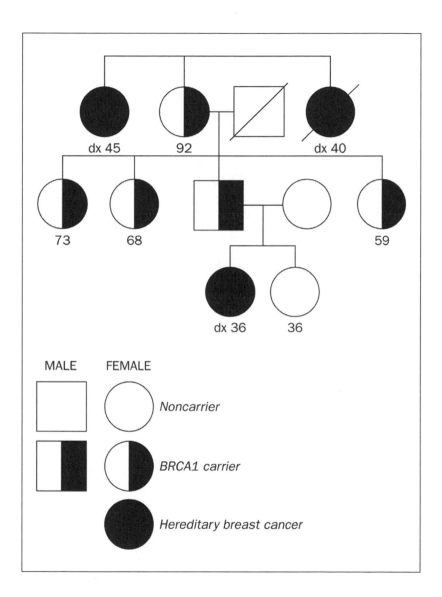

MALE   FEMALE

Noncarrier

BRCA1 carrier

Hereditary breast cancer

Figure 14.1 Example of pedigree for patients with a familial risk for hereditary breast and ovarian cancer. It demonstrates the incomplete penetrance of this gene mutation. There is a premenopausal onset of breast cancer in three family members and an example of paternal transmission of the familial gene mutation. The woman, diagnosed with breast cancer at age 36, who inherited the *BRCA1* mutation from her father, should look to her great-aunts for evidence of breast cancer in her family. Several women, including the 92-year-old grandmother, are carriers of the familial mutation but do not have breast cancer.

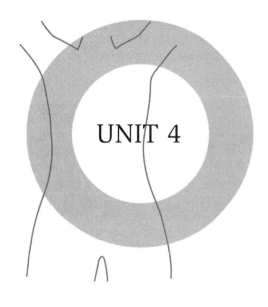

UNIT 4

Contraceptive Devices

The FemCap™

CHAPTER 15

Rebecca Koeniger-Donohue

I. **The FemCap explained: The FemCap is ideal for women of childbearing age who cannot or do not want to use hormonal contraceptives or an intrauterine device (IUD) and may be interested in using a female barrier contraceptive, especially one that requires no involvement by the male partner.**
   A. The FemCap is a nonhormonal, latex-free female-controlled barrier contraceptive.
   B. Available by prescription.
   C. Comes in three sizes. Proper size selection based on a woman's obstetric history based on the fact that pregnancy and delivery are the two major factors that have the greatest impact on the elasticity of the vagina and the size of the cervix.
   D. Approved by the U.S. Food and Drug Administration (FDA) in March 2003.
   E. Unique design: brim designed to flare outward like an inverted funnel—flaring of the brim is met by the physiological inward concentric contraction of the vagina. Unlike the former Prentif cervical cap, which had to be snug over the cervix, the FemCap is held in place by the vaginal contraction, which allows the vagina to hold and support the FemCap in place without causing any pressure over the cervix.
   F. Reusable for more than 1 year.
   G. Does not interfere with the menstrual cycle, libido, or pleasure for either partner.
   H. Easy to insert and remove.
   I. Designed to cover the cervix completely, delivers spermicide on

271

the cervical—and most important—on the vaginal side, to meet the sperm head on.

J. It is effective in preventing unintended pregnancy when used as directed and is safe to use, with no systemic side effects.

II. Overview of cervical caps.

A. The cervical cap dates back more than 150 years, with a longer history of contraceptive use than the diaphragm.

B. Before FDA approval of the FemCap, the only cervical cap available to women in the United States was the Prentif cavity rim cervical cap, which was manufactured by Lamberts Ltd. of London and is now off the market.

C. Cervical caps differ from diaphragms in that they are designed to cover the cervix only; they are not placed to fit in the entire vagina.

D. Cervical caps have been touted as one of the best-kept secrets of the modern age. However, they have never been used on a large scale in North America, because of lack of clinician interest and lack of access.

III. Description of the FemCap.

A. Made of soft, durable, hypoallergenic, silicone rubber.

B. Its shape resembles a sailor's hat with an upturned brim that lies against the vaginal walls around the cervix (see Figure 15.1).

C. The design conforms to the anatomy of the cervix and the physiologic changes of the vagina that occur during sexual arousal. The dome of the FemCap fits over the cervix "like a glove," covering it completely.

D. Complete cervical coverage prevents sperm from entering the cervix and the uterus.

   1. The rim of the cervical cap provides a snug fit into the vaginal fornices and covers the vaginal vault, and the brim covers the vaginal walls surrounding the cervix.

   2. The brim is longer posteriorly to conform to the unique anatomy of the vaginal walls.

   3. The out-flaring of the brim facing the vaginal opening has a unique groove that acts as a trap for sperm and a reservoir for any spermicide, or any microbicidal/spermicide that will soon be developed in the future, to reinforce the mechanical barrier of the FemCap.

   4. The FemCap is held in place by the muscular walls of the vagina and does not have to be snug around the cervix or hinge behind the pubic bone.

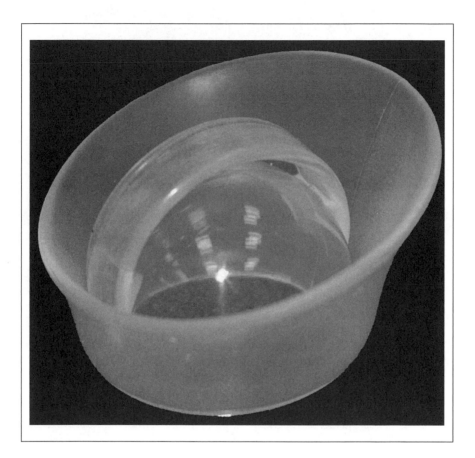

Figure 15.1 The FemCap shape resembles a sailor's hat with an upturned brim that lies against the vaginal walls around the cervix.

E. The FemCap has a strap over the dome to facilitate removal of the device and provides added protection to the vaginal walls and cervix from possible fingernail abrasions during removal.

F. When the FemCap is placed correctly, users should rarely, if ever, be aware of its presence. During the several clinical trials fewer than 2% of women and 22% of men reported a sense of awareness of the FemCap and it did not interfere with their sexual pleasure.

G. The anatomical design and the nonallergenic material of the Fem-Cap offers an additional benefit when compared with the latex diaphragm. Unlike the diaphragm, the FemCap reduces the likeli-

Advantages and Disadvantages of the FemCap   **BOX 15.1**

Advantages

- Ease of use
- Few local effects and no systemic side effects
- Silicone rubber has longer shelf life than does latex rubber
- Safe for latex-allergic women or for partners with a latex allergy
- Can be left in place for up to 48 hours
- Cannot be punctured by fingernails
- Does not break down with petroleum-based products or extremes of temperature
- Does not absorb odors; easy to clean
- Immediately reversible if and when pregnancy is desired
- *Compared with diaphragm*—Associated with fewer UTIs, needs less spermicide, more comfortable
- *Compared with IUD*—Less invasive
- *Compared with hormonal contraceptives*—Does not have systemic or serious side effects, does not change the menstrual cycle, does not decrease libido
- *Compared with male condom*—Does not interrupt spontaneity or reduce sexual pleasure for either partner, is under the woman's control

Disadvantages

- Requires a prescription and a pelvic exam
- Necessitates that a woman touch her genitalia, which may be culturally or personally unacceptable
- Theoretical risk of toxic shock syndrome

STI = sexually transmitted infection; UTI = urinary tract infection; IUD = intrauterine device.

hood of contracting a urinary tract infection (UTI). It is occlusive for the cervix, and yet, unobtrusive to the vagina and urethra.

H. The FemCap can be cleansed easily with hand soap and water.

I. It does not deteriorate from exposure to heat, body fluids, or petroleum-based products. It is reusable for about 1 year without any deterioration.

J. To avoid the theoretical risk of toxic shock syndrome, it must not be used during menstruation.

K. Box 15.1 lists advantages and disadvantages of the FemCap.

IV. **Size selection.**

A. Selecting the correct size is based on obstetric history and pelvic exam.

B. The pelvic exam is essential to estimate the size of the cervix

FemCap: Contraindications

BOX
15.2

- Adhesions between the cervix and the vaginal walls
- Third-degree uterine prolapse
- Flat cervix
- Acute cervicitis
- Cancer of the cervix
- Active pelvic inflammatory disease
- History of toxic shock syndrome
- Cut or tear in the vagina or cervix visualized on pelvic exam
- Allergy to spermicide
- Women who are adverse to touching their genitals (cultural norms or personal preference).

and to exclude women who have contraindications such as cancer, laceration, infection, or a flat cervix.

Box 15.2 summarizes contraindications.

C. Available in three sizes:

1. Small (22 mm internal diameter) for nulligravida women.
2. Medium (26 mm) for women who have been pregnant but have had a miscarriage, therapeutic abortion, or delivered by Cesarean section.
3. Large (30 mm) for women who have had at least one full-term vaginal delivery.
4. If in doubt about the fit it is safest to use the 26-mm size.

D. Cost: One device costs $66 and a two-pack costs $88. Each kit comes with an instructional videotape, illustrated color brochure, and FDA package insert.

E. It is recommended that the FemCap be replaced every year (or sooner if it shows signs of deterioration)

F. For information and orders please visit: *www.femcap.com.*

V. **Protection against STIs (sexually transmitted infections) and HIV/AIDS.**

A. Using the FemCap with spermicide, the diaphragm with spermicide, or Lea's shield with spermicide have *not* been shown to protect against STIs.

B. No studies have yet demonstrated a protective effect against HIV by limiting access to cells in the cervix.

C. Nonoxynol-9 alone does not provide protection against HIV, chlamydia, and gonorrhea.

D. Frequent use of spermicide alone can cause disruption of the sin-

> ## Seven Requirements for Perfect Use of the FemCap
>
> **BOX 15.3**
>
> 1. Motivation for consistent and correct use of the FemCap.
> 2. Viewing of instructional video provided with the FemCap prior to use.
> 3. Use of backup method of contraception during the learning phase.
> 4. Insertion of the FemCap before any sexual arousal.
> 5. Application of a small amount of spermicide; checking the FemCap's position before each use.
> 6. Leaving the FemCap in place for at least 6 hours after the last act of intercourse.
> 7. Use of emergency contraception (morning-after pill) if the FemCap was not used or if it was used incorrectly.

gle-layer endocervical columnar epithelium. This disruption creates microabrasions or ulcerations that, at least in theory, could *increase* susceptibility to HIV transmission.

VI. Efficacy and acceptability.

    A. The typical failure rate (Pearl index) of the second-generation FemCap was estimated to be 7.6 per hundred women per year.

    B. Effectiveness of the FemCap varies, depending on the motivation of the user and on whether she uses the device correctly and consistently.

    C. Labeling recommends the use of an emergency contraceptive pill if a woman uses the FemCap incorrectly or fails to use it during an act of intercourse.

    D. Seven requirements for perfect use of the FemCap are listed in Box 15.3.

VII. Candidate selection.

    A. Clinicians can enhance correct and consistent use of the FemCap by discussing the following key points:

        1. Emphasizing motivational and lifestyle factors.

        2. Establishing a habit or routine of contraceptive use.

        3. Keeping two FemCaps on hand (one for home and one for travel).

        4. Inserting the FemCap before sexual arousal to ensure proper fit and to avoid interruption of spontaneity.

        5. Maintaining a diary to record dates of insertion, removal, and menstrual cycles.

        6. Strongly advising emergency contraception as soon as possible if the woman did have unprotected intercourse or used the FemCap incorrectly.

VIII. FemCap protocol for clinicians. One can request information on the FemCap, as well as request a kit, by logging on to www.femcap.com.
  A. The clinician should
    1. Schedule a 30- to 45-minute visit for cap fitting and instructions.
    2. Perform a pelvic examination to exclude any anatomical or pathological contraindications.
    3. Discuss the advantages and disadvantages and reinforce the importance of compliance with its use.
    4. Provide the woman with her FemCap size, according to obstetrical history (one of three sizes).
    5. Provide her with the package insert and videotape.
    6. Allow her privacy and time to practice inserting and removing the FemCap, making sure she can identify and cover her cervix with the cap.
    7. Encourage her to practice insertion and removal several times.
    8. Practice should be continued until she can successfully insert, remove, and recognize proper placement of the cap.
    9. Have the woman leave the cap in place for clinician to recheck for proper fit by digital examination.
    10. Speculum examination (if needed for further confirmation).
    11. Use only a plastic disposable speculum as it has blunt tips and allows good lighting.
    12. Insert halfway into the vagina and open it enough at this point to be able to see the FemCap covering the cervix without dislodging it.
    13. Some comments:
      a. Unlike the diaphragm the bulk of the spermicide is stored in the grooved area between the dome and brim of the FemCap, facing the opening, to expose sperm to the spermicide upon deposition into the vagina.
      b. The FemCap does not require measurement for custom fitting like the diaphragm.
      c. The woman can insert and remove the FemCap in a squatting position on her own much easier and faster than any clinician can insert it for her, no matter how skillful.
IX. Directions for use.
  A. Insertion.
    1. Place 1/2 teaspoon of spermicide in the groove between the dome and the brim of the FemCap and 1/4 teaspoon of the spermicide in the bowl of the device.

2. Spread a thin layer all over the brim of the FemCap except for the spots where the finger and the thumb are holding the device.
3. Squeeze and flatten the device, insert it into the vagina with the bowl facing upward and the long brim entering first.
4. The FemCap is inserted downward toward the rectum and then downward and back as far as possible in the vagina to be sure the cervix is covered.
5. It is important to ensure that the FemCap is not part way between the vaginal opening and the cervix.
6. With repeated acts of intercourse check the position of the FemCap and add more spermicide (without removing the device).
7. If the FemCap is placed correctly, the woman should not be aware of its presence during intercourse or daily activities. It should fit comfortably over the cervix, with the rim fitting snugly to the vaginal fornices and the brim adhering to the vaginal walls.
8. It *must* be placed in the vagina **before** any sexual stimulation and may be worn for up to 48 hours maximum. The device should remain in place for at least 6 hours after sexual intercourse, but no longer than 48 hours altogether.

B. Removal
   1. The woman should squat and bear down, which will bring the removal strap closer to the fingers, facilitating removal of the device.
   2. The device can then be rotated and removed comfortably by pushing the tip of the finger against the dome of the FemCap to dimple it. This will break the suction and allow room for the finger to be inserted between the dome and the removal strap and then it can be pulled out gently by hooking a finger into the removal strap.
   3. Woman should develop a routine for insertion and removal, such as after her daily shower.

C. Detailed instructions are provided by the manufacturer in both the video or DVD and in written materials included in the FemCap kit.

X. **Care of the FemCap.**
   A. The FemCap should be washed with antibacterial soap and rinsed thoroughly with tepid tap water and air dried or patted dry with a clean soft towel.
   B. It should be stored in the plastic container supplied with it and kept in a cool, dry place. Do not use powder.

C. It should never be placed in a microwave or cleaned by synthetic detergents, organic solvents, or sharp objects.

D. This process is 99.9% effective in eliminating all bacteria and viruses.

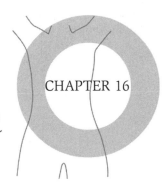

CHAPTER 16

The Diaphragm

Helen A. Carcio

I. **The diaphragm explained.**
   A. The diaphragm is an effective form of contraception.
      1. It is considered a barrier method, which means that it provides a barrier between the ejaculated sperm and its entrance into the uterus.
      2. The anterior rim fits securely behind the pubic bone, and the posterior rim fits behind and below the cervix, covering the cervix with the spermicidal jelly-filled cup.
      3. Correct fitting, consistent use, and proper insertion are critical to the success of the use of the diaphragm.
   B. Mechanism of action.
      1. The diaphragm prevents contraception by eliminating the possibility of the sperm fertilizing the egg.
      2. It forms a mechanical barrier to prevent sperm from entering the cervical canal.
      3. It acts as a receptacle for the spermicide, which immobilizes the sperm.
   C. Historical perspective.
      1. The diaphragm has been used ever since the beginning of recorded history.
      2. There are early references to use of honey, spice, oils, sticky plugs, and other substances for birth control.
      3. The actual diaphragm was invented in late 1800s, although it was not well promoted.
   D. Use today.
      1. Has fallen in and out of vogue over the last 10 to 20 years.

    2. Has been replaced by the more effective and easier-to-use cervical cap (see chapter 15).

E. Advantages.

    1. It offers the woman a large degree of control over her body, which women are seeking.

    2. Acts as a barrier to many sexually transmitted diseases when used with contraceptive jelly, foam, or cream. (This feature is under investigation.)

    3. Provides a local contraceptive effect, rather than a systemic effect, such as that provided by oral contraceptives or Depo-Provera.

    4. It is inexpensive.

    5. The diaphragm is durable, easy to care for.

    6. Serious side effects are rare.

    7. No data as yet regarding effect on transmission of human immunodeficiency virus (HIV).

F. Disadvantages.

    1. User dependent: depends on the motivation of the user.

    2. It cannot be bought over the counter, such as contraceptive foam.

    3. Requires that the woman see her practitioner for proper sizing and prescribing.

    4. May interfere with the spontaneity of lovemaking because spermicide must be added after each act of intercourse. (The woman may teach her partner to insert the diaphragm as part of the ritual.)

    5. Spermicidal cream or jelly is perceived as being messy.

    6. The partner may feel the diaphragm. A different size or type of diaphragm might help.

    7. The diaphragm may be uncomfortable if it is fitted improperly.

    8. It is difficult to conceal its use.

    9. The woman's partner may object to the taste of spermicide. Suggest the diaphragm be insert after oral sex.

    10. There is expense related to the use of spermicide if intercourse is frequent.

    11. Women need to feel comfortable with touching their own bodies.

    12. One needs time and privacy for insertion and removal of diaphragm.

    13. Prolonged retention can cause vaginal irritation.

    14. Possibility of toxic shock syndrome. Most research today states that the incidence of this syndrome is rare.

Contraindications to Diaphragm Use   BOX 16.1

Allergy to rubber, spermicide, or both—may try changing brands

Inability of patient or partner to learn insertion technique

Inability to physically hold diaphragm and insert into vagina

Prolapsed uterus

Large cystocele

Markedly shallow pubic arch

Vesicovaginal fistula

Full-term delivery in past 12 weeks

Acute pelvic inflammatory disease or cervicitis

Undiagnosed vaginal bleeding

Abnormal Pap smear

Recent cervical procedure

---

15. Not all women can use the diaphragm. See Box 16.1 for a list of contraindications.

G. Effectiveness.
   1. The diaphragm is 97% effective.
   2. It is nearly as good as the birth control pill, but not as effective as Depo-Provera and the intrauterine device (IUD).
   3. A major factor that increases the effectiveness of the diaphragm is the ability of the user to use it consistently.

II. **Description.**
   A. The diaphragm is a small rubber cup, with a firm rim stabilized by a rubber-covered steel spring.
      1. The diaphragm fits behind the pubic bone within the vaginal vault.
      2. Saucer-like disc made of latex with a flexible rim.
   B. Types. There are many different types of diaphragms, the choice of which depends on the woman's pelvic muscle tone, as well as the anatomic shape of the vagina and the pubic bone, which holds the diaphragm tightly in place. (See Table 16.1 for comparison of various types.)
   C. Sizes.
      1. Sizes range from 50 to 105 mm in diameter, in increments of 2.5 to 5 mm.
      2. Most women use between size 65 and 80 mm.

Table 16.1   **Comparison of Types of Diaphragms**

	Diaphragm Type	Strength	Indications
Flat spring	Thin rim with gentle strength	Normal vaginal tone	Shallow pubic arch
Coil spring	Intermediate strength	Good muscle tone	Deep recess behind pubic arch
Arcing spring	Strong, firm double spring	Vaginal delivery	Poor vaginal muscle tone

    D. Use of spermicide.
      1. Diaphragms must be always used with spermicide.
      2. Spreading the cream on the edge of the diaphragm may ease insertion but may also make the diaphragm more slippery, thus possibly making insertion more difficult.
      3. Spermicide is usually effective for 6 hours.
        a. Some clinicians believe that 2 hours should be the cutoff point for intercourse after spermicide application
        b. Probably best to err on the side of caution; therefore, the recommendation is that if more than 2 hours have elapsed since insertion, additional spermicide should be added vaginally with subsequent intercourse.
      4. Warn the woman never to substitute petroleum jelly or other lubricants for spermicide.
        a. Other lubricants lack spermicidal effects.
        b. Petroleum jelly can deteriorate the latex in the diaphragm.

III. Indications for use.
    A. The diaphragm is well liked by many women, but not every woman can use a diaphragm.
    B. It is an appropriate method for a couple in a monogamous relationship who are motivated to work together to prevent pregnancy.
      1. The failure rate decreases with increasing age and duration of use.
      2. The failure rate increases with single status and increased coital frequency.
    C. The diaphragm is an excellent choice for the woman who is comfortable with touching her genitals and who is committed to using the device every time she has intercourse.

IV. The fitting procedure.
   A. Timing of fitting.
      1. Fitting of the diaphragm can occur at any time of the month.
      2. It is best to wait until at least 6 weeks after delivery of a child.
      3. Menses makes the fitting more uncomfortable for the patient.
      4. If any infection is present or there are abnormal findings on the woman's Papanicolaou (Pap) smear, wait until condition resolves.
   B. Fitting kits.
      1. Fitting kits can be obtained from the companies that produce the diaphragm.
      2. The kit should be available in the examining room.
      3. Fitting diaphragms are better to use than fitting rings.
   C. Health history.
      1. Inquire about contraindications listed in Box 16.1.
      2. Ask about the woman's success with other methods of contraception.
      3. Assess comfort with and use of tampons.
         a. Address woman's comfort with touching her genital area.
         b. Help in learning how to use the diaphragm if the woman has prior experience with tampons.
   D. Before insertion, review.
      1. Printed instructions.
      2. Effectiveness.
      3. Insertion and removal technique.
      4. Discuss when to insert and remove.
      5. Explain that the diaphragm comes in many sizes and that the woman may have to try two or three different ones to get the right fit.
      6. Explain that she will be allowed time to practice in the examination room, taking the diaphragm in and out a few times.
   E. Perform the pelvic examination.
      1. Note the size and position of the uterus
      2. Check for irritation or infection.
         a. Observe the cervix for any signs of infection.
         b. Perform a wet mount, if indicated, and treat any diagnosed infection.
      3. Have woman bear down to determine if a cystocele is present. Measure depth of the pubic arch.
         a. Normal pubic arch: choose coil spring.

      b. Shallow pubic arch: choose flat spring.

      c. Markedly shallow pubic arch: Consider an alternate method.

F. Fitting the diaphragm.

  1. Explain each step of the procedure, eliciting feedback from the patient.

  2. Move the tips of the examining fingers into the posterior fornix of the vagina.

  3. Make note of where the hand comes in contact with the pubic bone.

  4. The rim of the fitting diaphragm should extend from the tip of the middle examining finger to just in front of the point noted on the examining hand.

  5. The average sizes used are 70, 75, and 80.

      a. Start with one of those three sizes and adjust up or down as needed.

  6. Grasp the edges of the diaphragm, and squeeze the edges together rim to rim.

  7. While holding labia apart, insert diaphragm deep into the vagina, sliding it posteriorly under the cervix and tucking the anterior rim behind pubic bone (see Figure 16.1).

  8. Checking for proper fit:

      a. If the woman can feel the diaphragm, it may be too big or improperly placed.

      b. The diaphragm should not be able to move from side to side or from front to back.

      c. The rim should not be buckled.

      d. One should only be able to get the tip of one finger between the rim of the diaphragm and the pubic bone.

      e. The fit should be on the snug side because the vagina expands with sexual excitement.

  9. Once the diaphragm is inserted:

      a. Have woman cough or bear down.

      b. Allow time for the woman to walk around the room, sit down, and stand up a few times.

      c. Give the woman privacy to practice insertion and removal two or three times.

      d. Ask her to leave the diaphragm in place.

  10. Recheck position and proper size.

      a. Evaluate whether the diaphragm still covers the cervix and is tucked behind the pubic bone.

  11. Remove the diaphragm and check for any tears.

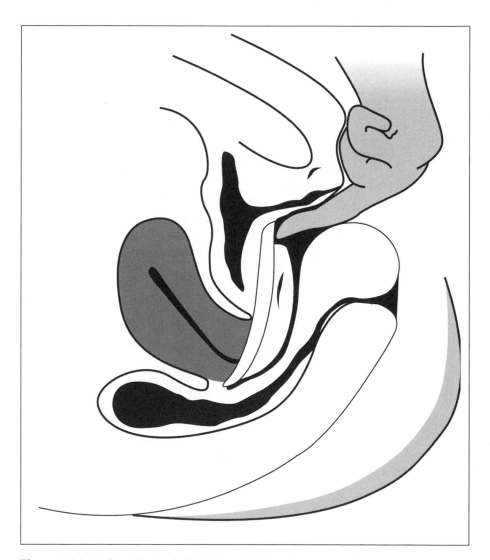

Figure 16.1 Tucking the rim behind the pubic bone for a proper fit.

G. Document
1. Size and type of diaphragm.
2. Perceived patient comprehension.
3. Fit.
4. Demonstration and redemonstration.

V. **Patient education.**
   A. Review causes of method failure.
      1. Dislodgment during coitus particularly with:
         a. Change in coital position.
         b. Use of the female superior position.
         c. Expansion of the vagina with sexual excitement.
      2. If the diaphragm is too large the woman will experience:
         a. Lower back and/or rectal pain.
         b. Lower abdominal pain.
         c. Difficulty voiding.
         d. Cramps in thighs.
      3. If the diaphragm is too small:
         a. It moves out of proper position.
      4. Failure to insert before every occasion of coitus.
      5. Failure to tuck the rim of the diaphragm behind the pubic bone, allowing the penis to override the diaphragm.
      6. Failure to check coverage of cervix.
   B. Discuss adjustment period.
      1. It does take a period of time to become adjusted to using the diaphragm.
      2. Use of the diaphragm soon becomes much easier once it becomes more habitual.
   C. The woman should call the health center or return to the office should:
      1. Pain or discomfort occur with the diaphragm in place.
      2. A change in vaginal discharge occurs.

VI. **Instructions to the woman for use at home.**
   A. Initial trial.
      1. Practice insertion and removal every night.
      2. Use backup method until return visit.
      3. Return in 2 to 4 weeks with the diaphragm in place.
   B. Before insertion:
      1. Hold diaphragm up to the light and observe for any holes or cracks, especially near the rim.
      2. Rinse off any powder.
      3. Make sure your fingernails are short so that there is no possibility of tearing the diaphragm.
      4. Box 16.2 summarizes the insertion and removal techniques.
      5. If the diaphragm is left in for more than 24 hours, be alert for signs and symptoms of toxic shock syndrome (Box 16.3).

Inserting and Removing a Diaphragm

BOX
16.2

Insertion

- The diaphragm is inserted up to 2 hours before intercourse.
- Apply spermicidal jelly or cream to rim and inside of dome.
- Holding dome down, squeeze rim until sides touch.
- Stand with one foot propped, squat, or lie down.
- Spread labia, insert folded diaphragm deep into vagina.
- Push diaphragm back as far as possible, then tuck front rim up behind the pubic bone inside the vagina.
- Check for placement; feel for cervix covered with rubber dome.
- For repeated intercourse, add more spermicide without removing diaphragm.
- Leave diaphragm in place for 6 to 8 hours after last intercourse.

Removal

- To remove diaphragm, place index finger behind front rim; pull down.
- If suction is tight, insert finger between pubic bone and rim to break suction, then pull down.
- Clean diaphragm with soap and water, rinse, and dry. Dust with cornstarch or unscented powder; perfumed powders can damage rubber or irritate tissue.
- Store diaphragm in plastic container in cool, dry place.
- Check diaphragm before and after every use for tears and holes.
- Do not use petroleum jelly because it causes deterioration of rubber.

C. Care of the diaphragm.
   1. The diaphragm can last for years, as long it has been carefully maintained.
   2. After use, the diaphragm should be washed with warm water, using a mild soap, and allowed to air dry.
   3. The diaphragm should be powdered with corn starch, which will help absorb excess moisture and odors. (Talc should not be used because its use has been linked to cervical cancer.)
   4. Corn starch should be washed off before the next use.
   5. Always be sure to hold the device up to the light to observe for any tiny cracks and holes, particularly around the rim.
   6. A diaphragm that has been tucked away in a drawer should be checked carefully.
   7. Store in a plastic container in cool dry location.
   8. Do not:
      a. Store in alcohol, because it will ruin the diaphragm.

Reducing the Risk of Toxic Shock Syndrome   **BOX 16.3**

Toxic shock syndrome (TSS) can occur with the use of the diaphragm and cervical cap.

To reduce the risk of TSS with these contraceptives, you should do the following:

- Wash your hands thoroughly with soap and water before insertion or removal.
- Never leave in place for more than 24 hours.
- Never use during your menstrual period or if you have any vaginal bleeding or spotting.
- Wait 12 weeks before using a contraceptive after a full-term pregnancy.
- Watch for TSS danger signs:

  - Fever (temperature 101°F or more)
  - Diarrhea
  - Vomiting
  - Muscle aches
  - Rash (similar to sunburn)

- Remove the contraceptive right away if you develop these signs, and see your health care provider.
- Choose a different type of contraceptive if you have ever had TSS.

        b. Put the device in the microwave for sterilization. The metal ring will ruin the microwave.

    D. Common errors.

        1. Inserting diaphragm into the anterior fornix, above the cervix.

        2. Failing to tuck the diaphragm behind the pubic bone, which allows the penis to override the diaphragm during penetration.

    E. The follow-up visit.

        1. Return in 2 to 4 weeks.

        2. Have the diaphragm in place.

        3. Use an alternate form of birth control (i.e., condoms), until you become comfortable with the diaphragm.

VII. The return visit.

    A. Inquire about any difficulty with:

        1. Insertion technique. Checking fit over the cervix.

            a. A critical aspect.

            b. Some women do not check because they feel uncomfortable touching their own genitals.

2. Removal.
3. Cleaning.
4. Use of spermicide.
5. Partner satisfaction.

B. Perform the pelvic examination.
1. Check for proper position of the diaphragm over the cervix.
2. Recheck for proper size.
3. Remove the diaphragm. Check for any tears.
4. Observe the cervix for any signs of infection.
5. Check for vaginal irritation.

C. Educate the woman as to when the diaphragm must be refitted.
1. With change in weight of plus or minus 20 pounds.
2. Postpartum.
3. After any pelvic surgery.
4. If it has been more than a year since it was used.
5. If another form of contraception is desired.
6. Occurrence of stress incontinence.
7. If the diaphragm is damaged or deteriorating.

D. Call or return with any concerns listed previously.

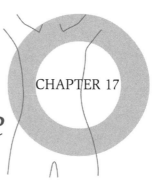

CHAPTER 17

The Intrauterine Contraception

Mimi Clarke Secor and Marcia Denine

I. **The intrauterine device (IUD and IUS) explained.**
   A. Definition: The IUD is a plastic contraceptive device that is inserted into the uterine cavity through the cervical canal.
      1. There are two kinds of intrauterine devices available in the United States: Both types have a 2-strand, polyethylene monofilament string that protrudes from the os.
         a. ParaGard (IUD). Internet source www.paragard.com.
         b. Mirena (IUS). Internet source www.mirena.com;
            Table 17.1 compares and contrasts the two types of IUDs.
      2. IUD/IUS is for contraceptive use only. No intrauterine device is intended to offer any protection against STD (sexually transmitted disease) transmission
      3. Efficacy equivalent to sterilization yet reversible.
      4. Cost-effective.
   B. The ParaGard T380A is a copper-releasing intrauterine contraceptive.
      1. Manufactured by Duramed Pharmaceuticals.
      2. One size; fine-copper wire wound around vertical limb of T.
      3. Releasing free copper and copper salts, affecting the endometrium.

4. Advantages
   a. Is the longest acting contraceptive method available.
   b. Metabolically neutral.
   c. Can remain in place for 10 years.
   d. Has the lowest expulsion rates.
   e. Can be inserted into nulliparous women.
   f. Safety and efficacy has been established in women over 16 years of age (Package insert, 2009).
5. Contraindicated in women with known allergy to copper or a diagnosis of Wilson's disease.
6. Disadvantage: May alter bleeding pattern and increase menstrual flow as well as increase cramping associated with menses.

C. The Mirena IUS is a levonorgestrel-containing intrauterine contraceptive.
   a. Manufactured by Bayer HealthCare.
   b. Progestin-only hormone-releasing device with 20 µg time-released every 24 hours.
   c. The progestin is contained in a vertical limb that releases low-dose progestin locally into the endometrial cavity.
   d. Offers continous contraceptive protection for 5 years.
   e. Cumulative 5-year failure rate is 0.5–0.7 per 100 women.
   f. Thins endometrial lining.
   g. Thickens cervical secretions.
   h. Decreases menstrual flow.
   i. Reduces dysmenorrheal and menstrual blood loss. After 8 months 50% of women have no menstrual bleeding, only monthly spotting. Twenty percent of women have amcnorrhea in the first year.
   j. Indications include contraception and for treatment of heavy menstrual bleeding for women who choose to use intrauterine contraception as their method of contraception (Package insert, 2009).
   k. Recommended for women who have had at least one child (Package insert, 2009).
   l. Appropriate for parous women or nulliparous women with dysmenorrhea or menorrhagia.
   m. Contraindications (see Box 17.3).

D. Historical perspective (listed in chronologic order).
   1. The first intrauterine device was a ring-shaped device described in 1909 by a German gynecologist, Ernest Grafenberg.

2. During the 1960s and 1970s, 10% of women in the United States who used contraception chose the IUD.
3. The Dalkon Shield was introduced in 1970.
    a. Within 3 years, a high incidence of pelvic inflammatory disease (PID) was recognized.
    b. It was documented that the braided multifilamented tail of the Dalkon Shield provided a pathway for bacteria to pass through the protective cervical mucus and ascend into the uterus.
    c. A large number of women sued the manufacturer.
    d. The number of IUDs used decreased in proportion to the increase in IUD litigation.
4. The controversy and litigation surrounding the Dalkon Shield tainted the image of all IUDs.
5. Additionally, two studies in the mid-1980s reported that the use of IUDs was associated with infertility, further frightening women.
6. Many IUDs were removed from the market in 1986 because of the concern regarding medical liability, giving the message that IUDs are unsafe.
7. Women become distrustful because they remember the Dalkon Shield.
8. The number of women using IUDs in the United States declined by two thirds from 1981 to 1989.
9. Today, manufacturers have taken great strides to protect the product.
    a. Package materials include an informed consent.
    b. Strict patient-selection criteria are listed.
    c. Appropriate doctor–patient dialogue is strongly encouraged.
    d. Label comes with extensive warnings.
10. Despite the above-mentioned measures, IUCs (intrauterine contraception) now account for less than 1% of the contraception used in the United States.
11. Worldwide, IUC is the most popular method of reversible contraception.

E. Some comments and considerations regarding selection of contraception.
    1. The prescription of any contraception needs to be individually tailored.
    2. Patient selection and proper insertion technique is vital.
    3. Factors influencing a woman's choice of contraceptive.

Table 17.1   **FDA-Approved Intrauterine Devices**

Device	Description	Sizes	Length (mm)	Width (mm)	Description of Tail
Copper T	T of white polyethylene. Fine copper wire wound around vertical limb of T	One size	36	32	Blue (2 strands; polyethylene)
Mirena IUS	T-shaped polyethylene frame with white body embedded with levonorgestrel	One size	32	32	Brown 2-strand polyethylene threads

       a. Sexual lifestyle.

       b. Number of partners and frequency of coitus.

       c. Status of marriage or relationship.

       d. Cultural or religious beliefs.

       e. Motivation of the woman and her partner.

       f. Degree of comfort with one's body.

       g. Lactation status.

       h. Confidence in the method.

       i. Effectiveness.

       j. Safety.

       k. Access to health care.

       l. Convenience.

       m.Temporary or permanent nature of the method.

       n. Previous experience or experience of others.

       o. Educational and cognitive status.

       p. Cost.

       q. Health concerns.

    4. Box 17.1 summarizes the recommended profile of the IUC user.

  F. Advantages of the IUD in general.

    1. It is safe, highly effective, and economical.

    2. Offers long-term protection with little compliance.

    3. Does not require daily dosing, such as oral contraceptives, or frequent clinic visits for injections, such as with Depo-Provera.

Recommended Patient Profile for Use of the Intrauterine Device (IUD)   **BOX 17.1**

1. Multiparous
2. Stable, mutually monogamous relationship
3. Negative history of pelvic inflammatory disease
4. A desire for longer term reversible contraception
5. Poor or limited success with other forms of contraception
6. Not to the point of permanent sterilization
7. Unable to use hormones owing to conditions such as breast cancer, smoker over age 35
8. Older age (older than 25); the older the patient, the lower the risk for acquiring sexually transmitted diseases
9. A good choice for a woman with diabetes mellitus

Common Misconceptions About the IUS   **BOX 17.2**

Acts primarily as an abortifacient

Causes pelvic inflammatory disease

Increases the risk of ectopic pregnancy

Causes infertilitiy

4. Does not require coital-dependent maneuvers.
5. Is cost-effective over time.

II. **Common misconceptions (Box 17.2).**
   A. IUDs increase the risk of PID.
      1. Largely related to the Dalkon Shield (relative risk with Dalkon Shield was eight times the risk of contemporary device).
         a. Wicking action of the Dalkon Shield tail caused ascension of bacteria into the uterine cavity.
         b. New IUDs changed the tail filament to a monofilament.
      2. The risk is greatest immediately following insertion, when new bacteria are present in the uterine cavity.
         a. Endometrial cultures that are taken within 30 days after insertion are negative.
         b. No increased incidence of PID found after the first 20 days of use (World Health Organization).
      3. In a recent study, the incidence of PID was 1.6 cases per 1000 women and did not increase over time.

---

*Absolute Contraindications to Use of IUD**   BOX 17.3

1. Acute PID
2. Postpartum or postabortal endometritis, or septic abortion in past 3 months
3. Current cancer of the cervix or uterus
4. Known or suspected pregnancy
5. Known or suspected untreated chlamydia, gonorrhea, or mucopurulent cervicitis
6. Active liver disease or liver tumor (benign or malignant) (Mirena)
7. Unexplained abnormal vaginal bleeding
8. Current breast cancer or history of < 5 years (Mirena)
9. Current DVT or PE withut adequate anti-coagulation (Mirena)

---

*WHO (2009) Contraceptive Eligibility Criteria Categories
1 = a condition for which there are no restrictions;
2 = a codition where the advantages of using the method generally outweigh the theoretical or proven risks;
3 = a condition where the theoretical or proven risks usually outweigh the advantages of using the method;
4 = a condition whidh represents and unacceptable health risk if the contraceptive is used.

---

    4. The clinician can decrease incidence with proper screening.
    5. Conclusion.
        a. The incidence of PID reflects the lifestyle of the user.
        b. Development of PID after the first 20 days is related almost entirely to STDs.
        c. There is no evidence that the IUD will protect against STDs.
        d. Should PID occur, only potential infertility would be affected.
  B. IUDs increase the risk of ectopic pregnancy.
    1. Conflicting thoughts exist on this issue because those using IUDs are more likely to have an ectopic pregnancy but are less likely to become pregnant.
    2. Copper devices contribute to lower rates of ectopic pregnancy than the progesterone type of IUD.

III. Contraindications.
  A. Absolute contraindications (see Box 17.3).
  B. Relative contraindications. Need to determine if risks outweighs the benefits (See WHO, 2009 for complete guidelines).
    1. Migraine with aura at any age, risk may outweigh the benefits particularly continuation of IUS/IUD use. If a new or

more severe headache than usual occurs, clinical evaluation is imperative.

2. HIV-positive status is not a contraindication and the IUS/IUD has not been found to increase risk of HIV patients transmission nor contribute to HIV disease progression.

3. AIDS and clinically well on antiretroviral therapy, benefits of IUS/IUD may outweigh the risks, but patients should be monitored carefully especiall for PID and STIs.

4. Among women with heart valve abnormalities the risk of bacterial endocarditis following IUD insertion or removal is unknown but thought to be extremely low. Therefore, current research and new American Heart Association Guidelines suggests antibiotic prophylaxis is NOT recommended, however, this is still somewhat controversial.

5. Anticoagulation therapy.

6. Blood coagulation disorder or blood dyscrasias.

7. Cervical stenosis.

8. Endometriosis.

9. History of ectopic pregnancy or a known condition that may predispose the patient to an ectopic pregnancy.

10. Prior problems with IUDs such as expulsion, pregnancy, and ectopic pregnancy.

C. Conditions that may interfere with insertion technique.

1. Distorted uterine cavity.
   a. Fibroids.
   b. Endometrial polyp.

2. Uterine contour.
   a. Antiverted, antiflexed.
   b. Retroverted, retroflexed.
   c. Small uterus (sounds less than 6 cm).

3. Cervical os.
   a. Stenosis of the cervical os.
   b. Cervical polyp.

D. Conditions that may interfere with satisfaction of user.

1. Prior normally heavy menses and cramping.
   a. The IUD may increase menstrual flow, particularly in the first 2 months after insertion.
   b. The clinician should offer Mirena, which decreases menstrual flow.

2. Established anemia, which may worsen with increased menses.

3. Impaired ability to check for IUD string.

    4. Previous IUD expulsion, which may occur again if uterine conditions are not right.

  E. Conditions that require review or consult:

    1. History of heart disease such as subacute bacterial endocarditis, valvular disease, or arrhythmias, because these patients are more prone to developing bacterial endocarditis.

    2. Some sources believe that IUDs should not be used in women at increased risk for bacterial endocarditis. These women include those with:

      a. Previous endocarditis.

      b. Rheumatic heart disease.

      c. Presence of a prosthetic heart valve.

    3. The presence of cervical stenosis, which may require dilation. Refer if uncomfortable with this procedure.

IV. The insertion.

  A. Timing of insertion. Controversial.

    1. Can occur at any time as long as contraindications and potential pregnancy have been ruled out.

    2. Insertion during menses.

      a. Insertion may be easier—cervical canal is lubricated with menstrual blood.

      b. Relatively sure that the patient is not pregnant.

      c. Os is slightly dilated.

      d. The disadvantage is that menstrual blood may provide a medium for bacterial growth. The infection rate and expulsion rate are higher when the IUD is inserted during menses.

    3. Insertion at midcycle.

      a. Cervical os is dilated.

      b. Must have used protection the previous week.

    4. Insertion immediately on the removal of another IUD.

    5. Following delivery or abortion. May be inserted following these procedures. Expulsion rate is lower if the clinician waits until 4 to 8 weeks' postpartum visit.

  B. Preinsertion visit, with IUD insertion at next visit.

    1. Complete history.

      a. Emphasize contraindications (see Box 17.3).

      b. Inquire about previous episode of syncope.

      c. Focus on the patient's history of heart disease.

      d. Note date of last menses, length, flow, and any associated pain. Document.

Sample Patient Consent Form

**BOX
17.4**

I have read this brochure in its entirety and discussed its contents
with my clinician. My clinician has answered all my questions and has
advised me of the risks and benefits associated with the use of ParaGard® T
380A, with other forms of contraception, and with no contraception at all.
     I have considered all these factors and voluntarily choose to have the
ParaGard® T 380A inserted by _____ on
date _____

Clinician _____

Patient Signature _____

     The patient has signed this brochure in my presence after I counseled
her and answered all her questions.
_____   _____

Clinician _____   Date _____

This ParaGard® T380A is scheduled for removal on _____

Distributed courtesy of Ortho Pharmaceutical Corporation.

    e. Ask if any odor or change in vaginal discharge is present.
    f. Inquire about any signs of pregnancy.
    g. Determine past and present sexual partners.
    h. Assess behavioral risk of STDs.
  2. Pelvic examination, including bimanual examination.
    a. Inspect vulva, vagina, and cervix, noting any signs of infection or cervical stenosis.
    b. Note size, shape, contour, and position of uterus or any tenderness or masses on palpation.
    c. Establish absence of infection, pregnancy, or neoplasia.
  3. Use a wet mount to assess for vaginitis, if indicated.
    a. If WBCs (white blood cells) are present, culture for gonorrhea and chlamydia. Delay insertion of the IUD until after treatment if culture is positive. Explain the risks.
    b. If bacterial vaginoses is present, the condition must be treated first.
  4. Counseling regarding disadvantages and advantages.
  5. Encourage questions.
  6. Explain procedure.
  7. The patient may read and sign informed consent, or she may bring to next visit (Box 17.4).

8. Explain the necessity of proper protection against pregnancy until insertion visit.
9. Laboratory tests.
    a. Hemoglobin and hematocrit measurement recommended, particularly if the patient has a history of heavy menses.
    b. Pap smear, if it has been more than a year since one was taken. If the results are abnormal, explore the cause and treat.
    c. Sedimentation rate if history of PID.
    d. Routine urinalysis and urine pregnancy test as needed.
    e. Chlamydia and gonorrhea screening.
10. Discuss analgesia. Prostaglandin inhibitor such as ibuprofen for discomfort.
    a. Take nonsteroidal antiinflammatory drugs (NSAIDs) one half hour before appointment (Motrin, 400 mg; or Aleve, 1 tab).
11. Discuss use of antibiotics.
    a. No consensus as to effectiveness of use of antibiotics in reducing postinsertion infection.
    b. Probably not necessary for women in long-term, mutually monogamous relationships.
    c. If subacute endocarditis is present, most clinicians do not recommend use of IUD.
C. Insertion visit.
    1. If irregular or absent menses are noted, perform sensitive (within 10 days' postovulation) pregnancy test.
    2. Review laboratory results.
    3. Obtain signed consent if this was not done at the previous visit.
    4. Allow time for any questions.
D. Some comments and considerations.
    1. Move slowly and gently during all phases of IUD insertion to minimize chance of perforation and vasovagal reaction.
    2. Use strictest sterile technique.
    3. Always read the manufacturer's instructions included in the IUD package because they vary slightly.
    4. The withdrawal technique may minimize risk of uterine perforation.
    5. Explain the procedure carefully to help the patient relax.
    6. Show the IUD, and review the insertion technique.
    7. Vasovagal reactions are more common in women who:
        a. Have not been pregnant for many years.

    b. Are nulliparous.

    c. Are very nervous and fearful.

    d. Have an empty stomach.

    e. Have a history of previous episodes of fainting.

    f. Reactions are usually transient and spontaneously subside.

  8. Slow manipulation with the instruments decreases occurrence of syncope.

  9. Patient discomfort.

    a. The woman may feel menstrual-type cramps during the sounding of the uterus and the actual insertion of the IUD.

    b. The tenaculum may cause a pinching sensation.

E. Equipment.

  1. Sterile gloves.

  2. Bivalve speculum.

  3. Ring forceps.

  4. Six to eight cotton balls.

  5. Single-toothed tenaculum.

  6. Uterine sound.

  7. Antiseptic solution.

  8. Rectal swab (four).

  9. Sterile IUD in unopened package.

  10. Scissors to trim string after insertion.

  11. Optional: Paracervical block tray.

F. Technique of the examination.

  1. Perform a bimanual examination to reassess the position of the uterus (although this was done previously). Perforations occur most often in an anteflexed or retroflexed uterus that was not diagnosed before the IUD was inserted.

  2. Visualize the cervix, and wash the cervix with an antiseptic solution. If iodine is present in the antiseptic solution, rule out an allergy to iodine.

  3. A topical local anesthetic (Hurricaine) may be used at this point during the insertion process, over the area where the tenaculum is to be placed.

  4. Grasp the anterior lip of the cervix with a tenaculum about 1.5 to 2.0 cm from the os. Close the single-toothed tenaculum slowly, one notch at a time. (Use of a tenaculum is not always necessary, although it is generally recommended.) Apply gentle traction to stabilize the uterus and straighten the canal.

a. Warn that the woman may feel a pinching sensation.
b. The tenaculum should avoid areas of blood vessels on the cervix.
  (1) If the cervix is anteverted, apply tenaculum at the 2 and 10 o'clock positions.
  (2) If the cervix is retroverted, apply the tenaculum to the cervix at the 4 and 8 o'clock positions

5. Sound the uterus slowly and gently until the resistance of the fundus is felt, to determine depth, direction, and configuration of uterus.
6. Measure the depth of the fundus by sounding.
  a. Place a cotton swab at the cervix when the sound is all the way in.
  b. Remove sound and swab while holding swab against sound.
  c. Measure distance between end of swab and end of sound.
  d. If the distance is less than 6 cm, expulsion, bleeding, pain, and perforation are more likely.
  e. If the distance is greater than 10 cm, decreased contraceptive effectiveness (increased cavity surface) may occur.
  f. No resistance may indicate perforation.
  g. Leave sound in place for a few seconds to dilate the cervix.
7. Load the IUC device into the inserter barrel under sterile conditions. IUD and IUS loading instructions differ in how the T-shaped plastic frame is loaded into the inserter. ParaGard IUD folds the ends of the wings down into the inserter, whereas the Mirena IUS folds the wings up into the inserter as they are pulled through with a gentle tug on the threads. Check the loading instructions with the product packaging before loading the device.
8. Inserter may be slightly bent to conform to the shape of the cervical canal.
9. Apply steady gentle traction on the tenaculum with nondominant hand.
  a. If it is anteverted, pull downward and outward.
  b. If it is retroverted, pull upward and outward.
10. Introduce the inserter barrel through the cervical canal until the top of the fundus is reached. (The tip of the inserter may be lubricated with sterile, water-soluble jelly.)
11. Release the IUC device from the inserter only after placement at the top of the fundus is confirmed by feeling the fun-

dal walls. (This correct position is essential to maximize protection against pregnancy and minimize the risk of expulsion.)

12. Withdraw the inserter tip 1/2 inch, enough to allow for release of the IUD's transverse arms from the tube.
13. Transfer the inserter to the nondominant hand that is also holding the tenaculum.
14. Extract the plunger while gentle pressure is placed on the inserted tube to ensure that the IUC device remains at the top of the fundal cavity. Be careful to prevent impingement of the tail as the tube is removed.
15. Withdraw the inserter tube and the tail of the device, allowing for proper placement.
16. Remove the tenaculum, and observe for any bleeding.
17. If suspected perforation occurs at any point, stop the procedure immediately.
18. Withdraw the plunger, then the barrel of the inserter.
19. Remove the tenaculum. Be careful to note any bleeding.
20. Trim string.
21. Remove the speculum.
22. Perform bimanual examination to feel for any protrusion of device through the uterine wall.
23. Trim the string. Leave 3–5 cm. Remember that it is always possible to trim the string at a later date.
24. Possible causes of disappearance of strings.
    a. Drawing up of strings into the cervical canal or uterus.
    b. Cut too short during insertion.
    c. Rotation of the device within the uterus.
    d. If the problem occurs, try to grasp strings with uterine forceps (no further than 1 inch) and pull them down into the vagina.
25. Assist the woman to a sitting position.
26. Observe for a syncopal episode.
27. Allow her to rest if necessary.
G. Postinsertion instructions.
    1. Teach the patient to feel for the string of the IUD before leaving the examining room.
       a. She should be instructed to feel for the IUD string similarly after each menses.
       b. May use a mirror to show the placement in the os.
       c. Instruct the woman how to feel for the string.
          (1) Wash hands.

        (2) Assume a comfortable position, either lying down with knees on her chest, standing with one leg on a chair, toilet or stool, or sitting on the toilet.

        (3) Insert fingers into the vagina, and feel backward toward the cervix.

        (4) Call the clinician if no string is felt. It may simply be curled up in the cervix.

        (5) Avoid tugging on the string.

  2. Call the clinician if moderate to severe uterine cramps occur.

    a. Mild cramping occurring over 1 to 3 days is normal. Treat the patient with NSAIDs.

    b. May normally occur 1 to 3 months after insertion.

  3. Avoid use of tampons for the first 48 hours.

  4. Avoid sexual intercourse for the first 24 hours.

  5. Call the clinician if you miss a period—can occur normally with the Mirena device.

  6. Always use condoms with a new sexual partner.

  7. Chances of accidental pregnancy, although low, are highest during the first month. The patient may use additional contraception but it is usually not necessary.

  8. A follow-up visit after the first menses is recommended.

  9. Keep a careful menstruation calendar.

10. Warn the patient that initially bleeding may normally be heavy for the first few periods.

11. Reinforce that the first month is the period of greatest risk of infection.

    a. Patient should observe for early signs of PID, and return immediately if present.

    b. Report increased and abnormal vaginal discharge, fever, or lower abdominal pain.

12. Review need for barrier methods should a chance of any exposure to STDs arise.

H. Postinsertion documentation. Clearly document the following:

  1. Teaching and counseling provided.

  2. Uterine contour.

  3. Depth of uterine sounding.

  4. Type of IUC device used.

  5. Ease of insertion.

  6. How patient tolerated the procedure.

  7. Length of string.

  8. Any pregnancy test results.

  9. File signed consent form.

V. **Management of side effects.**
   A. Increased cramping. If this should occur:
      1. Avoid strenuous exercise, and rest when possible.
      2. Hot water bottle or heating pad placed on lower abdomen may be helpful.
      3. Use analgesics. (Ibuprofen as needed.)
      4. Call provider if concerned.
   B. Partner feels string. Return for evaluation:
      1. String too long: cut.
      2. String too short: Remove IUC device and replace.
   C. Missed menses. Return for a pregnancy test. May normally occur with Mirena.
   D. Increased vaginal discharge. Perform infection check.
   E. Heavy menses, anemia. Monitor.
      1. Prescribe ferrous sulfate (300 mg) daily.

VI. **Follow-up visit.**
   A. Schedule after next menses.
      1. Assess satisfaction with IUD/IUS.
      2. Review menstruation calendar.
      3. Check for the strings (may have to trim).
         a. If no strings are visualized, they can be extracted from the cervical canal by rotating two cotton-tipped applicators or a Pap smear cytobrush in the endocervical canal.
         b. If further maneuvers are required, the clinician needs to refer the patient to a gynecologist.
      4. Return 1 year for annual exam, prn (as needed), or with concerns.
   B. Elicit information regarding the presence of:
      1. Foul-smelling vaginal discharge.
      2. Low backache.
      3. Menorrhagia.
      4. Dysmenorrhea.
      5. New sexual partner(s).
   C. Perform wet mount if infection is suspected.
   D. Patient instructions:
      1. Reinforce previous teaching.
      2. Return for annual examination.

VII. **Removal.**
   A. Reasons for removal:
      1. Patient wishes.
         a. Desire to switch to alternative method of contraception.

       b. Desires pregnancy.

       c. Contraception is no longer required.

       d. Uncomfortable with side effects.

    2. Possible medical indications.

       a. Accidental pregnancy.

       b. Severe anemia resulting from persistent bleeding.

       c. PID—controversial.

       d. Excessive cramping and bleeding.

       e. Development of a malignancy.

       f. Pain with intercourse.

       g. Partial expulsion of the device.

       h. Cervical or fundal perforation.

       i. Finding of actinomyces on Pap smear—controversial.

         (1) May leave the device in place with treatment.

B. Technique.

    1. Insert speculum and visualize os.

    2. Grasp tail with ring forceps.

    3. If the IUD is embedded, the patient may require hysteroscopy.

    4. Apply gentle, steady traction, being careful not to break the strings, and remove.

    5. If gentle traction does not lead to IUD/IUS removal, refer to gynecologist.

    6. Remove the speculum.

    7. Examine the device for unusual discharge.

    8. Instruct woman to remain sitting on the table for a few minutes. Observe for any dizziness.

VIII. Management of side effects and complications.

    A. Pelvic inflammatory disease.

       1. Positive cultures and IUD/IUS in place with no symptoms—treat without removal.

       2. If PID, treat per CDC, but if *not* improved within 72 hours, the device should be removed. Prudent clinical judgment must be used.

    B. Bacterial vaginosis—treat the patient with oral antibiotics to prevent BV-associated endometritis; the IUD/IUS may remain in place.

    C. Endometritis. If uterine tenderness is the only finding, administer doxycycline 100 mg po bid for 14 days.

    D. Pregnancy.

       1. Risk of pregnancy is very low.

Table 17.2   **IUD Reimbursement and Coding**

Reimbursement and Coding	*ICD-9* Code
Insertion of IUD	58300
General Counseling and Advice	V25.0
Removal of IUD	58301
Checking, reinsertion, or removal of IUD	V25.42

2. Irregular menses commonly occur. Lack of menses is no longer an indicator of pregnancy.
3. Routine pregnancy testing is not necessary.
4. Testing indicated in a patient who has an abrupt change in bleeding patterns or who develops symptoms of pregnancy.
5. Women who conceive need to have ultrasonographic localization of the gestational sac to rule out ectopic pregnancy.
6. In pregnancy the IUD should be removed because the risk of miscarriage, sepsis, premature labor, and delivery increase.

E. Actinomyces.
   1. Actinomyces may be found on the Pap smear in up to 30% of IUD/IUS users. May be normal colonization (not infection).
   2. If the patient is asymptomatic and the clinical exam indicates no infection, then no treatment is needed and the clinician may leave the device in place.
   3. If the patient is symptomatic, the device should be removed and oral antibiotics should be given. Penicillin 500 mg orally four times a day for 1 month is recommended.
   4. May replace device after repeat culture performed 3 months later shows absence of actinomyces.

IX. **Expulsion.**
   A. Removal of partially expelled IUD/IUS.
      1. Grasp the string or tip with ring forceps.
      2. Evaluate the patient for infection or pregnancy.
      3. Reinsert another IUD/IUS if the woman desires.

X. **Reimbursement and coding. See Table 17.2.**

Contraceptive Implants

Nancy Gardner Dirubbo

I. **Etonogestrel (Implanon) explained.**
   A. Implanon is a progestin-only, single rod, subdermal implant effective for up to 3 years.
      1. Over 3 million implants have been inserted worldwide in over 30 countries since 1998.
      2. Etonogestrel was approved by the FDA in the United States in 2006.
      3. Single rod 4 cm long by 2 mm in diameter with a rate-controlling membrane of 40% ethylene vinyl acetate (EVA) and 60% etonogestrel (68 mg).
      4. Etonogestrel is released at a rate of 60–70 micron grams initially and then decreases to 25–30 micron grams by the third year.
      5. Is a long-acting, low-dose, quickly reversible, progestin-only method of contraception.
      6. Average retail cost ranges from $600–$850 for the device and insertion charges range from $125 to $200.
      7. Many private insurers cover all or some of the cost of the device as well as insertion and removal. Organon-Schering-Plough offers clinicians a program that will investigate individual patient's insurance policies to determine coverage and copays.

8. Many state Medicaid programs cover the device and insertion and removal in full.
9. Careful and correct subdermal placement is key to successful insertion and facilitates removal.
10. All providers must complete a free educational program on Implanon provided by the manufacturer per FDA require ments before inserting or removing these implants. For information about training programs go to www.implanonusa.com

B. Effectiveness.
1. Six pregnancies were reported in 20,648 cycles. Each conception was likely to have occurred before removal or within 2 weeks after removal.
2. Cumulative Pearl Index is 0.38 pregnancies per 100 woman-years of use.
3. No clinical data are available concerning efficacy and overweight or obese women.

C. Mechanism of action.
1. Primarily inhibits ovulation.
2. Secondarily increases viscosity of cervical mucus.

D. Indications: Implanon can be used by any woman who:
1. Seeks a safe, highly effective, long-term, reversible form of contraception.
2. Cannot take estrogen because of contraindications or intolerance of side effects.
3. Is breastfeeding.
4. Has a history of poor compliance with other methods of contraception.
5. Does not desire future pregnancies but is unsure of permanent sterilization.
6. Because of health problems or medication use should not become pregnant.

E. Advantages.
1. Does not contain estrogen so can be used for effective hormonal contraception in women who cannot use estrogen.
2. Can be used postpartum in breastfeeding women. Less than 0.2% estimated absolute maternal dose is excreted in breast milk. Does not affect production or quality of breast milk.
3. No significant effects or differences in physical or psychomotor development of infants who were breastfed by mother's using Implanon.
4. Effective immediately when inserted at the proper time (see manufacturer's insert).

5. Stabile hemoglobin levels with use. Patients do not develop iron-deficiency anemia because menstrual blood loss is less than that of menstruating women who are not on hormones.
6. Safe, highly effective method that requires little user compliance.
7. Rapidly reversible.
8. Free 2- to 3-hour training program to learn product insertion and removal.
9. Method is paid for upfront. If patient's financial or insurance status changes in those 3 years contraception is already paid for.

F. Disadvantages.
   1. Predictably unpredictable bleeding patterns throughout the duration of the 3 years of use.
   2. Weight changes may occur in women who use Implanon. Some women gain weight and some women lose weight. The number who gain is about equal to the number of those who lose. Total weight gain is minimal, that is, less than 2 to 3 lbs. per year.
   3. Mandatory 3-hour training program for insertion and removal must be completed by the clinician before he or she can insert and remove Implanon.
   4. Cost can be a disadvantage for some women as all the costs for this method are paid upfront.
   5. Some women do not like that they cannot start or stop this method without the assistance of a clinician and so feel less in control.
   6. Some women do not like the idea of a foreign object being inserted into their bodies.
   7. Some women may be able to see the implant slightly under the skin.
   8. Implant offers no protection from sexually transmitted infections

G. Irregular bleeding.
   1. Bleeding is the most common reason for removal. Patient needs to be educated that this is to be expected and that it is normal. If patient is intolerant of irregular bleeding she may not want to choose implants.
   2. Counsel patient that bleeding can be light or heavy, last for a few days or many days in a row; amenorrhea lasting for several months can occur.
   3. Bleeding patterns are not necessarily similar to other proges-

> ## Contraindications of Implanon Use
> BOX 18.1
> 1. Known or suspected pregnancy
> 2. Current or past history of thrombolytic disease
> 3. Hepatic tumor or active liver disease
> 4. Undiagnosed genital bleeding
> 5. Known, suspected, or past history of breast cancer
> 6. Hypersensitivity to any components of etonogestrel implant

tin-only methods of contraception. Patient's experiences with other methods of progestin-only contraception do not predict what her experience with Implanon will be like.

    4. Typically the mean bleeding days per 90-day reference time shows that women using Implanon had fewer total bleeding and/or spotting days than women not using any hormones.

H. Contraindications are summarized in Box 18.1.

I. Drug interactions.

    1. Women who take drugs that are potent inducers of hepatic enzymes should not use etonogestrel, as these drugs potentially can decrease the efficacy of etonogestrel and therefore may result in an unintended pregnancy.

    2. Examples of these drugs include griseofulvin, barbiturates, rifampin, phenylbutazone, phenytoin, carbamazepine, felbamate, oxcarbazepine, topiramate, and modafinil.

II. Implanon insertion—Providers must complete a training program provided free by the manufacturer per FDA regulations before clinicians can insert or remove Implanon. To inquire about training, visit www.implanon-usa.com.

A. Counseling:

    1. Appropriate counseling is essential for proper selection of implants for contraception.

    2. It is best to do this during a visit separate from product insertion.

    3. Explain what it is, how it works, its advantages and disadvantages, bleeding patterns, what to expect at insertion and removal, contraindications, and costs.

    4. Informed consent may be obtained at this visit or at time of insertion.

B. When to insert. *Pregnancy must be excluded before insertion.*

    1. If patient is not using any hormonal contraception, it can be inserted on day 1–5 of her menstrual cycle.

2. If patient is switching from combined oral contraceptive, Implanon can be inserted any time within 7 days from the last dose of active hormone pill.
3. If patient is switching from a progesterone-only pill and has not skipped any pills that month, Implanon can be inserted at any time.
4. If patient has an intrauterine device or intrauterine system, Implanon can be inserted the same day as the device's removal.
5. If the patient has an Implanon that is due for removal and wishes to continue with Implanon, a new one can be inserted right after removal through the same incision.
6. If the patient is switching from medroxyprogesterone acetate injections, Implanon can be inserted during the 2-week window when the next injection would have been due.
7. Implanon can be inserted within the first 5 days after a first-trimester abortion.
8. Implanon can be inserted 3–4 weeks after childbirth or a third-trimester abortion.
9. Implanon can be inserted after the fourth week postpartum if the patient is breastfeeding exclusively.
10. If Implanon is inserted according to the preceding guidelines, it is effective immediately.
11. If Implanon is being inserted outside these guidelines, pregnancy must be excluded first and patient should be advised to use a backup form of nonhormonal contraception for 7 days.

C. Equipment required.
1. Implanon comes in a sterile, disposable, preloaded applicator.
2. A comfortable table with support for the patient's arm (a pillow works well) is needed.
3. Sterile gloves, antiseptic solution, local anesthetic, sterile gauze, skin closures, paper tape, and elastic bandage are needed.

D. Insertion procedure.
1. Nondominate arm is used.
2. Insertion site is between the biceps and triceps muscle, in midline 4 cm from the medial condyle of the humerus.
3. Insertion is always subdermal.
4. No incision is necessary as insertion is via the trocar.
5. Experienced clinicians can insert Implanon in 2 to 3 minutes.

Circumstances for the Removal of Implanon   **BOX 18.2**

Implanon should be removed:

1. If the patient wants to conceive
2. If patient wants to change to another form of contraception
3. Three years after insertion; if patient wants to continue with etonogestrel implant, a new rod can be inserted at the time of removal of initial rod, at the same site

  6. Correct placement must be confirmed right after insertion.
  7. Careful and correct subdermal insertion is necessary for successful placement and will facilitate removal.
E. Postinsertion complications.
  1. Pain at insertion site occurred in fewer than 3% of women.
  2. Redness, swelling, and hematoma were reported in fewer than 1% of women.

III. **Implanon removal procedure.**
A. When to remove: The Implanon should be removed at the patient's request or when the time period has expired (Box 18.2).
B. Patient education points.
  1. Most removals take about 5 to 10 minutes.
  2. Minor to no discomfort is experienced at the time of removal.
  3. Postremoval the patient may have some bruising and tenderness at the site.
C. Changing to another method of contraception.
  1. Another method of contraception can be initiated immediately postremoval without loss of contraceptive efficacy, that is, oral contraceptives, contraceptive ring or patches, or IUD/IUS.

IV. **Patient and provider resources.**
A. The manufacturer has a comprehensive program for provider and patient education and support that can be accessed by calling 1-677-467-5266 or by visiting: www.implanon-usa.com.
B. For full prescribing information see the package insert available on the manufacturer's Web site.

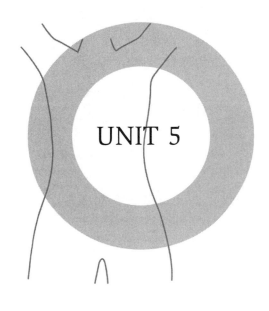

UNIT 5

Assessment
of Women at Risk

CHAPTER 19

The Sexual-Assault Victim

Karen Kalmakis

I. **Sexual assault explained.**
  A. Sexual assault is an invasive, traumatic crime that is accompanied by both legal and health concerns. All women are at risk regardless of age, socioeconomic status, ethnic background, and race.
    1. Twenty-nine percent of female rape victims experience their first rape between the ages of 18 and 24. The Federal Bureau of Investigation (FBI) has identified sexual assault as the most rapidly increasing violent crime in America.
    2. Only 26% of rape victims receive medical care postassault.
  B. Many emergency departments are well equipped with a rape crisis team, which includes sexual-assault nurse examiners (SANE).
  C. The legal definition of rape varies from state to state, but all definitions share similar components:
    1. Nonconsensual sexual penetration involving intimidation, or the use or threat of force.
    2. Legal definition of penetration: Invasion of the vulva, mouth, or anus (not necessarily the vagina).
    3. Legal definition of lack of consent:
      a. Assumed when a weapon or brutal force is used.
      b. When the victim is a minor.
      c. When the victim has physical or mental limitations or is under the influence of alcohol or other substances.

Table 19.1   **Explanation of Terms Used in Sexual Assault**

Term	Definition
Stranger rape	Victim is assaulted by an unknown assailant for unknown purpose.
Acquaintance rape	Assaulted by an acquaintance who the victim has met previously during a nonthreatening social encounter—not considered a friend.
Date rape	Occurred during a date or encounter in which the victim agreed to accompany the perpetrator. May occur after an initial encounter or after many dates of a nonthreatening nature.
Intimate or partner rape, or marital rape	Sexual assault perpetrated by an intimate partner.
Aggravated assault	Sexual assault of a victim who is disabled (mentally or physically) or elderly. Associated with excessive force to cause physical injury.
Incest	Sexual assault by a blood relative who is a close family member.
Statutory rape	Sexual intercourse with a minor, defined by the state in which the incident occurs. It may be with or without consent.

D. College students are at higher risk for sexual assault. Alcohol is associated with 72% of these assaults.

E. Table 19.1 lists the definition of terms often used with a sexual assault.

II. Some reasons why women may not report sexual assault.

A. Embarrassment.

B. Feelings of self-blame that they are somehow at fault.

C. Fear of retribution, especially if perpetrator is a known or close acquaintance.

D. Lack of faith in the medical or legal system.

E. Lack of knowledge concerning their legal rights.

F. Lack of access to health care.

G. Concerns about confidentiality.

H. The victim may not believe that date rape constitutes true sexual assault.

Recommended Medication Regimens	**BOX 19.1**

Ceftriaxone 125 mg IM (intramuscular) in a single dose
PLUS
Azithromycin 1 g orally in a single dose
OR
Doxycycline 100 mg orally twice a day for 7 days
AND
Plan B (emergency contraception)
1 orally now, repeat in 12 hours if at risk of pregnancy

  I. The person may have financial constraints.
  J. The person may be unsure where to go for help.

III. The forensic examination.
   A. Best performed by a specially trained SANE nurse or an emergency department physician.
   B. Examinations must be done within 5 days of the assault. The victim may come to the primary care office hours, weeks, or months after the incident.
   C. Once a history of an assault has been identified the practitioner should follow recommended guidelines.

IV. Guidelines for the primary care provider following sexual assault.
   A. Facilitate emotional stability and safety of the victim.
   B. Determine time elapsed since the sexual assault, **if fewer than 5 days and patient consents to forensic evidence collection,** refer to the emergency department for a sexual-assault examination.
   C. If greater than 5 days, or patient declines forensic evidence collection:
      1. Obtain history of the assault using patient's own words when possible.
      2. Gather information about the victim's prior medical history, particularly her gynecologic history and risk for or presence of pregnancy.
      3. Document all injuries.
      4. **If 5 days or less since assault**, offer prophylaxis against sexually transmitted diseases and pregnancy (Box 19.1).
      5. Recommendations for HIV assessment of adolescent and adult patients **72 hours** postsexual assault.
         a. Assess risk for HIV infection.

    b. Consult with a specialist in HIV treatment, if PEP (postexposure prophylaxis) is being considered.

    c. If the patient appears to be at risk for HIV transmission from the assault, discuss antiretroviral prophylaxis, including toxicity and lack of proven benefit.

    d. If the patient chooses to start antiretroviral PEP, give enough medication to last until the next return visit; reevaluate 3 to 7 days after initial assessment and assess tolerance of medications.

    e. If PEP is started, perform CBC (complete blood count) and serum chemistry at baseline (initiation of PEP should **not** be delayed, pending results).

    f. Perform HIV antibody test at original assessment; repeat at 6 weeks, 3 months, and 6 months.

  6. Arrange follow-up care, including mental health counseling and physical exam.

  7. Complete mandatory report forms as appropriate.

  8. Discuss with the patient the possibility of reporting the assault to police.

  9. Discharge patient with written instructions to increase adherence to plan of care, including medication regime.

  10. Send the victim home in the care of family or friends.

  11. Provide a list of community resources for support, including a referral to mental health counseling.

V. Management.

  A. Follow-up examinations with a health care provider are recommended at 4 to 6 weeks postsexual assault in cases where the patient received prophylactic medications. This follow-up examination should take place in 1 to 2 weeks if no prophylaxis was provided.

    1. Vaginal wet mount for microscopy examination.

      a. Trichomoniasis.

      b. Bacterial vaginosis.

    2. Gonorrhea culture from throat, cervix, and rectum as deemed appropriate from patient report of the assault.

    3. Chlamydia culture.

    4. Human immunodeficiency virus (HIV) antibody screening (complete at 6 weeks, 3 months, and 6 months).

    5. Hepatitis B surface antigen with Hepatitis B immunizations as needed.

    6. Other interventions and care as clinically indicated (i.e., herpes lesions).

   7. Provide ongoing counseling and support, determine need for additional mental health counseling and referrals.
   8. Pregnancy test if no menses.
B. Additional follow-up should be scheduled for testing of diseases that have a long incubation period before they are discernible in the serum.
   1. Test for syphilis at 12 weeks.
   2. Test for HIV at 3 and 6 months.
   3. Continued mental health counseling as needed.

CHAPTER 20

Domestic Violence

Helen A. Carcio

I. Violence and abuse explained.

  A. Violence and abuse that is directed at women by their intimate partners is an enormous health problem in the United States.

  B. The prevalence of violence ranges from 9.7 to 29.7% over a woman's lifetime.

  C. Definition: Violent or controlling behavior that is directed at a woman by a person who has or had an intimate relationship with that woman.

  1. The overwhelming majority of violence and abuse is perpetrated by men against women.

  2. Violence does occur in same-sex relationships.

  3. There is a small proportion of women who are abusive to men.

  D. The many forms of abuse include:

  1. Destructive criticism.

  2. Guilt tripping.

  3. Disrespect.

  4. Emotional withholding.

  5. Economic control.

  6. Isolation.

  7. Harassment.

  E. Violence may also take many forms including:

  1. Intimidation.

    2. Destruction of pets or property.

    3. Sexual violence.

    4. Physical violence (slapping, biting, punching, burning, stabbing, shooting, kicking, and choking).

    5. Threatening with weapons.

F. Violence against women interferes with the health of the woman, even during pregnancy and in the postpartum period.

G. Violence and abusive behavior can lead to:

    1. Increased unintended pregnancies (especially among adolescents).

    2. An increase in sexually transmitted disease.

    3. Possible interference with breastfeeding, which is associated with child abuse and substance abuse.

H. Many organizations have adopted policies and guidelines to address the problem of violence.

    1. *Healthy People 2000* (www.healthypeople.gov/) has included objectives related to a decrease in the incidence and prevalence of violence against women.

    2. The American Nurses Association, the American College of Nurse Midwives, the American Academy of Nursing, and other national nursing organizations all support the notion of assessing all women for violence and abuse and providing the appropriate supports.

    3. Gradually, through the efforts of the women themselves and responsive health care providers, a point has been reached where it is believed that every provider in contact with any woman should assess that woman for past or present violence and abuse.

    4. Because of the work of many in the nursing profession, the powerful myths in our society (which make woman abuse a private and shameful matter) have been questioned and largely exposed.

I. The relationship with the primary care provider.

    1. We are now close to providing careful, sensitive, and safe assessment for violence and abuse in all women in all settings. However, for many reasons, many women in practice settings are still not routinely assessed for abuse in an appropriate manner. This problem is due more to a lack of knowledge on the part of the provider than to a lack of caring.

    2. Violence and abuse against women is given very little time in curricula; many providers do not understand how severe a health problem it is.

Abuse Assessment Screening Questions   **BOX 20.1**

1. Do you feel emotionally abused by your partner?
2. Has your partner ever hit, slapped, kicked, or otherwise physically hurt you?
3. Are you afraid of your partner?
4. Do you feel that your partner tries to control you?
5. Has your partner ever forced you into sex that you did not wish to participate in?

3. Some providers are afraid women will be insulted if they ask about abuse, whereas other providers worry that the woman will disclose violence and the provider will not know how to intervene.

II. Principles related to assessment of violence and abuse.

A. First, it is helpful to understand that it is very important to assess for violence and abuse in women's lives.

B. Violence and abuse is a serious health problem. If the woman does disclose information on abuse, encourage her talk about the specifics of the violence as much as you can. Your careful attention to her story is intervention.

C. Some principles of assessment for abuse are the following:

1. Because abuse may be emotional or sexual, merely observing for signs of physical abuse during a routine visit may not be sufficient to rule out abuse. If there are obvious signs of what might be physical abuse, the provider can say something like, "Often when I see marks like this on women, it is because someone is hurting them. Is anyone hurting you?"

2. Always screen for abuse when the woman is alone. She should never be asked questions about violence and abuse in front of anyone else.

3. Screening questions should be direct. If you merely ask about her relationship, the woman may not disclose information because she might feel that being abused is a shameful thing—too shameful for the health care provider to even ask about. (See Box 20.1 for some suggested screening questions. These questions were developed by the Nursing Research Consortium on Violence and Abuse [King, 1989].)

4. Screen all women. Abuse occurs in lesbian relationships also. The abuse assessment screening questions you decide to use should be gender neutral.

5. Always screen for abuse orally. Women respond more accurately to oral screens than to written screens. Engage the woman, and ask the questions slowly and directly.
6. The health care provider should be the one to screen for abuse. Do not delegate this task to anyone. As a health care provider, you are working to establish trust with your client; assessing for abuse at each visit is part of this trust.
7. If you do not speak the same language as the woman, you must obtain a professional interpreter to screen for violence and abuse. It is obvious that you should not ask *any* family member or friend to translate for you.
8. If you are going to assess all women routinely, then you must know the referral options in your agency and community. Your local shelter for abused women will be able to supply you with brochures or cards that you can leave in a woman's examination room or give to women. The shelter staff will also be willing to counsel women and provide legal advocacy.
9. Assessing women for abuse can function as primary prevention as well as lead to intervention and referral.
   a. If a woman is not abused, the provider now has a "teaching moment" to talk about the prevalence of abuse, how serious a health problem it is, and how all health care providers are screening routinely.
   b. The woman can be given the brochure from the shelter in case she has a friend or a relative who might need the information.
   c. This health education about violence and abuse against women is a form of primary prevention.
   d. If the woman is abused, you have demonstrated that you are a provider who cares about abuse and perhaps she will disclose information at a later visit.
   e. If she is not abused, then you have made one more person aware of the incidence and severity of violence and abuse against women and let that person know that help is available.
10. If the provider is planning a pelvic examination, then the woman should definitely be asked about past or current sexual abuse. It is almost negligent to ask a woman to undergo a pelvic examination if she has been previously sexually abused. Again, this question must be asked directly because women do not respond to it readily on written intake forms.

11. If a woman discloses abuse, ask her what she wants to do.
    a. The woman herself knows how safe she is and if she wants to leave the situation.
    b. Leaving the abusive partner may not be the solution, or even an option, for many women.
    c. Health care providers can be misled into a "rescue fantasy," and subtly pressure the woman to leave.
    d. The time immediately after a woman leaves her abuser is potentially the greatest period of risk for homicide.
    e. Do not encourage the woman to leave her abuser unless she wants to. Instead, listen to the woman, provide her with referrals, tell her how courageous she is, provide her with a safety plan, and have her come back and see you. These actions are interventions.
12. Pregnant women should be screened for past abuse and abuse during the current pregnancy. Pregnancy protects some women from physical abuse, whereas for some women, the abuse may start during pregnancy or become more severe if the abuse was present before the pregnancy.
13. Establish a violence and abuse against women interdisciplinary task force.
    a. Such task forces provide a venue for further education about violence and abuse and for the establishment of standards of care, policies, and protocols.
    b. These elements of an infrastructure ensure that screening is universal and standard practice by all clinicians.

III. Some concluding comments.

A. There now exists a solid body of literature about violence and abuse of women as a health problem.
B. Many communities have community roundtable discussions related to violence against women.
C. Most states have some type of protective orders to protect women from their abusers; some are good, and some are not. The courts in most states try to prosecute the perpetrators.
D. Every state has a grassroots organization that provides services for abused women, although these organizations are woefully underfunded.
E. Violence and abuse against women by their partners has become a more obvious problem.
F. Health care professions are slowly understanding the enormity of this health problem.

G. Safe, kind, intelligent universal screening with appropriate referrals is almost a reality.

CHAPTER 21

Sexually Transmitted Infections

Mimi Clarke Secor

I. Sexually transmitted infections explained.

  A. Statistics and trends.

  1. Previously known as sexually transmitted diseases now referred to as sexually transmitted infections (STIs).

  2. Approximately 19 million new infections occur each year in the United States per Centers for Disease Control (CDC; www.cdc.gov/std/ststs07/trends.htm).

  3. Nearly 50% affecting 15- to 24-year-olds.

  4. One in four teens has one or more STIs.

  5. One in two African American teens has one or more STIs.

  6. STIs are twice as common in African American populations.

  7. Significant physical and psychological consequences resulting from STIs.

  8. Direct costs of managing STIs estimated at $14 billion in 2006.

  9. Reportable STIs include gonorrhea, chlamydia, and syphilis.

  10. STIs not reportable include HPV (human papilloma virus) and HSV (herpes simplex virus).

  11. Biological factors place women at greater risk than men for acquiring STIs and suffering from more severe health consequences associated with STIs.

B. Epidemiology.
1. Chlamydia is the most common *reportable* STI:
   a. With an estimated 3 million new cases each year.
   b. More than half of the new cases remain undiagnosed and unreported.
   c. Leading cause of PID (pelvic inflammatory disease) and infertility in United States.
2. Gonorrhea is the second most common *reportable* STI:
   a. Estimated 358,366 reportable cases in 2006, underdiagnosed and underreported.
   b. Likely twice as common as reported numbers.
   c. More common in southern and western United States.
   d. More common in MSM (Men having sex with men).
   e. Increases susceptibility to HIV three- to fivefold.
   f. Widespread fluoroquinolone-resistance among MSM and heterosexual populations.
3. Genital herpes is the most prevalent STI.
   a. Affecting one in five Americans, 25% women, and 1 out of 3 women affected is over 30 years old.
   b. Most transmission occurs when patients are asymptomatic.
   c. Most symptoms are atypical.
   d. When signs do occur, they typically appear as one or more painful blisters in the urogenital area or rectum. The fluid filled blisters soon break, leaving tender ulcers (sores) that may take two to four weeks to heal if it is the primary outbreak.
   e. HSV Type 1 accounts for up to 35% of primary genital infections but rarely causes recurrences after one year.
   f. HSV Type 2 is associated with the highest shedding and recurrence rate the first year with up to 1 in 3 days associated with asymptomatic or symptomatic shedding. Recurrences and/or asymptomatic shedding may continue over a lifetime, waxing and waning in variable ways per individual.
4. HPV is the most common STI with the highest incidence among young populations:
   a. Ubiquitous exposure among the sexually active young population.
   b. Usually transient infection, clearing within 9 to 12 months.
   c. HPV is the cause of cervical cancer and this is a rare complication associated with persistent HPV infection with high-risk subtypes, including 16, 18, 31 and others.

   d. More than 100 different strains or subtypes exist, 30 of which are sexually transmitted.

   e. HPV can infect the genital area of men and women including the skin of the penis, vulva, anus and the vagina, cervix and rectal mucosa.

  5. Syphilis rates have increased in recent years:

   a. Rates six times higher in MSM than among heterosexual women.

   b. This is a decade-long trend:

   (1) Ten years ago rates were equal among men and women.

   c. Recent 11% increase in women, reason unclear.

   d. Known as "the great imitator" because the signs and symptoms are indistinguishable from those associated with other STIs.

 C. Complications associated with STIs.

  1. Chlamydia and gonorrhea, often asymptomatic and undiagnosed, if untreated, may lead to PID, ectopic pregnancy, chronic pelvic pain and infertility.

  2. Long term complications of chlamydia are much more serious in women.

  3. Many STIs increase risk of acquiring HIV including gonorrhea, herpes, bacterial vaginosis, and syphilis.

  4. Several STIs are associated with preterm labor including trichomoniasis and bacterial vaginosis.

  5. Cervical cancer is a rare complication from persistent HPV infection.

   a. HPV is the cause of cervical cancer.

 D. Female considerations.

  1. Women are more susceptible to STIs due to the extensive mucous membrane tissue lining the female genital area.

  2. Many STIs in women are asymptomatic, and most cases go undiagnosed.

  3. Chlamydia is three times more common in women than in men.

  4. HIV is increasing more rapidly in heterosexual women than in any other group.

  5. Women may be reinfected if their partners are not diagnosed and appropriately treated.

II. Clinical evaluation of female.

 A. History.

  1. Symptoms:

   a. Onset, duration, severity, course.

b. Past history of same problem, symptoms, diagnosis, management.

c. Self care to present.

d. Associated symptoms with review of symptoms (ROS):

  (1) Constitutional; malaise, fatigue, myalgia, chills, fever, weight loss, anorexia.

  (2) HEENT (HSV 1, gonorrhea).

  • Sores, lesions, oropharnygeal erythema, exudate, tenderness.

  (3) Respiratory (Tb).

  • Wheezing/rhonchi, rales, reduced breath sounds, pain with breathing.

  (4) Cardiac (syphilis).

  • Murmurs, irregularity, other abnormal findings.

  (5) GI (hepatitis, PID, HIV).

  • Abdominal, pelvic pain (PID), back pain (Pyelonephritis), upper right quadrant pain (liver), bloating, indigestion, nausea, vomiting, diarrhea, anorexia, weight loss.

  (6) GU (HSV 2, gonorrhea, chlamydia, trichomoniosis, bacterial vaginosis).

  • Urinary symptoms of frequency, urgency, dysuria, hematuria, odor, abnormal color to urine, back pain.

  • Genital itching, sores, tears, lesions, burning, pain, discharge, odor, dyspareunia.

  (7) Neuro (syphilis).

  • Mental status changes.

  (8) Skin (syphilis, gonorrhea, HSV).

  • Sores, lesions, blisters, rashes, tattoos, branding, body piercings, icterus (hepatitis).

  (9) Extremities (gonorrhea, syphilis).

  • Arthralgias, joint stiffness, pain, swelling.

2. Gynecologic history.

  a. Pregnancy history summary including gravida, parous:

  (1) Abortions; spontaneous, medical, surgical, miscarriage.

  b. Menstrual history.

  (1) Last menstrual period: was it normal, late, lighter than normal?

  (2) Age of first period or menarche: how often, how many days; dysmenorrhea, new onset or worsening of dysmenorrhea; abnormal bleeding; bleeding after intercourse; type of protection used: tampons and/or pads.

  c. STI history.

    (1) Record all STIs, including vaginal infections; dates of infections, how previously diagnosed and treated, inquire about any incomplete treatments; record follow-ups, partner notification, and subsequent treatments.

    (2) Date last tested, what tests done, and results.

  d. Sexual history.

    (1) Record sexual partner, partners, gender, date of most recent sexual encounter, behaviors involved, frequency of sexual activity; daily, weekly, weekends only; dates of first penile/vaginal intercourse or coitarche, total number of sex partners, male, female, history of new partner in past 1-2 months, stated sexual orientation/preference.

    (2) Risky behaviors:
- Unprotected vaginal, anal, oral, (receptive, expressive), use of condoms (percent), sex with money exchange, IV drug use, tattooing, body piercing, branding, violence, rape, abuse including violent sex play, using dirty sex toys, etc.
- High-risk partner/s:
  - Exposure to HIV, hepatitis B, C, chlamydia, gonorrhea, IV drug use, sex worker, male having sex with men (MSM), bisexual, group sex, abusive, controlling, partner with unknown history or suspected high-risk history.

    (3) Contraceptive history:
- History of unprotected intercourse, consenting, rape, reluctant consent, access to plan B (emergency contraception)
- Current contraceptive method, methods used in past, dates, problems, satisfaction with current method, problems, complaints, and compliance with method of choice.

    (4) Pregnancy history.

    (5) Infertililty.

  e. Gynecologic surgery, procedures, problems.

  f. Personal hygiene.

    (1) Douching; may increase risk of recurrent vaginal infections (i.e., BV).

        (2) Tampon or pad use; deodorant tampons, synthetic, or cotton, note brand, use of panty liners; frequency of wear (daily versus with menses only).

        (3) Type of underwear (i.e., thong underwear associated with vaginal infections).

        (4) Hygiene practices:
- Including poor hygiene, not wiping front to back, not washing after anal intercourse, not washing sex toys, poor oral hygiene, not washing hands or genitals before sex.
- Use of soap, type, amount used, bubble baths, feminine hygiene sprays, other chemicals.
- Baths versus showers.

        (5) Clothing; tight clothing, workout clothing, pantyhose, bathing suit, duration of wear; particularly extended hours.

  3. Social history.
- **a.** History of sexual, physical, and verbal abuse.
- **b.** Lifestyle history; diet, exercise, sleep, stressors, occupation, and recreation, etc.

  4. Medical history.
- **a.** Medical conditions: past and present, stable or unstable.
- **b.** Immunization status including Tb, Hepatitis A, B.
- **c.** Date of last tuberculosis test and results.

  5. Medications.
- **a.** Prescription: borrowed, or self-medication.
- **b.** Medication allergies.
- **c.** Over-the-counter medications.

  6. Family history.

B. Examination.
  1. Vital signs.
  2. Skin:
- **a.** Lesions, rashes, ulcers, palmar or foot sole rash (syphilis), tattoos, piercings, brandings.

  3. Oral:
- **a.** Erythema, tenderness, sores, lesions; warts, exudate, plaques, etc.
- **b.** Foul odor, gum disease, plaque, dental caries, poor hygiene.

  4. Respiratory
- **a.** Determine if there has been exposure to Tb or if there are symptoms.

5. Cardiac.
  a. Tertiary syphilis.
6. Abdominal.
  a. Absence of bowel sounds or increased bowel sounds.
  b. Masses, enlargement:
    (1) Lower abdominal mass consider PID with tubo-ovarian abscess/TOA.
    (2) Right upper abdominal mass, consider hepatitis.
    (3) Inguinal nodes swelling and/or tenderness, consider HIV, pelvic, genital infection.
  c. Tenderness:
    (1) CVA tenderness with pyelonephritis.
    (2) Right upper quadrant, consider hepatitis.
    (3) Lower abdominal, consider PID, cystitis.
7. Pelvic examination.
  a. External genitalia.
    (1) Inguinal node tenderness or enlargement.
    (2) Erythema, lesions, urethral discharge, fissures, tears, tenderness.
    (3) Bartholin gland areas at 5 and 7 o'clock of vaginal introitus.
    (4) Skene's glands at 3 and 9 o'clock of urethral meatus.
  b. Vagina.
    (1) Introital erythema (focal or diffuse), lesions, tenderness, particularly between labial folds (displace tissue to fully visualize tissue).
    (2) Erythema, lesions.
    (3) Discharge:
      • Color, quality; flocular, creamy, coaty, clumpy, frothy; amount.
    (4) Vaginal pH, amine KOH test; foul-fishy odor is positive.
    (5) Vaginal microscopy/wet mount (Chapter 10).
  c. Cervix.
    (1) Redness, cervical erosion, ectropion, mucopus, friability, bleeding.
    (2) Cervical os, size, shape, mucopus from os, quantity.
    (3) Cervical motion tenderness; mild, moderate, severe or positive chandelier test suggestive of PID.
  d. Bimanual exam of uterus and adnexae:
    (1) Tenderness; mild, moderate, severe, rebound, localized, masses, mobility.

          (2) Uterus size, shape, mobility, firmness, tenderness.

          (3) Ovaries:

            • Palpable or nonpalpable.

            • Tenderness; mild, moderate, severe.

            • Fullness or masses.

      e. Rectal:

          (1) Lesions; sores, blisters, warts, tags, fissures, tears, hemorrhoids.

          (2) Erythema, hemorrhoids, lesions, tenderness, discharge.

  8. Extremities.

      a. Joint swelling, tenderness, increased heat, reduced range of motion.

C. Diagnostic testing per CDC.

  1. Chlamydia testing.

      a. Yearly screening of all sexually active women under age 26 years old.

      b. Screen women over 26 years old, if new or multiple sexual partners, or history of high-risk behaviors.

      c. Retesting 3 months after treatment to prevent reinfection.

  2. Gonorrhea testing:

      a. Men having sex with men, bisexual, heterosexual females with sex partners of unknown risk, or who have high-risk partners, females not using condoms, new partner.

      b. History of STIs.

  3. Genital herpes:

      a. Cultures if fluid-filled blisters or very moist lesions.

      b. Polymerase chain-reaction (PCR) culturing is four times more accurate than non-PCR, therefore nonblistering lesions may be tested with greater accuracy.

      c. Herpes Select Serology type 1 or 2 specific IGG antibody testing is the gold standard diagnostic test for nonprimary HSV testing.

          (1) Nearly 100% seroconversion within 4 months of infection.

          (2) Initial negative test indicates probable primary infection with recent acquisition of infection.

          (3) There is no type specific immunoglobulin M (IGM) antibody test and therefore IGM should not be ordered.

  4. HIV.

      a. MSM, bisexual, IV drug use, high-risk partner.

      b. Possible false-positive rate with point-of-care salivary test-

ing (orasure), confirmatory serology testing should be
done.

5. Hepatitis B.
   a. MSM, bisexual, IV drug use, high-risk partner.
6. Hepatitis C.
   a. MSM, bisexual, IV drug use, high-risk partner.
7. Syphilis.
   a. MSM, bisexual, IV drug use, high-risk partner.

III. Table 21.1 summarizes and compares STI in the female.

Table 21.1   **Sexually Transmitted Infection Assessment of the Female**

Infection	Cause	Prevalence	Symptoms	Diagnosis
Chancroid	Hemophilus ducreyi, gram negative bacillus	More common in populations exchanging sex for money.	Women are often asymptomatic, single painful genital ulcer in men.	Culture + for *H. ducreyi*, rule out more common HSV, also HIV, Syphilis by RPR
Chlamydia	Obligate intracellular parasite susceptible to antibiotics	Most common reported STI, 3 million new cases a year Leading cause of preventable infertility.	Often asymptomatic in women, so need for widespread screening < 26 years old.	Universal screening if < 26 years old; Urine PCR or cervical testing.
Genital Herpes	Type 1 or 2 herpes virus, both can infect genitals	Estimated 55 million Americans infected.	Most asymptomatic, most transmission when asymptomatic. Symptoms may include painful genital lesions, 1st infection most severe, recurrences most common with HSV 2, widely variable symptoms.	Classic symptoms suspect HSV. Culture if lesions, PCR culture more sensitive, expensive; type-specific serology IGG/HerpesSelect, 98% seroconversion 4 months post-HSV acquisition.
Genital Warts	Nononcogenic HPV, 6 11	1 million visits yearly, HPV affecting up to 80% of sexually active young women in US.	Single or multiple, soft, fleshy, non-tender, cauliflower-like lesions in genital area including vulvovaginal, anal, or cervix.	By exam, HPV DNA testing not recommended; RPR to rule out condylomata lata of syphilis; colposcopy and/or biopsy of atypical lesions.

(continued)

Table 21.1 *(continued)*

Infection	Cause	Prevalence	Symptoms	Diagnosis
Gonorrhea	*Neisseria gonorrhoeae,* gram-neg diplococcus bacteria	Second most common STI in US esp. among MSM.	Women commonly asymptomatic, or abnormal vaginal discharge, dysuria, abnormal menses.	Gram stain, culture, NAAT of cervical secretions; Urine NAAT an option too.
Pelvic Inflammatory Disease, (PID)	Polymicrobial, various combinations, *N. gonorrhoeae, C. trachomatis,* Anerobes, and others	1 million new cases yearly, leading cause of female infertility.	Many have no symptoms or atypical symptoms. Symptoms include pain/tenderness lower abdomen, uterus, ovaries, fever, chills, elevated WBCs/ESR, associated with menses.	High index of suspicion, low threshold for diagnosis, + cultures, CDC criteria, pelvic exam tenderness, mucopus, WBCs on vaginal microscopy.
Syphilis	Treponema pallidum spirochete	Increasing among MSM, Unusual in women, unless risk factors, higher rates in SW.	Primary: Classic chancre is painless, indurated ulcer in genital area, at site of exposure, may evade diagnosis if vaginal. Secondary: variable skin rash, may involve palmar hands, soles of feet. Latent: Few clinical symptoms, CNS changes.	Primary; Darkfield exam of chancre, with RPR serology. Secondary/ Latent; RPR serology.

(continued)

Table 21.1 *(continued)*

Infection	Cause	Prevalence	Symptoms	Diagnosis
Trichomoniasis	Motile protozoan	Most common curable STI in US and worldwide, 3 million US women infected yearly. May be asymptomatic for years.	Excessive, frothy, yellow-green vaginal discharge, exam findings variable, sometimes with genital erythema, swelling and pruritus.	Vaginal microscopy for typical motile trichomonads and WBCs; Pap should be verified with culture or microscopy; Various vaginal cultures may also be used.

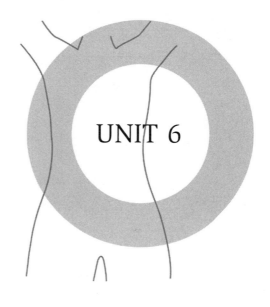

UNIT 6

Evaluation of the Menopausal Woman

CHAPTER 22

Assessment of Menopausal Status

Mimi Clarke Secor

I. **Menopause explained.**
   A. Menopause is the permanent cessation of menses after 12 consecutive months of amenorrhea, or when follicle stimulating hormone (FSH) levels (> 30 mIU or mIU/mL) are consistently elevated in the absence of other obvious pathologic causes.
      1. This event usually results from loss of ovarian follicular function due to aging or can be induced by medical intervention such as surgery (hysterectomy), chemotherapy, or radiation.
      2. On average, natural menopause occurs around age 51 but may range between 40 to 58 years of age.
   B. There will be 52 million postmenopausal women in the United States by 2010, and numbers are rapidly increasing as baby boomers reach midlife and beyond. This includes approximately 2 million women who have undergone total hysterectomies.
   C. The menopause transition represents the time when menstrual cycle, endocrine and central nervous system changes occur. Menopause-related definitions are summarized in Table 22.1. The menopause transition may be further divided into stages according to the STRAW nomenclature summarized in Table 22.2.

Table 22.1   **Menopause-Related Definitions**

Perimenopause = Menopause transition	Occurs around menopause, beginning in the early transition, ending 12 months after the final menstrual period (FMP) (includes stages −1, −2).
Premature menopause	Natural menopause occurring at < 40 years of age
Early Menopause	Natural menopause occurring well before the average age, equal to or less than 45 years of age. Includes premature menopause.
Menopause	Permanent cessation of menses after 12 consecutive months of amenorrhea, or consistently elevated FSH (greater than or equal to 30 mIU) in absence of other obvious pathologic causes.
Postmenopause	From FMP (natural or induced) extending through late menopause ending with death (includes states +1, +2).

Table 22.2   **STRAW (Stages of Reproductive Aging Workshop) Stages of Menopause**

-2 Stage = Early perimenopause	Onset of menstrual variability
-1 Stage = Late perimenopausal transition	Significant menstrual variability until FMP 2 or more missed menses, or cycle greater than 60 days
+ 1 Stage = Early postmenopause	FMP through next 5 years
+ 2 Stage = Late postmenopause	From 5 years post FMP until death

II. Physiology of menopause.

A. The menopause transition, also referred to as perimenopause, is associated with fluctuating hormone secretion causing irregular menstrual cycles and finally permanent cessation of menses.

B. Accelerated follicular atresia (egg death) occurs in perimenopause and by menopause only a few hundred to a few thousand follicles remain.

C. A year before the final menstrual period (FMP) a marked increase in FSH (> 30 mIU/mL) occurs and plateaus within 2 years of the FMP. This is due to the rapid loss of follicles, resulting in reduced inhibin B, which increases FSH levels.

D. For a brief period, higher levels of FSH produce more follicles causing overproduction of estradiol. This may cause a range of perimenopausal symptoms, including irritability, bloating, mastalgia, menorrhagia, growth of fibroids, and endometrial hyperplasia.

E. Irregular cycles and reduced fertility are associated with the menopause transition. However, pregnancy is possible until menopause occurs (12 months since FMP).

F. The ovary is the major source of estrogen (during the reproductive years), with reductions occurring in the late menopausal transition, and major reductions in estrogen secretion throughout the first year of postmenopause (first 12 months after FMP). After this, a gradual decline occurs over the following several years.

III. Menopause introduction and related concerns and risks.

A. Symptoms attributed to menopause include only vasomotor symptoms, painful intercourse, and possibly sleep disturbances.

  1. Vasomotor-related symptoms include hot flashes, flushing, and night sweating.

  2. Other common symptoms associated with perimenopause include menstrual changes with eventual cessation of menses.

  3. Less common physical and psychological symptoms associated include moodiness, anxiety, memory changes, depression, urinary symptoms, and sexual concerns (i.e., desire, arousal, and orgasm), hair and/or skin changes, weight gain, and joint pain.

  4. Symptoms and potential concerns are summarized in Box 22.1.

  5. Disease risks including cancer risks and modifiable risk factors should be identified by the clinician and addressed with the patient.

  6. Vasomotor symptoms explained:

   a. Vasomotor symptoms (VMS) is a global term referring to both hot flashes and night sweats. Considered a hallmark of menopause, VMS are experienced by up to 75% of all perimenopausal women in the United States.

   b. Fluctuations in estrogen and progesterone occurring in perimenopause and early menopause are commonly associated with vasomotor symptoms.

   c. Hot flashes are transient, recurrent symptoms of flushing and a sudden sensation of heat usually involving the upper body and face.

    (1) Frequency of hot flashes varies widely among

Symptoms Related to Menopause	BOX 22.1

- Vasomotor symptoms of hot flashes, night sweats, flushing
- Weight changes with weight gain most common
- Skin changes—dry skin, gray hair
- Cardiovascular concerns
- Urinary problems including incontinence and overactive bladder
- Atropic vaginitis, dyspareunia
- Pelvic pain
- Decline in fertility
- Pregnancy
- Sexual function effects, notably reduced libido, lubrication, and dyspareunia
- Alterations in sleep patterns
- Headache
- Cognition challenges
- Psychological concerns such as moodiness and anxiety
- Arthritis
- Dental and oral changes
- Ocular changes
- Hearing problems

women, ranging from occurring multiple times an hour, hourly, daily, weekly, or monthly. Within a 24-hour period, the greatest number of hot flashes occur during the early evening hours.

(2) Individual episodes of hot flashes usually range from 1–5 minutes

(3) Most hot flashes are mild to moderately severe; however, 10 to 15% of women have severe and/or very frequent hot flashes.

d. Night sweats are VMS occurring during sleep hours and are often associated with excessive perspiration, feeling overheated and disrupted sleep.

e. VMS are thought to result from fluctuations in estrogen and progesterone, but the precise mechanism and trigger of these symptoms is still not fully understood.

f. Frequency of VMS usually increases in perimenopause, peak during the first 2 years of postmenopause, then decline over time.

(1) The duration of time when VMS episodes occur ranges from 6 months to 2 years, but less commonly, symptoms may persist for 10 years or longer.

Factors That Contribute to the Occurrence and Severity of Vasomotor Symptoms

BOX 22.2

- History of PMS, PMDD
- Lower socioeconomic status
- Lack of exercise
- Caffeine
- Alcohol
- Stress
- Warmer room temp of bedroom
- Spicy foods
- Higher BMI
- Cigarette smoking
- Climate
- Roles and attitudes
- Other unconfirmed and/or unknown factors

---

    (2) VMS persisting for many years or that present as new onset in later menopause may indicate underlying cardiovascular disease and therefore a thorough evaluation is warranted.

    (3) VMS may occur or worsen once hormone therapy is stopped.

  g. VMS may negatively impact quality of life, be associated with physical complaints, and can result in a host of biopsychosocial complaints including; sleep problems, fatigue, anxiety, irritability, and other emotional problems. Work, home, relationships, and sexuality may be negatively impacted.

  h. Prevalence varies among ethnic and racial groups as follows: African American (46%), Hispanic (35%), Caucasian (31%), Chinese (21%), Japanese (18%) prevalence.

  i. Surgically induced menopause is associated with potentially severe and frequent VMS. This is due to the sudden drop in estrogen from removal of the ovaries.

  j. Many factors may exacerbate the occurrence and severity of VMS (see Box 22.2). Teaching should be initiated around measures to reduce VMS.

  k. VMS is common during menopause. It is important to rule out other medical conditions that may mimic VMS and not be associated with menopause (see Box 22.3).

  l. Clinical evaluation of VMS should be conducted as a part

Differential Diagnosis of Vasomotor Symptoms **BOX 22.3**

- Hyperthyroidism
- Epilepsy
- Autoimmune disorders
- Cancer
- Hypertension (new onset)
- Cardiovascular disease (new risk)
- Medications such as tamoxifen, raloxifen
- Tuberculosis, infection, lymphoma

of the clinical evaluation of the menopausal patient described below.

IV. **The goal of the clinical health evaluation is to identify menopause and age-related health issues, provide preventive care, anticipatory guidance, education, counseling, support and to diagnose and manage health problems.**

  A. A comprehensive menopause health questionnaire to assist clinicians in assessing the menopausal patient is available at The North American Menopause Society (NAMS) Web site: www.menopause.org/edumaterials/questionnare.pdf.

  B. Regular health examinations are recommended and should include:

  1. Comprehensive health, medical, social, family history.

  2. Complete physical examination including vital signs, height, weight, thyroid, breast, pelvic and rectovaginal examinations.

  3. Laboratory testing as indicated.

  C. Comprehensive history.

  1. Symptom history:

  a. Menopause related symptoms should be elicited and evaluated regarding frequency, severity, and duration. Also, note any associated symptoms.

  b. Ask detailed questions about symptoms such as vasomotor symptoms of hot flashes, night sweats, flushing, and sleep disturbances.

  c. Other symptoms, both menopause and age related, may include: moodiness, anxiety, depression, urinary symptoms, sexual issues such as low libido, dyspareunia, hair/ skin changes, weight gain, joint pain, and memory problems.

  d. Ask about management to present (i.e., self-care, medications, over-the-counter medications, level of coping)
2. Gynecologic history:
  a. Menstrual history, age of menarche, menses pattern over the years, perimenopausal menstrual pattern, LMP (last menstrual period), FMP (first menstrual period), abnormal vaginal bleeding, vaginal discharge or pruritus, urinary symptoms.
  b. Gynecologic problems, including a history of ovarian cysts, polycystic ovarian syndrome (PCOS), fibroids, infertility, endometriosis, PMS (premenstrual syndrome), PMDD (premenstrual dysphoric disorder), STIs, Pap history, DES (diethylstilbestrol) exposure in pregnancy, and gynecologic surgery.
  c. The dates of last breast and Pap exams, and other screening tests, including mammogram, bone density, and most recent lab results.
  d. Sexual history:
    (1) Sexual history should not assume a heterosexual bias and should be conducted in a supportive, nonjudgmental, confidential manner
    (2) Include sexual orientation (gender of sex partner/s), date of last sexual activity/ coitus, sexual concerns, low libido, dyspareunia, use of birth control, history of unprotected sex, orgasm issues.
  e. Contraceptive history: If LMP less than 12 months ago
    (1) Unprotected coitus, including hormonal options and current use of contraceptives; duration of use, doses, effectiveness, side effects, reason for stopping.
3. Obstetric history:
  a. Number of pregnancies, full-term births, premature babies, abortions, living children, age of first birth, complications during pregnancy or childbirth, age of children currently.
4. Medical history:
  a. Emphasis on CVD (cardiovascular disease), DM (diabetes mellitus), cancer, osteoporosis, and other relevant significant medical conditions, including hospitalizations.
  b. Identify modifiable risk factors (see Box 22.4) and educate regarding measures to prevent or decrease symptoms of menopause.
  c. Assess for potential risk of developing medical conditions

Complications of Menopause	**BOX 22.4**

Gallbladder disease
Cardiovascular conditions such as heart attack or stroke
Asthma
Cancers of the reproductive tract
Sexually transmitted infections
Pregnancy/Infertility
Incapacitating VMS symptoms
Diabetes mellitus—metabolic syndrome
Adverse effects of traditional and alternative therapies

that may be exacerbated during menopause (Box 22.4). Screen where appropriate.

5. Surgical history:
   a. Include all surgeries.
   b. Hysterectomy; note with or without oophorectomy.
6. Medication history:
   a. Current prescription medications (doses and timing).
   b. Over-the-counter medications, supplements (e.g., black cohosh, ginkgo, etc.).
   c. Complementary therapies.
   d. Medications or any allergies.
7. Psychological history:
   a. History of psychotherapy, mental health issues especially depression, anxiety, sleep issues, mood-related conditions, PMS, PMDD, postpartum depression, personality type, coping skills.
   b. Developmental challenges include: adolescent and/or college-aged children, empty nest, midlife crises, aging parents, retirement, grandchildren, changing spousal relations and roles, etc.
   c. Attitude and beliefs about menopause.
8. Social history:
   a. Occupation, marital status, living situation, financial status, and abuse, including current or past history of verbal, physical, or sexual abuse.
   b. Nutritional history:
      (1) Calcium, vitamin D, fruit, vegetable, protein, carbohydrate intake including fiber, junk food, high fat, types of fat, omega-3 fatty acid intake, alcohol, soda, artificial sweeteners, herbal preparations, and vitamins.

    c. Lifestyle:

       (1) Exercise, sleep, work, recreation, stressors, spirituality, complementary and alternative therapies and network of family and friends.

  9. Family history:

    a. Age of menopause in female relatives such as mother, older sisters, and aunts.

    b. Osteoporosis, heart disease, cancers, Alzheimer's disease, coagulopathies, and other significant conditions.

10. Review of system update with focus on menopausal health concerns.

11. Diagnostic and laboratory testing.

    a. Note: Menopause is a clinical diagnosis based on cessation of menses for 12 months (FMP). Laboratory confirmation is unnecessary unless natural menses is interrupted by hormonal contraceptives.

    b. Hormonal evaluation:

       (1) FSH is recommended if using hormonal contraceptives that interfere with normal menses. Test day 7 of pill-free interval. If results unclear, repeat 1 month after discontinuing contraceptive.

       (2) Recommend condom use until lab results are known.

       (3) FSH > 30 mIU/mL suggests menopause.
           • Not necessary to diagnose menopause.

       (4) Effective contraception should be used for an additional 12 months at which point FSH should be repeated. If still elevated then contraception may be discontinued and the patient is considered menopausal.

       (5) Estradiol < 20 pg/mL suggests menopause.
           • Not necessary to diagnose menopause.

       (6) Testosterone.
           • Indicated if rapidly virilizing symptoms, or suspected tumor, or pathology.
           • Not indicated for routine menopausal screening or for low libido.

    c. Routine diagnostic tests.

       (1) Fasting lipid profile.

       (2) Pap test (Until age 65 if not risk factors).

       (3) Thyroid testing.

       (4) Blood glucose.

       (5) Urine screening.

Modifiable Lifestyle-Related Risk Factors   **BOX 22.5**

- Weight gain
- Substance use and abuse
- Cigarette smoking
- Caffeine intake
- Alcohol consumption
- Prescription drug abuse
- Lack of exercise
- Sleep problems
- Stress
- Suboptimal nutrition
- Abuse (physical, sexual, mental)

---

    d. Age and risk-related screenings.
       (1) Bone density.
       (2) Mammogram.
       (3) Skin assessment.
       (4) Colon cancer screening.
       (5) Appropriate cultures or smears with suspicion of infection.
       (6) Glaucoma.
       (7) Hearing testing.
    e. Other testing as appropriate for the evaluation of health concerns.
       (1) Endometrial biopsy if irregular menses and heavy bleeding should occur, particularly if it has been more than a year since last menses (see chapter 33).
    f. Screening for risk factors (see Box 22.5).
       (1) Has C-reactive protein.
       (2) Homocysteine.
       (3) Lipoprotein.
D. Physical examination of the menopausal patient.
    1. Height.
    2. Weight and BMI (refer to chapter 8, Assessment of Obesity for chart).
    3. Blood Pressure.
    4. HEENT (head, eye, ear, nose, and throat).
    5. Lungs.
    6. Cardiac/neck for carotids/extremity pulse evaluation.
    7. Breast exam.
    8. Abdomen.

  a. Note tenderness, rebound, and other abnormalities.
9. Pelvic examination.
   a. External genitalia.
      (1) Thinning and/or graying of hair, loss of landmarks, tissue pallor, erythema, lesions, fissures, tenderness, urethral caruncle (see chapter 24, Pelvic Organ Prolapse), introital shrinkage or laxity, cystocele, and rectocele.
   b. Vagina (see Unit 6, chapter 23, Atrophic Vaginitis).
      (1) Introital laxity and loss of tone with Kegel and Valsalva maneuver (note cyctocele, rectocele, and grade of condition; see chapter 24).
      (2) Erythema, pallor, flattening of rugae, abnormal discharge (scant to variable), infection, lesions, shortening of vagina, loss of elasticity, and tenderness.
   c. Cervix.
      (1) Erythema, lesions, friability, bleeding, tenderness, flattening, and shortening, and stenosis of cervical os (small).
   d. Uterus.
      (1) Size, shape, especially asymmetry (associated with fibroids that usually shrink in menopause), diffuse enlargement associated with pregnancy or pathology such as hyperplasia, tenderness, sometimes fibroids, etc.
   e. Pelvic floor.
      (1) Note cystocele, rectocele, introital tone with Kegel and Valsalva maneuver (see chapter 24).
   f. Ovaries.
      (1) In menopause, ovaries should not be palpable.
      (2) If ovaries are palpable a work-up is indicated.
10. Colorectal evaluation.
    a. Rectocele, lesions, hemorrhoids, bleeding, tarry stools, guaiac testing.
11. Extremities.
    a. Including feet.
12. Skin.
    a. Note new or changing lesions.
    b. Evaluate yearly, especially with a history of excessive sun exposure.

CHAPTER 23

Atrophic Vaginitis

Mimi Clarke Secor

I. **Atrophic vaginitis explained.**
   A. Statistics.
      1. Statistics indicate that 45 million women are menopausal and that this number is growing as baby boomers reach menopause and beyond.
      2. Three years after the onset of menopause, almost 50% of women will experience vaginal dryness.
   B. Some facts.
      1. Symptoms of atrophic vaginitis are commonly associated with menopause as estrogen levels drop causing thinning of the vulvovaginal epithelium.
      2. Urogenital atrophy is the most inevitable consequence of menopause.
      3. Atrophic changes are reversible with the estrogen therapy.
      4. Conditions associated with low estrogen are summarized in Box 23.1.

II. **Pathophysiology.**
   A. Urogenital changes occur during perimenopause, often well in advance of cessation of menses. Vaginal mucosal tissues contain many estrogen receptors which are commonly affected by reductions in estrogen.
   B. As the wall of the vagina become thin, there is a decrease in the

---

| *Causes of Urogenital Atrophy* | **BOX 23.1** |

Antiestrogen medications
- Lupron
- Clomid
- Provera
- Synarel
- Nolvadex
- Danocrine

Postpartum   Absence of placental estrogen

Breastfeeding   Antagonistic action of prolactin on estrogen

Premenopausal   Premature ovarian failure

Extraneous causes
- Surgery (oophorectomy)
- Chemotherapy
- Radiation
- Menopause

Other milder forms
- Heavy smoking (reduced estrogen absorption)
- Reduced sexual activity
- Inadequate systemic estrogen replacement therapy

---

support for the pelvic organs and the muscles that are adjacent to it.

C. The drop in estrogen causes a decrease in glycogen reducing lactobacilli which leads to an increase in vaginal pH (from acid to alkaline). This often leads to overgrowth of various pathogenic bacteria such as Gardnerella vaginalis, mycoplasma, streptococci, and others (see Figure 23.1).

D. Reduced estrogen may also result in a reduced blood flow, loss of collagen, elasticity, and muscle tone. Thinning of the urogenital epithelium or atrophism leads to various symptoms associated with atrophic vaginitis including dyspareunia and pruritus.

E. Similar tissue changes may also occur in the urinary tract contributing to dysuria, incontinence, urinary frequency, and increased risk of urinary tract infections.

F. Symptoms and signs of genitourinary atrophy may develop slowly, over many months or years, or may have a more rapid onset.

G. Symptoms vary and are affected by many factors such as an individual's estrogen levels and response to these levels.

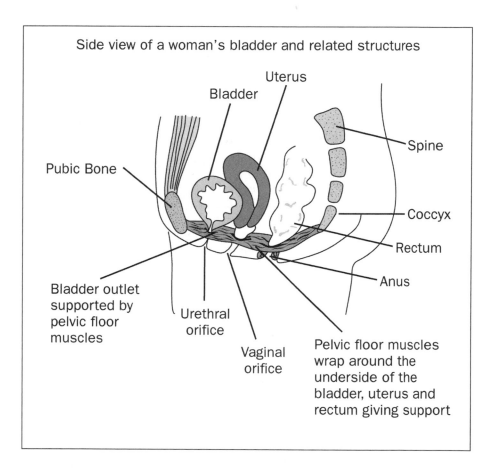

Figure 23.1 Side view of bladder and related structures.

III. Indications for evaluation.

A. The complaint of urogential symptoms is an indication for a thorough work-up.

IV. Assessment.

A. A history of symptoms may include the following:

  1. Vulvovaginal symptoms.

     a. Vulvar dryness, lack of lubrication, pruritus, irritation, and vaginal discharge.

  2. Vaginal bleeding.

     a. Due to tissue thinning and friability, vaginal spotting is of-

ten the first symptom a patient presents with. The source
of bleeding must be determined and if necessary, a biopsy
and/or ultrasound should be performed.
   b. Bleeding may be noticed after sex or after wiping with toilet tissue.
3. Dyspareunia.
   a. Also known as painful intercourse, this condition may result from stretching or tearing of the thin narrowed introital mucosa, or from stretching of the dry, less elastic, shorter vagina causing dyspareunia.
   b. These changes are less likely to occur if sexual relations are maintained during perimenopause and beyond (the "use it or lose it" phenomenon).
4. Low libido and other sexual complaints such as lack of lubrication, dyspareunia, and distress related to atrophic and/or sexual complaints.
5. Urinary symptoms.
   a. The lower urinary tract and pelvic musculature are under the influence of estrogen and share a common embryologic origin with the vagina.
   b. Squamous epithelium of the trigone and urethra thin and blood flow decreases.
   c. Urinary symptoms related to low estrogen levels include dysuria, hematuria, frequency, nocturia, urinary incontinence (usually stress type), sensation of a dropped bladder, and history of frequent urinary tract infections.
6. Hematuria is commonly associated with atrophism and must be thoroughly evaluated as it can, uncommonly, be a symptom of bladder cancer.
B. Gynecologic history may include:
1. Menstrual history including LMP, FMP, abnormal bleeding, history of hot flashes, night sweats, or flushing.
2. Age of biologic mother or sisters at menopause.
3. Date of last Papanicolaou test (Pap test), results, history of abnormal Pap, and management.
4. Sexual history including dyspareunia, dryness, sexual partner (gender), date of last sex, use of lubricants, distress related to symptoms.
5. Total hysterectomy is associated with atrophic vaginitis and symptoms may be severe due to the sudden reduction in estrogen levels.

V. **Medical, surgical, and family history, lifestyle, medications including use of AV (vaginal estrogen) over-the-counter preparations. (Box 23.2 summarizes the characteristic symptoms of AV.)**
   A. External genitalia exam.
      1. Note thinning of hair and tissues, pallor, erythema, lesions, fissures, loss of architectural landmarks, introital shrinkage, vulvar atrophy, pallor, erythema (diffuse versus focal), and tenderness.
      2. Vulvar dryness and/or positive "sticky glove sign," which occurs when the examiner's glove adheres temporarily and is thought to be diagnostic for atrophic vaginitis.
      3. Urethral caruncle.
         a. Small friable polyp of urethral mucosa which protrudes from the inferior border of the urethral meatus (Figure 23.2).
         b. Associated with symptoms of dysuria, frequency, and may be the cause of vaginal bleeding in the menopausal woman.
   B. Vaginal exam.
      1. Cystocele, rectocele, and grade (see Unit 7, chapter 24).
      2. Introital laxity, tension, loss of tone with Kegels, or Valsalva maneuver.
      3. Tenderness with palpation or during speculum insertion and/or exam.
      4. Note vaginal pallor, erythema, loss of rugae (flattening), lesions, shortening of vagina, loss of elasticity, tenderness.
      5. Discharge; which may range from scant to copious, be variable in quality ranging from thin white to thick, yellow/green and malordorous.
      6. Abnormal discharge may mimic trichomoniasis or other STI associated discharge.
      7. Cervix.
         a. Erythema, lesions, friability, bleeding, tenderness, flattening and shortening, stenosis of cervical os (small).
   C. Bimanual exam.
      1. Uterus.
         a. Size, shape especially asymmetry (associated with fibroids that usually shrink in menopause), diffuse enlargement associated with pregnancy or pathology such as hyperplasia, tenderness, sometimes fibroids, etc.
      2. Pelvic floor (see chapter 24).

Summary of Characteristics of Urogenital Atrophy

BOX 23.2

Labia (majora and minora)

- Less prominent, flattened
- Fusion of labia minora
- Lax and wrinkled (lack of subcutaneous fat)
- Thinning cell layer
- Prominent sebaceous glands
- Positive sticky glove sign
- Easily traumatized (fissures, excoriations)
- Irritation due to continuous use of pad for urinary incontinence

Clitoris

- Less prominent
- Retracts beneath the prepuce
- Slight atrophy

Subcutaneous fat

- Diminished

Pubic hair

- Thins
- Less coarse

Vaginal wall epithelium

- Thin (a few layers thick)
- Friable
- Shiny
- Small ulcerations
- Patches of granulation tissue
- Petechial spots (resemble trichomoniasis)
- Fissures
- Ecchymotic areas from exposed capillaries
- Loss of rugae
- Decreased vascularity (pale)
- Less lubrication (dryness)
- Loss of distensibility, elasticity
- Decreased discharge

Vagina

- Introital stenosis (< two fingers)
- Shortened
- Shrinkage of fornices
- Less elasticity
- Possible cystocele, rectocele or pelvic prolapse

Box 23.2 *(continued)*

Discharge

- Variable
- Watery to thick and cloudy
- May be serosanguineous from friable surfaces

Maturation Index

- Preponderance of parabasal cells

Cervix

- Shrinks, flattens into vaginal wall
- Os becomes tiny
- Squamo-columnar junction recedes up the cervical canal
- Atrophied crypts and ducts in canal

Uterus

- Smaller
- Endometrium thins—less glandular, atrophic
- Uterine stripe < 4mm
- Fibroids may shrink

Perineum

- Minor laceration at the posterior fourchette

Urethra

- Caruncle—red, berry-type protrusion
- Atrophy
- Polyps
- Prolapse/eversion of urethral mucosa

Pelvic Floor

- Muscle tone diminishes
- Cystocele
- Rectocele

Ligaments and connective tissue

- Lose strength and tone

Bladder mucosa and urethra

- Decreased tone

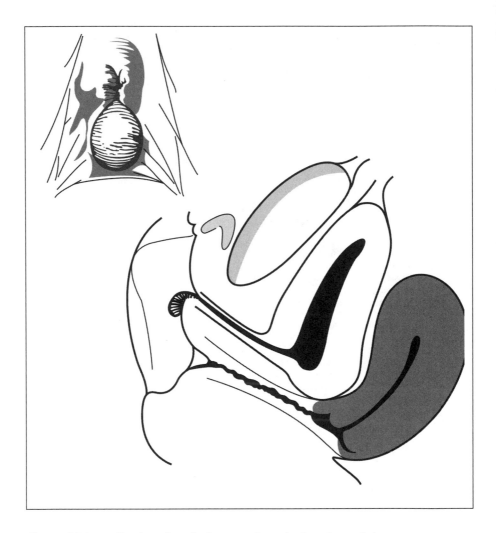

Figure 23.2 Small polyp of urethral mucosa in sagittal section and shown protruding from the inferior border of the urethral meatus.

        a. Note cystocele, rectocele, introital tone with Kegels, and Valsalva maneuver.
    3. Ovaries.
        a. In menopause, ovaries should not be palpable.
        b. If ovaries are palpable, a work-up is indicated.
VI. Diagnostic testing and differential diagnosis.
    A. Differential considerations (Table 23.1).

Table 23.1 **Differential Considerations in the Diagnosis of Atrophic Vaginitis**

Differential	pH	KOH	Microscopy
Atrophic vaginitis	≥ 5.0	Negative	Few LB, WBCs variable, Immature Epithelial Cells (ECs)
Trichomoniasis	≥ 5.0	Negative	Trich, WBCs, Immature ECs, Few LB
BV	≥ 4.7	Positive	Clue cells, few WBCs, few LB
Intermediate Flora	± normal	± positive	Grainy epithelial cells, reduced LB

Factors That Affect Vaginal pH   **BOX 23.3**

- Menses (pH 7.2)
- Semen (pH > 7)
- Cervical mucus, because it is alkaline
- Lubricant from speculum
- Intravaginal medications
- Lubricating jelly
- Tap water

---

1. Vaginal pH.
   a. Atrophic vaginitis is associated with a significantly elevated vaginal pH, usually above 5.
      (1) A normal vaginal pH (4.0 to 4.5) indicates normal circulating estrogen levels and rules out atrophic vaginitis.
      (2) A high pH is due to the lack of lactobacilli which make lactic acid.
   b. Many factors can alter the pH results (Box 23.3).
2. Amine testing with potassium hydroxide (KOH).
   a. If negative, BV (bacterial vaginosis) is unlikely, and atrophic vaginitis is possible, especially if vaginal pH is also elevated.
3. Vaginal microscopy (see chapter 10).
   a. Note reduced or absent lactobacilli (LB).
   b. Note immature epithelial cells indicating low estrogen.

    c. Rule out trichomoniasis. If microscopy is equivocal for the identification of trichomoniasis, a trich culture should be done. Trichomoniasis may be asymptomatic for decades reactivating in perimenopause or postmenopause. The clinical presentation may mimic that of atrophic vaginitis.

    d. Rule out genital herpes with herpes select serology IGG type 2 testing. HSV 2 (herpes simplex virus) may be latent and/or asymptomatic for decades, activating in perimenopause or menopause. Genital HSV 2 is very common, and prevalence increases with age, affecting 1 out of 3 women over 30 years of age. Adding to the diagnostic challenge most clinical presentations are atypical, further evading easy diagnosis.

    e. If WBCs (white blood cells), this is most likely related to atrophic effects resulting in secondary vaginal infection, which will resolve when local estrogen is administered and maintained. Initial treatment daily for 2 to 6 weeks, then may be tapered to 2 to 3 times a week depending on patient response. If symptoms recur, frequency of treatment may need to be increased to daily, then gradually decreased again after 2 to 6 weeks of daily treatment.

    f. STIs must be ruled out (chapter 21), especially if WBCs are noted. STIs are increasing in older adults, so to assess risk, consider clinical assessment (history and exam) and age of sexual partners.

  4. The "Maturation Index."

    a. The presence of estrogen promotes the maturation of the cells lining the vaginal mucosa.

    b. The "Maturation Index" monitors the differentiation of the immature squamous cells toward their most evolved forms, from parabasal to intermediate cells, to the mature superficial cells, each representing a cellular layer (Figure 23.3).

    c. Sample is obtained by scraping the lateral wall of the vagina.

    d. The index represents the relative number of each kind of cell per hundred cells counted. (See Box 23.4, which compares the type of cell in each cell layer.)

    e. Expressed in a ratio of parabasal to intermediate to superficial cells and read from "left to right."

      (1) 0:0:100—superficial cells—well estrogenized because there are all superficial cells present.

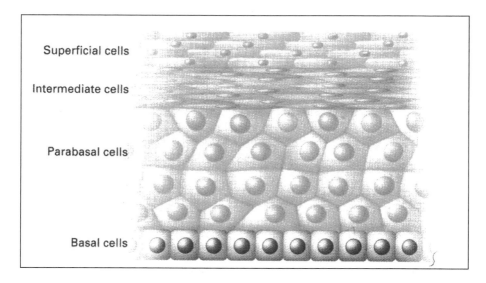

Figure 23.3 Layers of the vaginal epithelium.

Comparison of the Squamous Epithelial Cells of the Vagina	BOX 23.4
Parabasal	Lower layer
	Smaller, round cells with large nuclei comprising 50% to 75% of the total cell size
	Sparse cytoplasm
Intermediate	Middle layer
	Smaller nuclei with round cell
Superficial	Surface layer
	Small nuclei with rectangular cell membrane
	Nucleus comprises only 10% to 20% of the cell
	Abundant cytoplasm

(2) 0:100:0—intermediate cell atrophy—minimal atrophic vaginitis.

(3) 100:0:0—parabasal cell atrophy—marked atrophic vaginitis because there are no mature epithelial cells, only parabasal cells.

(4) Note: The presence of any parabasal cells on a wet mount may be considered documentation of atrophic vaginitis.

5. Endometrial biopsy, colposcopy (based on Pap and HPV results) and possibly an ultrasound should be considered for abnormal vaginal bleeding.

VII. Treatment considerations.

A. Local estrogen is preferred to systemic estrogen as it is more effective for the treatment of atrophic vaginitis and is thought to be safer due to lower systemic absorption compared to oral administration.

B. Systemic estrogen is not recommended for treatment of atrophic symptoms and if it is given for VMS (vasomotor symptoms) additional local estrogen may be necessary to adequately treat atrophic symptoms.

C. Only the intravaginal estrogen "FemRing" is effective for the treatment of both hot flashes and atrophic vaginitis.

D. Local estrogen therapy starts with daily intravaginal treatment for 2 to 4 weeks then may be tapered to three times weekly then twice a week as needed.

E. Applying a small pea-sized amount of local estrogen cream to the introital area may relieve dyspareunia. Daily application is recommended initially, then three or two times weekly as needed.

F. Less effective than estrogen, non-prescription over-the-counter (OTC) lubricants may help relieve dyspareunia and vaginal dryness.

G. If BV is present with atrophic vaginitis, either local estrogen alone may be used, or BV may be treated followed by treatment with local estrogen. If estrogen has been stopped and BV recurs, local estrogen should be restarted and used for a longer term to prevent BV. Estrogen supports the regrowth and maintenance of lactobacilli, which is thought to be protective against recurrent BV.

H. If vulvar skin lesions do not resolve within 6 weeks, a skin biopsy should be considered (see chapter 32).

VIII. Follow-up.

A. Follow-up visits may range from 2 weeks to 3 months based on the patient's problems, response to therapy, and clinician/patient preference.

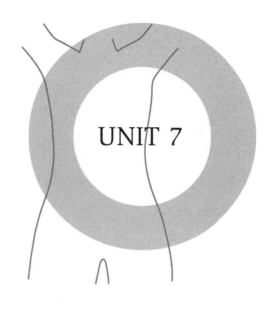

UNIT 7

Evaluation of the Pelvic Floor

CHAPTER 24

Pelvic Organ Prolapse

Helen A. Carcio

I. **Pelvic organ prolapse explained.**
  A. The pelvis lies at the bottom of the abdominopelvic cavity.
    1. It forms a supportive layer that prevents the pelvic organs from falling through the bony pelvis.
    2. It supports conception and parturition.
    3. It controls storage and evacuation of feces and urine.
  B. Mechanical principles in relation to prolapse of pelvic organs.
    1. The uterus and vagina lie suspended in a slinglike network of ligaments and fascial structures attached to the side walls of the pelvis.
    2. Levator ani muscles constrict forming an occlusive layer on which the pelvic organs may rest.
      a. They consist of strong striated muscle tissue, comprising the iliococcygeus, the pubococcygeus, and the puborectalis (Figure 24.1).
      b. They compress the rectum, vagina, and urethra against the pubic bone, holding them in position.
    3. As long as the pelvic floor musculature functions normally, the pelvic floor is closed and the ligaments and fascia are under no tension.
    4. Problems exist when the pelvic floor muscles relax or are damaged. Risk factors are listed in Box 24.1.
      a. The pelvic floor opens, and the vagina lies between the

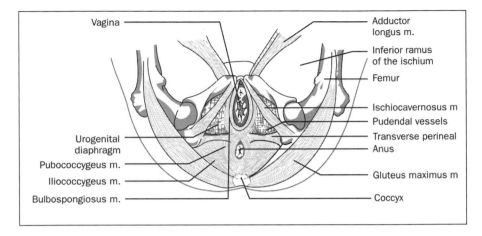

Figure 24.1 Muscles of the pelvic floor.

Risk Factors for the Development of Pelvic Floor Relaxation

- Chronic cough (due to asthma or chronic bronchitis)
- Heavy lifting (prolonged)
- High impact sports
- Obesity
- Pelvic malignancy
- High parity
- White skin color (higher incidence in this population)
- Large uterine or ovarian masses
- Advancing age (estrogen deficiency)
- History of traumatic birth
- Genetic predisposition (less collagen support)
- Previous pelvic or vaginal irradiation
- Multiple antiincontinence procedures
- Metabolic diseases that affect muscle function
- Failure to reattach the cardinal ligaments at hysterectomy
- Decreased pelvic muscle strength

high intraabdominal pressure and the low atmospheric pressure, where it must be held in place by ligaments.
b. Eventually, connective tissue will become damaged and fail to hold the vagina in place.

5. The increase in intra-abdominal pressure placed on the pelvic floor muscles and ligaments causes the development of a prolapse, rather than problems with the organs themselves.

C. Urinary continence.
   1. Depends on support of the urethra.
      a. Fascial structures supporting the urethra at the vesical neck.
      b. Active muscle contraction.
      c. Intact neuromuscular mechanisms.
   2. Ability of the urethra to remain closed.
   3. Note: Closure pressure of urethra must equal or exceed intravesical pressure.

D. Several factors influence the development of genital prolapse and urinary incontinence.

II. Diagnosis of pelvic organ prolapse.

A. The pelvic examination.
   1. Be sensitive to the fact that many of these women may be older and may not have had a pelvic examination in many years.
   2. They may have suffered for months or even years with symptoms and be anxious concerning the cause.
   3. If stress incontinence is present, the woman may be fearful that she will leak during the examination.
   4. It takes a while to develop assessment skills to diagnose correctly the type and extent of a prolapse. It is a good idea to examine all patients for a prolapse, regardless of whether or not they are symptomatic, in order to compare normal and abnormal findings.
   5. Reassure the patient that although pelvic relaxation is slowly progressive, it is unlikely to affect longevity.
   6. The clinician may use a hand-held mirror to explain pelvic findings.

B. Position.
   1. Place the patient in a comfortable lithotomy position, with her feet in the stirrups (may be difficult for older women).
   2. She may have to stand and bear down at some point in the examination.
   3. Drape the patient appropriately.

C. Vital steps in correctly diagnosing a prolapse.
   1. The examination must be made with the woman pushing down, as though she is straining at stool; the entire extent of the prolapse must be seen.

Table 24.1   **Grading Prolapse of the Uterus**

Degree	Description
Stage 1	Slight to moderate uterine descent with cervix still inside vagina to any distal point 1 cm above the hymen
Stage 2	Uterine descent to 1 cm above or below the hymen
Stage 3	Descent of uterus to a point beyond 1 cm distal to the hymen
Stage 4	Total eversion

  a. Sometimes, women are reluctant to follow through with this part of the examination because they are afraid that they may leak or pass flatus, which would be very embarrassing to them.
  b. It is useful to acknowledge what might occur and let the patient know that it is okay.
  c. It may be difficult to exert enough pressure in the lithotomy position; the clinician may have to ask the woman to stand and bear down while examining her.
  2. The clinician must examine each different structure independently.
D. Once the prolapse is visible, other structures need to be systematically assessed.
  1. Focus on the specific defects.
  2. Note the severity of the prolapse.
E. Identify the extent that the vaginal wall, cervix, and posterior walls have descended.
  1. Examine the anterior and posterior walls by retracting the opposite wall with the posterior half of a vaginal speculum so that a larger cystocele does not obscure a smaller rectocele.
F. Classification of the severity of a prolapse.
  1. Grading systems are varied and very subjective. Table 24.1 lists one form of classification.
  2. It is best to describe the size of a prolapse in terms of the distance the prolapse descends below or rises above the hymenal ring with the prolapse extended to its fullest. (e.g., "The cervix lies 2 cm below the hymenal ring.")
  3. Describe the diameter of the prolapse to help assist in assessing the severity. The greater the diameter, the more severe the prolapse.

    4. Types of prolapse.
        a. First-degree prolapse is without symptoms and is mildly descended.
        b. Second-degree prolapse is halfway into the vagina and is usually asymptomatic.
        c. Third-degree prolapse is at the level of the introitus and is usually symptomatic.
        d. Fourth-degree prolapse is out of the vagina, even at rest. Symptoms are severe.
G. Evaluating anterior wall support.
    1. Establishes status of urethral and bladder support.
    2. Urethra is fused with the lower 3 to 4 cm of the vaginal wall.
    3. Urethrocele.
        a. Diagnosed by descent of the lower anterior vaginal wall to the level of the hymenal ring during straining.
        b. Seen as a herniation between the urethra and vagina, as the urethra prolapses into the anterior vaginal vault, out of the correct angle with the bladder.
        c. Usually associated with stress incontinence and loss of urethral support.
        d. Often occurs with a cystocele.
        e. Difficult to grade.
        f. By itself, it is not usually an indication for use of a pessary.
    4. Cystocele.
        a. Defective support of the upper portion of the anterior vaginal wall or stretching of the vesicovaginal fascia because the bladder lies adjacent to this portion of the vaginal wall (Figure 24.2).
        b. Herniation occurring between the bladder and the vagina, with descent of a portion of the common wall between these structures.
        c. Occurs gradually with stretching, increased bladder capacity, and development of atrophic vulvovaginitis.
    5. Cystourethrocele—defective support of the entire anterior wall which is often manifested by descent below the hymenal ring, whether or not stress incontinence is present.
    6. Must include direct observation of the urethra while coughing in supine and standing positions.
H. Determine the position of the uterus and vagina.

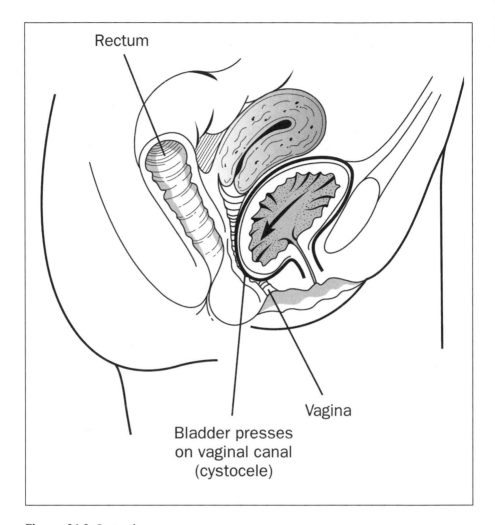

Figure 24.2 Cystocele.

1. Vagina and cervix are fused with one another.
2. If the cervix prolapses downward it brings the upper vagina along with it.
3. May be caused by:
   a. Stretching of the uterosacral and cardinal ligaments.
   b. Lacerations or damage to the levator ani and perineal body.

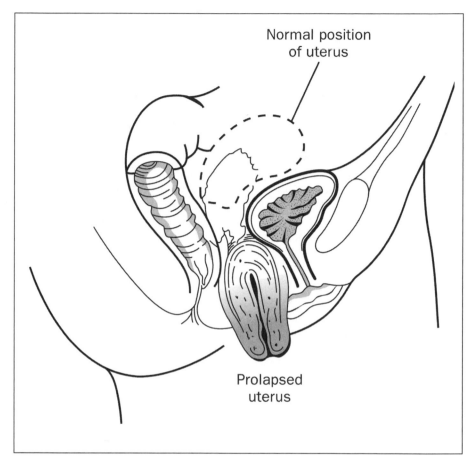

Figure 24.3 Prolapse of uterus compared to normal uterus position.

    4. Prolapse (or procidentia).
      a. Descent of the uterus below its normal level.
      b. As support of ligaments give way, the uterus moves backward to a retroverted or retroflexed position.
      c. Round ligaments stretch, failing to hold the body of the uterus in the anteverted position.
      d. Uterus next aligns itself with the long axis of the vagina.
      e. An increase in intra-abdominal pressure causes the uterus to descend down the vaginal canal (similar to the action of a piston in a cylinder) (Figure 24.3).

  5. Measured by the location of the cervix relative to the hymenal ring.
     a. Important. Cervix may not be visible behind a cystocele or rectocele and must be palpated as the patient bears down.
     b. May also test the extent to which the cervix and uterus descend by either of the following methods:
        (1) Have the patient stand. Using a mirror placed between her legs, have her observe for descent, as she is asked to bear down.
        (2) Grasp the cervix with a tenaculum to assess, while gently pulling the cervix toward the vaginal opening. (This is certainly the more invasive maneuver.)
     c. If the cervix descends to within 1 cm of the hymenal ring, there is considerable loss of support. Cervical elongation is common in women with a prolapse.
  I. Posterior vaginal wall.
     1. Rectocele (see Figure 24.4).
        a. Protrusion of the anterior rectal wall and posterior wall of the overlying vagina.
        b. May protrude below the hymenal ring to form a bulging mass originating from the posterior vaginal wall, causing the anterior rectal wall to balloon down through the vaginal ring.
        c. Causes.
           (1) Disruption of the rectovaginal fascia during childbirth.
           (2) Chronic fecal constipation and straining.
     2. Enterocele.
        a. The cul-de-sac becomes distended with intestine, and bulges the posterior vaginal wall outward.
        b. Hernia of the fascia of the posterior vagina above the rectovaginal septum and below the cervix.
        c. Sometimes mistaken for a rectocele.
        d. A large enterocele may protrude through the vagina.
        e. Requires correction only if symptomatic.

III. **The diagnosis.**
   A. Assess pelvic muscle tone.
      1. Ask patient to squeeze around your two examining fingers while palpating the levator ani muscle (Table 24.2).
      2. Note the patient's ability to sustain constriction and deflection of finger or fingers upward with a good squeeze. No deflection indicates weaker muscles.

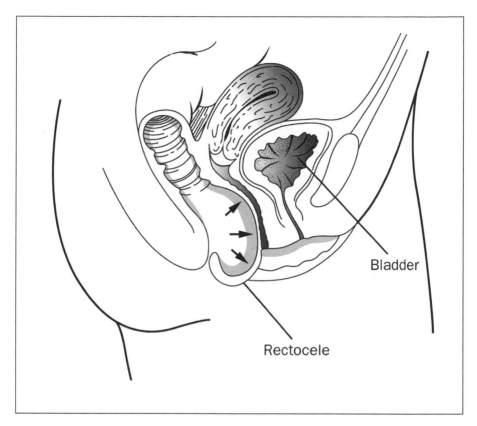

Figure 24.4 Rectocele (sagittal section showing relative position of uterus and bladder).

Table 24.2   **Assessment of Pelvic Muscle Strength**

	0	1	2	3
Pressure	None	Weak	Moderate	Strong—fingers compressed
Duration	None	Less than 1 second	1 to 3 seconds	More than 3 seconds
Displacement	None	Slight incline	Noticeable incline	Fingers drawn in

3. Constriction lasting a few seconds indicates weakening.
4. Stress incontinence protocol.

B. Provocative stress test.
   1. Ask the patient, when she has a full bladder, to stand and cough.
   2. Observe for small spurts of urine that escape simultaneously with each cough. (May place pad between legs to catch and observe any urine released.)
   3. If urine escapes, place one finger on either side of the urethra.
   4. Ask the patient to cough again.
   5. If there is no loss of urine during the cough, the test is considered positive for stress urinary incontinence.

C. Assess the neuronal support to the sacral dermatone, S2, S3, and S4.
   These dermatones innervate the micturation reflex.
   1. Lightly stroke the skin area innervated by the dermatones.
      a. Note response to light touch.
      b. Compare contralateral sides.
   2. Bulbocavernosus reflex.
      a. Stroke or gently squeeze the clitoris.
      b. Note contraction of the bulbocavernous muscle around the clitoris.
   3. Anal reflex (so-called anal wink).
      a. Lightly stroke the skin lateral to the anus.
      b. Note contraction of the anal sphincter.

D. The cotton-tipped swab (Q-tip) test (see chapter 25).

E. Digital rectal examination.
   1. Assess for any fecal impaction.
   2. Note sphincter muscle tone.

F. Assess vulvovaginal area for estrogen status (see also chapter 23).
   1. Observe the vagina for the presence of rugae, degree of moistness, and color.
      a. These features decrease during menopause.
   2. Estrogen status of the vulva and vaginal is important.
      a. The presence of mature squamous epithelium indicates good estrogen nourishment.
      b. Estrogen thickens the layers of the vaginal wall, enhancing support of the bladder and rectum.

G. May refer the patient for a cystometrogram or urodynamic techniques.

       1. To assess for detrusor instability before surgery.

       2. To evaluate symptoms to determine need for anticholinergic medications.

  H. Assessment of urinary symptoms.

       1. Determine postvoid residual if any retention is suspected.

          a. Should be less than 200 ml.

          b. Culture, if pyuria is present.

       2. Urinalysis (see chapter 11).

  I. Referral as surgical candidates.

       1. Based on the particular situation and symptoms of the woman depending on:

          a. Size of the prolapse.

          b. Degree of symptoms.

          c. Any related physiologic complications.

          d. Patient's feelings and attitudes toward pessary or surgery.

IV. Symptoms of anterior wall prolapse and uterine prolapse. Note: Symptoms increase with advancing age and tissue atrophy during the postmenopausal years.

  A. Prolapse.

       1. Dragging sensation.

          a. Usually occurring in the groin and sacral and lumbar area.

          b. Caused by downward force on the uterosacral ligaments and fasciae that support the uterus and vagina.

          c. Discomfort improves when the woman lies flat, relieving the downward pressure.

       2. Sensation of peritoneal wetness probably caused by protrusion of moist vaginal walls rather than leakage of urine.

       3. The patient may complain of a sense of things falling out after prolonged standing.

       4. The patient may notice a mass protruding from her vagina, particularly after bearing down, heavy lifting, or prolonged standing.

       5. Erosions or ulceration of any mass that has protruded.

       6. Dyspareunia.

  B. Cystocele.

       1. Stress urinary incontinence caused by loss of urethral support of the lower vaginal wall.

       2. Difficulty emptying the bladder caused by loss of support of the upper anterior vaginal wall and bladder.

       3. Urinary urgency and frequency probably due to stretching of

the bladder base associated with the prolapse, which is often less pronounced when patient is supine.

4. Development of recurrent cystitis or a stone from stagnant urine if residual urine occurs.

C. Stress incontinence.

1. Occurs when intravesical pressure exceeds the maximum urethral closure pressure, in the absence of detrusor muscle contraction.

   a. Normally, the sphincter at the upper urethra is able to withhold urine.

   b. Inability of the sphincter to withstand increased pressure is caused by:

      (1) Changes in the angle of the bladder.

      (2) Anatomic descent of the proximal urethra.

      (3) Failure of the neuromuscular support.

      (4) Inability of sphincter to resist increased abdominal pressure, resulting in uncontrolled expulsion of urine.

2. Loss of support may also cause descent of the bladder neck, with the internal sphincter opening prematurely without voluntary compensation by the muscle surrounding it.

3. Often results from injury to the vesicourethral structure during childbirth.

4. The condition is defined as the involuntary loss of urine with a sudden increase in intra-abdominal pressure from physical activity, laughing, lifting, aerobics, coughing, or sneezing.

5. Often leaks only small amounts.

6. Need to rule out acute causes such as:

   a. Urinary tract infection (usually associated with dysuria, urgency, and frequency).

   b. Atrophic vaginitis (may be present but may not be cause of the incontinence).

   c. Dietary irritants such as coffee, aspartame (Nutrasweet), and alcohol.

   d. Medications such as doxazosin (Cardura).

   e. Diabetes (mellitus or insipidus).

   f. Pelvic mass pressing against the bladder or urethra.

   g. Chronic urethritis.

7. Urgency, frequency, nocturia, and dysuria do not usually occur.

8. Assess for other types of urinary incontinence or mixed disorders.

D. Rectocele.
   1. Feeling of rectal or pelvic pressure.
   2. Difficulty in emptying the rectum.
   3. Stool fills the rectocele the harder the patient strains.
   4. Must differentiate between true constipation (common in older women) and symptoms of a rectocele.
   5. A woman may state that she has to press between the vagina and rectum (to reduce the rectocele) or press in the vagina to help with defecation; further supports the diagnosis.

V. Pessary.
   A. Historical perspectives.
   1. Pessaries frequently appear in both Greek and Latin literature.
   2. The term usually refers to a mechanical device such as a ball, wool, or lint soaked in medicine. They were very dissimilar from the modern pessary. The earliest pessaries were stones.
   3. Most pessaries had string attachments to facilitate removal.
   4. More than 200 different types of pessaries have been used throughout history.
   5. Now pessaries are made of polyvinyl plastic or medical-grade silicone, replacing the traditional red rubber material.
      a. Nontoxic silicone does not absorb vaginal secretions or odors.
      b. Material is biologically inert; rare allergic reactions.
      c. This type of silicone material should not be confused with the silicone gel found in breast implants.
      d. The material can be autoclaved or boiled, or sterilized in Cidex.
   6. Ten to 20 years ago, use of the pessary was replaced by vaginal surgery.
   7. Pessaries are now increasing in use as baby boomers are aging and experiencing prolapse.
   8. The pessary offers a viable alternative to surgery.
   9. Different devices are often used to treat the same problem in different patients.
   10. The satisfaction rate with pessary use is high, with 72 to 95% reporting symptom relief.
   11. Pessary fittings and the device itself are reimbursed by Medicare.
   B. Purpose.
   1. To support the pelvic organs in close alignment to their

proper anatomic position in the treatment of second-through
fourth-degree prolapse.

2. To restore continence by stabilizing the bladder base.
3. To support an anterior-pointing cervix during pregnancy
   (Hodge pessary).
4. To support and correct retrodisplacement of the uterus in
   early pregnancy.
5. To provide an alternative treatment for women who are at a
   high risk for surgical repair of the prolapse.

C. Cornerstone of therapy for genital prolapse.
D. Proper management of a pessary is significantly less expensive
   and is safer than its surgical counterpart.
E. Goals.
   1. Can be used as a temporary measure for relief of symptoms
      while a patient delays surgery until a more opportune time,
      or until she decides whether to have surgery.
   2. Used as a permanent alternative to prolapse surgery, particu-
      larly in elderly women who are at surgical risk.
   3. Used as a diagnostic aid to determine whether there is relief
      of symptoms with prolapse replacement. It serves as a use-
      ful predictor of a successful outcome from surgical
      management.
      a. Can uncover urinary incontinence, which is masked by
         obstruction of the urinary outflow tract.
F. Some comments related to the role of the advanced practice
   clinician.
   1. When selecting a pessary, a clinician may be overwhelmed
      by the choices of pessary size and style, and may feel inse-
      cure regarding which to choose for which condition.
      a. The three or four sizes in the middle are most commonly
         used.
      b. Most pessary wearers do well with the most common
         sizes.
   2. Modern use is a function of the clinician's experience and
      training, along with the availability of the device.
   3. With knowledge and practice, an advanced practice clinician
      can become adept at fitting and caring for the supportive va-
      ginal pessary.
   4. As the elderly population increases, knowledge and skill in
      the use of pessaries in lieu of or as an adjunct to surgery
      should be considered.
   5. Most pessaries come with printed material from the manufac-

---

Reasons for Discontinuing Pessary Use   **BOX 24.2**

- Inconvenient to use
- Inadequate relief of symptoms
- Uncomfortable
- Elected for surgery
- Unable to remain in place
- Difficulty urinating
- Incontinence increased

---

turer that gives instructions regarding the insertion and care of a specific device.

6. Clinicians soon develop favorite types that they become familiar with.

G. Coitus.

1. Coitus is possible with many pessaries that are not vaginally occlusive.

2. The woman must have the dexterity to remove and reinsert the pessary.

3. Never assume that because a patient is elderly that she is not sexually active.

4. Sexual intercourse is not possible with the following types of pessaries:

   a. Gellhorn.

   b. Doughnut.

   c. Shatz.

5. The inflato ball and cube: Intercourse is not possible with them in place; however, because they need to be removed daily, intercourse can occur after removal.

H. Pessaries are available in various sizes, shapes, and materials.

I. Uterine prolapse is the most common gynecologic problem that is corrected by pessaries.

J. If a pessary is made of latex rubber, the clinician needs to determine if the woman has a sensitivity to latex before fitting.

K. Not all women can use a pessary. Box 24.2 lists reasons for discontinuing use of a pessary.

VI. **General principles for fitting a pessary.**

A. Some comments.

1. Pessaries are generally fit by trial and error.

2. The pessary retention test. Insert two fingers in vagina and extend to both fornices. With fingers thus extended, pull

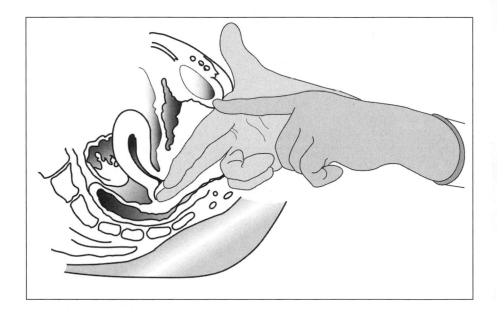

Figure 24.5 Measuring the vaginal canal for a pessary.

hand back through the introitus. If the fingers stay in the original extended position then it is unlikely that the woman will be able to retain a pessary because the vaginal introitus is too wide.

3. To measure for a pessary, once again insert the first two fingers deep into the vaginal canal. Fold thumb against the forefinger where it touches the introitus or use forefinger from other hand to measure. Withdraw hand and measure against the pessary or the fitting kit (Figure 24.5).

4. Inform the woman that two or three pessaries may be tried before proper fit is achieved.
   a. It may or may not be uncomfortable.
   b. Once the proper size is found the patient should be completely comfortable.

5. Have at least three sizes (often middle sizes) of a given pessary available during the fitting process.

6. A pessary fitting kit is available (Figure 24.6).

7. Many pessaries are difficult for the patient to remove and insert correctly, and she needs to receive routine follow-up care from her clinician.

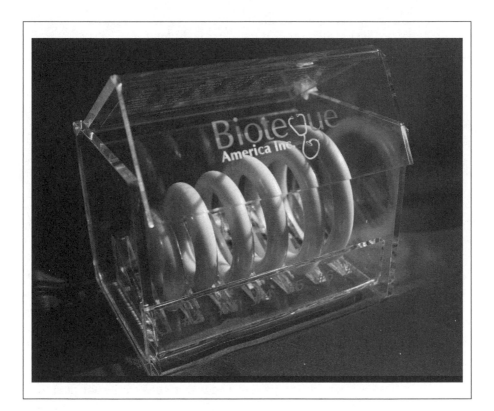

Figure 24.6 Pessary fitting kit.

8. Diaphragms are fit differently than most pessaries, except for the ring types.
   a. Ring types are fit in the same position; however, they have thicker rims.
   b. If diaphragm fitting rings are used, they will only give an approximation.
9. Inform the patient that it is not uncommon:
   a. To have to try a variety of pessaries during an initial fitting.
   b. To change the size on a subsequent visit (particularly after vaginal estrogenation).
10. Recommendations for follow-up vary. After initial visit, recommend:
    a. Routine return in 12 to 72 hours.
    b. Or return in 2 to 3 weeks.

    c. Must return sooner if:

      (1) Urination or defecation is difficult.

      (2) The pessary is uncomfortable in any way.

    d. Return visit is important to:

      (1) Recheck the size.

      (2) Question the patient regarding urination and defecation to assess status.

      (3) Observe for a tissue reaction such as discharge, irritation, or ulceration.

      (4) Reassure and support the woman.

      (5) Determine the presence of any discomfort. (If it is fit properly, the pessary should not be felt.)

11. Every woman with a pessary must be followed up closely by her clinician if she is not able to perform self-care.

    a. It is possible to forget or neglect a pessary. A list of pessary users within a given office must be kept and followed closely.

    b. Patient or clinician must routinely observe for any ulcerations or irritation from undue pressure (note, this is minimized by vaginal estrogen use).

    c. Return every 4 to 6 weeks (never more than 12 weeks) depending on individual considerations.

      (1) May alter follow-up plan. If odor develops at 12 weeks, the patient needs to return earlier for next visit.

      (2) Remember that a pessary is a foreign body and that there are limited nerve endings in the vagina and cervix. Therefore, a woman may not sense that any ulcerations are occurring.

12. A pessary should not be used in a noncompliant patient or a woman unable to care for herself unless her caregivers are well aware that the pessary is in place and that the patient will receive routine follow-up care.

13. Because many pessary users are elderly, it is important to keep in mind that a woman's status may change over the years (e.g., due to a stroke).

    a. Caregivers (such as nursing home personnel) may not be aware that a pessary is in place.

    b. A list should be kept with the expected routine for follow-up; contact the patient if visits are missed.

14. Estrogen therapy (see chapter 23).

    a. Recommend estrogen therapy, preferably via the vaginal

Contraindications to Pessary Use	BOX 24.3

- Active vaginitis
- Abnormal Pap smear
- Acute pelvic inflammatory disease
- Endometriosis (research varies)
- Noncompliant patient
- Woman with dementia without possibility of reasonable follow-up

route, 1 to 2 weeks before the necessary fitting in order to:

(1) Nourish the vaginal tissues.

(2) Mature squamous epithelial tissues.

(3) Increase pliability of submucosal connective tissue.

(4) Improve perineal muscle tone.

b. Routinely recommend as an adjunct to pessary use.

(1) May not be necessary in the postmenopausal woman receiving estrogen replacement therapy.

(2) May be in the form of estrogen cream, suppositories, or estradiol vaginal ring (Estring).

(3) If Estring is used, insert before the pessary and change every 3 months.

15. If any vaginal conditions are present:

a. Perform a wet mount and treat diagnosed condition.

b. If ulcerations are present, local estrogen therapy is recommended.

16. There are very few contraindications for pessary use (Box 24.3).

a. After seeing the various types of pessaries, some women have an aversion to such a "foreign-looking object" being inside of them.

b. Most patients view the pessary as a godsend.

17. Use the largest pessary a patient can accommodate comfortably.

18. Fit ring and lever pessaries snugly behind the symphysis pubis, posterior to the cervix.

19. If the pessary fits properly, the examiner should be able to sweep the tip of the finger around the pessary and the vaginal wall. This prevents the breakdown of tissue.

20. Many women who have had a hysterectomy are in need of a pessary.

        a. Although most pessaries fit up against the cervix, a cervix is not necessary to anchor the pessary.

        b. The vaginal wall works as well.

B. General insertion technique.

   1. Ask the patient to empty her bladder and rectum, and to position herself as mentioned earlier.

        a. If a large cystocele is present, the woman may need to be straight catheterized, and the bladder emptied.

        b. With incontinence pessaries, it is imperative that the woman void before leaving the clinical site because the knob of the pessary may obstruct the urethra. Some clinicians do not recommend voiding before fitting, to ensure that the woman has urine to void following the fitting.

   2. Wear gloves; an unlubricated glove makes handling of the pessary easier.

   3. Perform a pelvic examination to determine the size, shape, and position of the uterus and associated structures.

   4. Pessary Retention test.

        a. Insert 2 fingers in vagina and extend fingers to either side of the vaginal fornices.

        b. Keep fingers thus extended and pull back through the orifice.

        c. If you pull hand straight through without having to collapse the fingers, it is unlikely that a pessary will fit because the introitus is too wide.

   5. Approximate size by using fingers to determine the length and depth of the vaginal vault (generally can predict within one size either way).

        a. May use lubricant for a narrow or small introitus.

        b. May cause the pessary to be slippery and difficult to bend or hold.

        c. Best to lubricate only the entering edge.

   6. Spread the labia, and pull downward with the nondominant hand.

   7. Ask patient to bear down.

   8. Grade prolapse, as described in Table 24.1.

   9. Displacement of a prolapse.

        a. Insert two fingers into the vagina, push the uterine corpus out of the cul-de-sac, and anteflex it into or above the long axis of the vagina.

        b. With the opposite hand on the anterior abdominal wall, elevate the fundus and hold it in place while inserting the pessary into the vagina.

10. Fit for various pessaries as described under each section below.
11. Begin fitting with the largest size that will fit comfortably, allowing room for the fingertip to sweep around.
12. After insertion.
    a. Separate the labia, observing the introitus.
    b. Ask the patient to stand and bear down while being examined.
    c. The pessary should descend and become visible at the introitus but ascend with relaxation.
    d. The presence of the pessary should not be apparent to the user.
    e. Ask the patient to walk around the room, to sit, or to even use the toilet.
    f. Reassess fit.
    g. If the pessary has shifted, try a larger size.
13. A larger size may be necessary after using the pessary for a few weeks, due to an enlargement of the vault with the pessary in position.

VII. Description of the various types of pessaries.
A. Ring (Figure 24.7).
   1. Indications.
      a. First- and second-degree uterine prolapse.
      b. The administration of estrogen is advocated to improve tissue circulation and regain vaginal mucosal integrity.
      c. The folding ring pessary is especially useful for a patient who is sexually active because it can easily be inserted and removed, or it may remain in place during intercourse (as with a diaphragm).
      d. If a cystocele or rectocele is present, use the ring with support.
   2. Description: Comes with a porous diaphragm for additional support.
      a. Membrane helps support a mild cystocele that accompanies a prolapse.
      b. It is usually made of medical-grade silicone.
   3. Insertion technique.
      a. Fit similar to a diaphragm.
      b. Measure the length of the vaginal canal against the examining finger, measured against the pessary.
      c. Bend pessary in half at the notches.
      d. Insert the pessary with the folded arc concavity facing downward.

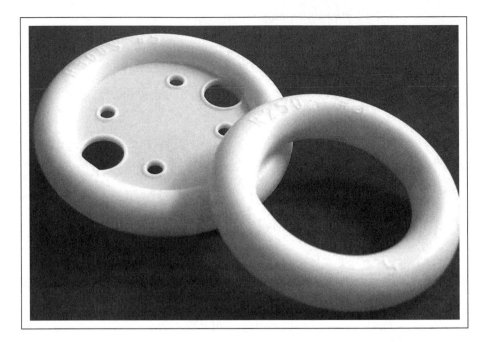

Figure 24.7 Pessary ring.

  e. Direct downward past the cervix into the posterior fornix.
  f. Place in the posterior fornix, allowing ring to spring open once it is in the vagina.
  g. Give a quarter turn to secure in position to prevent the pessary from falling in on itself and coming out of the vagina.
  h. When the pessary is placed properly, it will take up redundant vaginal tissue, forming a sling that will support and elevate the uterus, to flatten and support the cystocele.
  4. Removal.
    a. Palpate the notch, and rotate a quarter turn, gently pulling down and out to remove. It is nearly impossible to re-fold while it is inside the vagina.
    b. It is much easier to insert a pessary than to remove one.
  5. Available sizes.
    a. Available in 14 sizes, numbered 0 to 13.
    b. Correlate to a diameter of 4.44 cm to 12.7 cm.
  B. Lever pessary called Hodge or Smith.
    1. Indications.

    a. Uterine retroversion: Posteriorly displaces the cervix and the uterus is anteverted.

    b. Incompetent cervix in pregnancy.

    c. Mild uterine prolapse with retroversion.

    d. Diagnostic evaluation of patients with large cystocele or urinary stress incontinence demonstrates support of the anterior vagina.

    e. Provides support to the proximal urethra, promoting increase in urethral function length and closing pressure without causing obstruction.

    f. Useful for stress urinary incontinence, with or without prolapse

    g. If it is properly fitted, sexual intercourse is possible.

2. Insertion technique.

    a. First, manually elevate a retrodisplaced uterus.

    b. Fold the device along the long axis, with the curved end oriented toward the vaginal introitus.

    c. Push into the vagina by the index finger, advancing the posterior bar into the posterior vaginal fornix.

    d. Keep pressure on the posterior bar during insertion.

    e. Anchor the anterior bar under the symphysis pubis (similar to diaphragm insertion).

    f. Note: The long arm of the pessary should face anteriorly, so that the device straddles the rectum.

3. The Smith pessary has a narrower anterior limb for use in a patient with a deep symphysis and a well-defined, narrow pubic arch.

4. Hodge pessary.

    a. Border anterior limb prevents the pessary from turning.

    b. Used when there is minimal pubic support and the symphysis is somewhat shallow.

    c. The anterior notch prevents urethral impingement and obstruction.

    d. It comes with a support for correction of a concomitant cystocele.

    e. It is especially useful for patients with stress incontinence.

    f. Establishes a diagnostic means of predicting which patients would be responsive to surgical correction.

    g. The Hodge pessary with support is indicated for women with stress urinary incontinence, with a mild cystocele and a very small introitus.

5. Risser pessary.

      a. Modification of the Hodge pessary.

      b. The Hodge pessary has a wider bar and a deeper notch, which allows a larger weight-bearing region with a lesser likelihood of soft tissue-pressure necrosis.

    6. Available sizes.

      a. Ten available sizes (0–9), measuring width and length.

      b. Recommend stocking fitting sizes 2 through 4.

C. Gehrung pessary.

    1. Indications: Correction of a cystocele and rectocele.

    2. Description.

      a. Provides support to the anterior vaginal wall; arms or heels rest flat on the vaginal floor.

      b. Avoids pressure on the rectum while supporting the bladder.

      c. Does not interfere with douching or coitus.

      d. Arclike, flexible plastic.

      e. Bars may also flatten out a rectocele.

      f. May be underused.

    3. Insertion. Creates a bladder bridge.

      a. The unusual shape of the pessary may make the clinician uncomfortable with insertion.

      b. It is relatively simple to insert.

      c. Fold with the arch convexity oriented upward, with both heels parallel to the pelvic floor, left heel first.

      d. Hold the device on its side, and insert the lateral bar over the perineum and into the vagina.

      e. When it is positioned intravaginally, push one heel back and the other forward to complete a 90-degree rotation, so that the convex curved portion lies against the anterior vaginal wall.

      f. The back arch should be positioned over the cervix in the anterior fornix, and the front arch should be positioned behind the symphysis.

      g. Both heels should be resting on the pelvic floor, with the arches and cross-support forming a bridge to raise the bladder.

    4. Available sizes.

      a. Choice of nine sizes (0–9).

      b. Recommended stocking sizes: 3, 4, and 5.

D. Gellhorn pessary (Figure 24.8).

    1. Indications: Provides support of a third-degree uterine prolapse and procidentia.

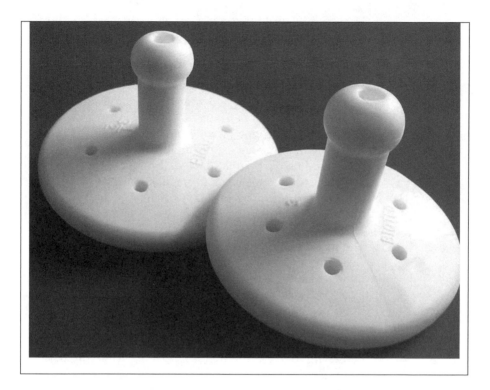

Figure 24.8 Gellhorn pessary.

2. Description.
   a. Most commonly used pessary for uterine prolapse (ring and doughnut pessaries also commonly used).
   b. Available:
      (1) Flexible silicone.
      (2) 95% rigid acrylic.
      (3) Rigid acrylic.
   c. Silicone can be boiled or autoclaved; acrylic should not be autoclaved or boiled because heat can alter the shape.
      (1) Needs to be disinfected in Cidex.
      (2) Never use alcohol because it will give the acrylic a shattered appearance.
   d. Provides less support for a rectocele because it fits superiorly and anteriorly, with less surface area to support the posterior segment.

  e. May be difficult to insert in women with a narrow introitus (e.g., virginal).
  f. Cervix rests against the flat base of the pessary, with the stem extending to the vaginal orifice.
    (1) Base of the pessary is large enough to support the tissue proximal to it, and rests above the levator muscles.
    (2) Its concave shape provides suction, helping to prevent spontaneous expulsion.
    (3) Stem fills the vagina, preventing the device from turning (requires a capacious vaginal vault).
  g. It is useful with intact (not lax) perineal body. If the patient is not successful, may progress to a cube.
3. Insertion.
  a. The main method of determining the proper size of the Gellhorn pessary is by trial and error.
  b. Lubricate the edge of the round disc.
  c. Insert sidewise, with the disc portion held parallel to the introitus.
  d. Apply downward pressure on the perineum with the nondominant hand.
  e. Be careful to avoid the urethral opening while the perineum is pushed downward.
  f. Push the pessary into the vagina using a corkscrew-like motion until the disc lies transversely beneath the cervix.
  g. Once the large disc is inside the vagina, push forward until the end of the stem slips within the orifice.
4. Removal.
  a. Grasp the knob and gently pull disc toward introitus.
  b. The clinician may have to reach behind disc to break any seal caused by suction. (May be difficult.)
  c. The knob may be slippery and may require use of a forceps for gentle traction.
  d. Use fingers to spread labia and turn the disc so that it is nearly parallel to the introitus.
  e. Push downward on the perineum to ease the pessary out of the vagina.
5. Available sizes.
  a. Comes in varying sizes of disc diameter, from 1-1/2 to 3-1/2 inches, increasing in quarter-inch increments.
  b. Choose from sizes 1 to 9.
  c. The recommended fitting size includes 2-1/4, 2-1/2, 2-3/4.

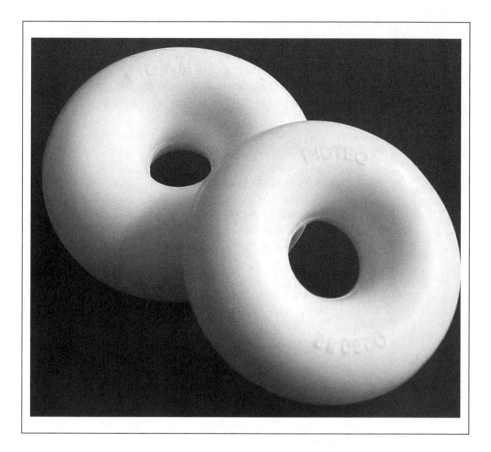

Figure 24.9 Doughnut pessary.

E. Doughnut (Figure 24.9).
   1. Indications: Occludes upper vagina and supports a uterine prolapse.
      a. Mass of the inflated pessary must be greater than the defect in the levator sling.
      b. It provides no support for the proximal urethra and can actually increase incontinence.
      c. Good for prolapse of the vagina after hysterectomy.
   2. Description.
      a. Useful for uterine prolapse, some recommend for third- to fourth-degree cystocele or rectocele.
      b. The hollow ring comes in two models of medical-grade silicone.

    c. Coitus is not possible with the pessary in place.

  3. Insertion technique.

    a. Similar to the ring pessary, but there is no notch, so internal rotation is not necessary.

    b. Once the labia is separated with nondominant hand, compress the doughnut. (It is somewhat rigid, so it does not compress too much.)

    c. With two fingers of the nondominant hand pressing down on the peritoneum, hold the pessary parallel, angle slightly, and slip past introitus into vagina.

  4. Removal technique.

    a. Hook finger inside on the center of the pessary (will not fit through hole, however).

    b. Compress the doughnut using the thumb and middle finger, and bring them parallel.

    c. Gently pull down and out through introitus. (The clinician may have to lubricate the pessary to remove it.)

  5. Available sizes.

    a. There is a choice of six sizes, ranging in diameter from 2 to 3-3/4 inches.

    b. Recommended stocking size includes 2 and 3.

F. Cube.

  1. Indications: Third-degree prolapse, cystocele, or rectocele, with or without vaginal tone.

    a. Often, this is the only satisfactory support for patients with complete prolapse complicated by cystourethrocele.

    b. Known as the pessary of last resort.

    c. It is excellent for vaginal wall prolapse in that it keeps the vaginal wall from collapsing by six pressure points.

  2. Description.

    a. Each side of cube has concave suction cups that adhere to the vaginal walls, helping to restore the anatomic vaginal support of the pelvic organs (Figure 24.10).

    b. Moist vaginal mucosa invaginates into the concavities owing to a slight negative pressure.

    c. Needs to be removed daily or requires regular follow-up care initiated by clinician or patient.

      (1) Requires highly motivated patient with good dexterity.

      (2) Difficult to remove (action of suction), so it may not be possible to be removed by the elderly client.

      (3) Remember that the longer the cube is left in place,

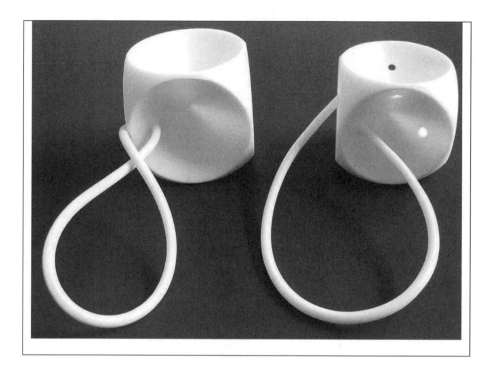

Figure 24.10 Cube pessary.

the stronger the negative pressure and thus the more difficult it is to remove.

(4) The cube completely fills the vagina and blocks off drainage of any secretions.

d. Some clinicians recommend its use in younger women who have incontinence with exercise.

(1) It can be inserted before vigorous exercise in young women to eliminate leakage.

(2) Other clinicians would recommend the ring with support for this condition.

3. Insertion.

a. It requires the compression of the cube before placement into the vagina.

b. The string should be oriented toward the vagina.

(1) Some clinicians recommend that the string be removed because it may be irritating.

(2) It should never be used to pull the pessary out because it may cause vaginal tears of the fragile mucosa.

c. Insert by compressing the cube as much as possible.

d. Spread the labia with the nondominant hand.

e. Push the compressed cube through introitus.

f. Place as high in the vagina as possible.

4. Removal.

   a. Removal may be difficult because of the suction that has been created.

   b. Suction must be broken before removal.

   c. Do not pull on the string to remove.

   d. Slide the fingertips between the vaginal mucosa and the pessary to break the seal.

   e. Compress the pessary and remove.

   f. If the woman is not able to remove the pessary, she needs to see her clinician immediately. If the pessary is firmly suctioned to the vaginal wall, the following technique may be necessary:

   (1) Insert 5 mL of lidocaine jelly.

   (2) Sweep the fingers around the cube to dispel the jelly.

   (3) Visualize the pessary.

   (4) Grasp the pessary with ring forceps.

   (5) Apply gentle traction, and pull down and out.

5. Available sizes.

   a. Eight sizes (0–7).

   b. The sizes correspond to 1 inch and 2 inches (25 mm to 50 mm).

   c. Recommend stocking sizes 2 to 4. Need a minimum of four sizes to fit a patient properly.

G. Inflato ball pessary.

1. Description. Rarely used today because it is made of latex.

   a. Support is adjusted by varying air pressure via the two-way valve.

   b. The patient can easily remove and clean this device herself; even with a stenotic introitus, it can be inflated and reinflated.

   c. Made of latex rubber. Cannot be used with any hormonal creams because they may rapidly deteriorate rubber.

   (1) The clinician must question the patient concerning latex allergy before insertion.

   (2) It absorbs vaginal secretions and should not be kept

in place more than 24 hours (as is recommended with
a diaphragm).

2. Indications.

   a. Genital prolapse.

   b. Extreme degrees of uterine prolapse.

   c. Prolapse of the vagina following a total hysterectomy.

3. Insertion.

   a. Approximate size by using fingers to determine the vaginal vault width.

   b. With the pessary deflated, hold it compressed between the thumb and forefingers.

   c. While it is deflated, insert the metal part of the bulb into the air vent.

   d. Insert the deflated pessary into the vaginal vault.

   e. Inflate the ball by squeezing the bulb.

   f. To close the air vent and maintain pressure within the ball, push the small bead at the tip of the stem 1 to 2 inches forward.

   g. Inflate the ball to a diameter large enough so that one finger can pass around the pessary and the vaginal wall.

4. Removal.

   a. Push the small bead in the direction opposite to its original position.

   b. Allow time for air to escape from the ball.

   c. Reach into vaginal vault, and squeeze the ball to deflate.

   d. Gently pull the deflated pessary through the introitus (do not pull on the stem).

5. Available sizes.

   a. Small, medium, large, and extra large.

   b. Corresponding to ball diameter of 2 to 2.5 inches.

   c. Recommended fitting sizes include medium and large.

6. Care should be performed frequently because rubber absorbs secretions and odors.

H. Incontinence ring pessary (Figure 24.11)

1. Description.

   a. Designed to stabilize the urethra and the urethrovesical junction.

   b. Woman must void following insertion before leaving the office to make sure the urethra is not obstructed.

2. Indication.

   a. Stress incontinence.

   b. Diagnostic test to assess the surgical outcome.

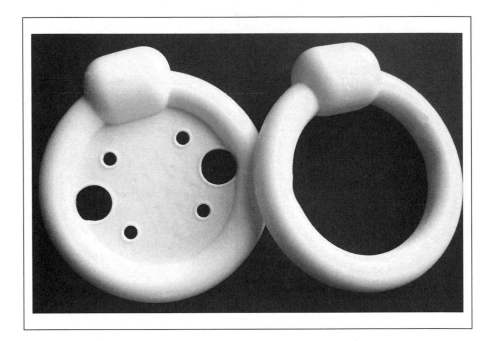

Figure 24.11 Incontinence ring pessary.

3. Insertion technique.
   a. Similar to the ring pessary without support.
   b. Must be fit properly because if it is too small, the knob may not remain in proper position, and if it is too large, it may obstruct the urethra and cause urinary retention.
   c. Insert the end without the knob first.
   d. Push the pessary up and behind cervix, with the knob resting behind the pubic bone.
4. Incontinence dish.
   a. Variations of the incontinence ring.
   b. It is indicated for stress urinary incontinence associated with a mild first- or second-degree prolapse.
   c. It is available in sizes of 55 mm to 85 mm in increments of 5 mm.
   d. Insert end without knob first. It is fitted with the knob behind the pubic bone.
5. Incontinence dish with support.
   a. Variation of dish with flexible membrane to support a mild cystocele.

b. It is indicated for stress urinary incontinence in conjunction with a first- or second-degree prolapse, or a mild cystocele. (Some clinicians recommend this type of pessary for second or third-degree cystocele because it provides additional support for the cystocele.)

c. It is available in sizes 55 mm to 85 mm, in increments of 5 mm.

d. It is fit with the knob behind the pubic bone.

VIII. Follow-up.

A. Must continuously monitor the woman for as long as the pessary is in place: although it is inert, it is still considered a foreign body.

B. Keep a list of all pessary users to make sure they are seen every 2 to 3 months. A forgotten pessary can cause serious complications. The woman can obtain a medic alert card at www.medid. com/phorm/phorm.php.

C. The pessary may require sizing alterations or a complete change in style at subsequent visits.

D. Discuss with the patient any possible problems.

    1. Coital discomfort (if intercourse is allowable).

    2. Disturbance in bowel or urinary function.

    3. Whether or not it remained in place.

    4. Overall comfort.

    5. Presence of any odor.

    6. Change in discharge.

        a. A yellow or white, or mild-to-moderate discharge is usually present.

        b. If the discharge increases during subsequent visits, question the patient's compliance with the vaginal care routine.

        c. The discharge should never be foul smelling.

           (1) Perform a wet mount, and treat any infection.

           (2) Replace the pessary after the infection is resolved.

E. At this point, one may discuss the possibility of the woman cleaning her own pessary.

    1. Particularly if she is used to touching her own genitals.

        a. Elderly women are not as familiar.

        b. If the woman has previously used a diaphragm, it may be easy for her to learn how to use a pessary.

        c. Observe dexterity.

        d. Evaluate compliance issues and ability to perform self-care.

    2. Most pessaries are difficult to insert and remove, so a woman must not feel that she has failed if she is unable to do it herself.

3. Do not even raise the possibility if it is obvious that the woman is unable to manage the pessary.

F. Provide instructions regarding:

    1. Use of lubricant.

      a. Estrogen cream may be used for insertion.

      b. Nonpetroleum-based lubricants are not caustic and can be used.

    2. Douching.

      a. No consensus has been presented as to its effectiveness.

      b. The woman should always consult with her clinician first.

      c. Mild vinegar may help to acidify the vagina.

    3. Use of estrogen.

      a. Vaginal estrogen, unless contraindicated, is recommended over systemic estrogen.

        (1) Vaginal creams or pill are inserted twice weekly.

        (2) Estring should be replaced every 3 months (should be inserted before pessary).

      b. May be used in conjunction with systemic preparations.

      c. The patient may have difficulty using the applicator and inserting the cream. (Many patients are elderly and have limited experience with devices such as tampons.)

      d. Will mature vaginal epithelium and improve perineal muscle tone.

    4. Use of Trimo-San.

      a. This is a cleansing, deodorant gel with a pH of 4 to maintain antibacterial acid environment.

      b. The patient should use one-half applicator two times per week.

      c. The active ingredient is oxyquinoline sulfate.

G. Pessary care and cleaning.

    1. If the patient is unable to remove the pessary, it should be removed and the patient should be observed for any excoriation, ulceration, or foul discharge.

    2. Clean the pessary in warm, soapy water; rinse thoroughly; and reinsert.

    3. Irrigate the vagina using a 20-cc syringe with an irrigating tip using warm water. A weak solution of betadine or vinegar may be used.

    4. Document type and amount of solution used and note character of discharge.

5. Replace the pessary if the old one shows signs of physical defects.
   a. It may become discolored, but does not need to be replaced.
H. Complications.
   1. Increase in vaginal discharge.
   2. Odor.
   3. Cytologic atypia from inflammatory changes that may occur.
   4. Poorly fitted or improper schedule of cleaning may cause ulcerations and excoriation.
   5. Incarceration—the cervix and uterus may herniate through the center of a poorly fitted ring pessary and become strangulated.
   6. In a neglected pessary, tissue may grow around it.
   7. There should be no evidence of serious problems with long-term wear of a well-maintained pessary.
I. Maintenance visits.
   1. Slight bleeding may be seen during removal of pessary; question the patient's compliance with estrogen therapy.
   2. If using the Estring, replace the ring every 3 months and insert before the pessary.
   3. Refit pessary if there has been a gain or loss of 20 pounds or more. (Discuss diet.)
   4. If heavy discharge:
      a. Perform wet mount to check for infection.
      b. If no infection is present, recommend vinegar and water douche.
         (1) One quarter cup vinegar to one quart of warm water.
         (2) Douche once to twice weekly.
   5. Reinforce use of Kegel exercises.
      a. Compliance is the key.
      b. Success rate of over 80% resolution of incontinence can be achieved in 4 to 8 weeks.
   6. Offer support groups.
J. Monitor urination.
   1. Ask woman to keep a voiding diary.
      a. Keep the diary for 1 week.
      b. Include frequency and quality of fluids.
      c. Note number and frequency of urination.
      d. Record which type of activities cause leaking.
   2. Note use of pads.
      a. Brand name.

Table 24.3 **Reimbursement Codes**

Procedure	Codes	Average Reimbursement
Pessary	A4562	$40
Pessary Insertion	57160	$35
Vaginal Irrigation	57150	$35

      b. How often has to wear (continuous versus intermittent).

      c. How often has to change if continuous.

   3. Kegel exercises.

      a. Inquire if the patient has done them in the past.

      b. Was she successful.

   4. Kegel exercise cones.

      a. These cones were designed as an aid to locating and identifying the correct pelvic floor muscle to be used during Kegel exercises.

      b. Begin by inserting the lightweight cone; the patient is unable to retain for 5 minutes while walking about.

      c. Work up to being able to retain the cone for 15 minutes twice a day while walking.

      d. Progress to the next heavier size, and continue.

      e. Patients with a prolapse or pessary cannot use cones.

 K. Reimbursment Codes (see Table 24.3).

IX. Pessaries in the 20th century.

  A. Newer devices to manage pelvic organ prolpase.

   1. Uresta.

      a. Uniquely shaped pessary that allows a woman to self-manage. Easy to remove and insert.

      b. The tissues compress the urethra and may reduce leakage.

   2. Colpexin Sphere.

      a. Round plastic sphere which is placed intravaginally above the levator ani muscle.

      b. Space-occupying properties allow support of the prolapse.

      c. Reflectively causes contraction of the pelvic floor muscle in an attempt to retain the sphere.

   3. Vaginal weights/cones.

      a. Five interchangeable cone-shaped plastic weights ranging from one to three ounces.

    b. Smooth, hypoallergenic.

    c. Used in conjunction with a home exercise program.

    d. Insert twice daily and wear for 15 minutes. Once the weight is able to be retained, increase to the next heavier cone.

B. Medications to increase contractility of the urinary sphincters.

  1. Have side effects.

    a. Rapid heart rate.

    b. Dry mouth.

  2. May be very useful if stress incontinence is associated with urge incontinence.

  3. Does not help most patients.

C. Biofeedback.

  1. Widely used worldwide to help patients regain control and awareness of pelvic muscles.

    a. Assists in the identification and strengthening of pelvic muscles.

    b. Is an audiovisual display of pelvic muscle activity.

  2. Useful for stress and mixed urinary incontinence.

  3. Usually, four to six treatments are needed.

  4. Many reliable studies show improvement of 87% in women with stress incontinence.

  5. Many nurses and physical therapists use this technique to re-train pelvic support.

D. Electrical stimulation of pelvic muscles.

  1. Low-frequency stimulation of the pelvic floor via a rectal or vaginal probe causes muscles of the periurethral and pelvic floor to contract.

    a. Uses an electrical probe, needle, or sensor to artificially contract the pelvic floor muscles.

    b. Causes pelvic muscle contraction with accompanying detrusor reflex inhibition.

    c. May cause some pain or discomfort.

  2. In the past, this method was used to treat urge incontinence and detrusor hyperreflexia.

  3. Recent indications include genuine stress incontinence.

  4. Clinical trials show an improvement rate of 89% after 6 weeks of treatment.

E. For more information on pessaries go to www.bioteque.com.

Acknowledgment

All pessary photographs are courtesy of Bioteque America, Inc.

CHAPTER 25

Urinary Incontinence

Helen A. Carcio

I. **Bladder dysfunction explained.**
   A. Statistics.
   1. Epidemiological studies suggest that 15% to 30% of all adults in the United States have some degree of incontinence.
   2. The actual frequency is probably much higher considering the significant underreporting of the problem because of patients' reluctance (Box 25.1).
   3. An estimated 75% of people affected are women.
   4. Demographic trends are changing the nature of the country and the health care landscape.
      a. The fastest growing segment of the population is the aging baby boomers; those between the ages of 45 and 65 have dramatically increased over the last 10 years.
      b. As the number of elderly increases, so will the need for incontinence services.
   5. Treatment of incontinence in not consumer driven. An astounding 50% of women affected never bring up the subject to their health care provider.
   B. Some thoughts.
   1. The most common form of incontinence is mixed incontinence, particularly among older women.

Common Reasons Why Women May Be Reluctant to Discuss Incontinence

BOX 25.1

- They believe incontinence is a normal part of aging.
- They are unaware there are conservative methods of treatment.
- They erroneously think that surgery is the only treatment option.
- They don't realize that they are not alone.
- They are afraid they will be put in a nursing home.
- They fear it is some form of cancer.
- They are able to rely on expensive incontinence products.
- They are not able to find resources to help with their problems.
- They are ashamed and embarrassed.
- They feel powerless and are resigned to their situation.

2. Aging itself does not cause incontinence, but the lower urinary tract does undergo some changes with age. These include:
   a. Diminished muscle tone, bladder capacity, and voided volume.
   b. The bladder is less compliant and less able to easily stretch with filling.
   c. Uninhibited bladder contractions and post void residual volumes increase.
   d. The function of the main pelvic floor muscle, the levator ani, deteriorates.
   e. The above changes are thought to be related to loss of estrogen to the cells and vascular insufficiency.
      (1) Symptoms include dysuria, incontinence, urinary frequency, and hematuria.
      (2) There is an increased risk of urinary tract infections.
      (3) These symptoms and signs of genitourinary atrophy may develop slowly, over many months or years, or may have a more rapid onset.
      (4) Urogenital atrophy is the most likely consequence of menopause.
   f. The lower urinary tract and pelvic musculature are under the influence of estrogen and share a common embryologic origin with the vagina.
      (a) Squamous epithelium of the trigone and urethra thins and blood flow decreases.

II. **Pathophysiology of the Lower Urinary Tract System (LUTS).**
    A. The bladder and the urethra make up the lower urinary tract.

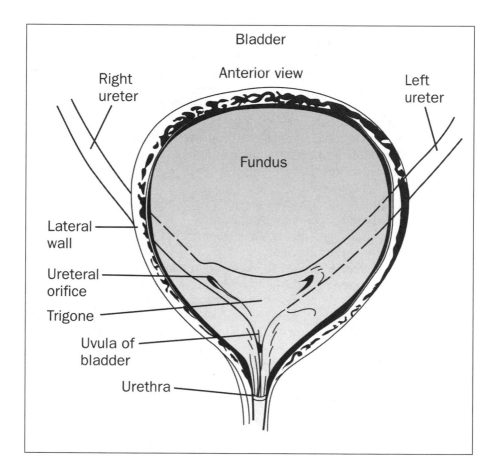

Figure 25.1 Anatomy of the bladder.

1. The bladder is both a holding tank and a pump.
   a. Stores urine.
   b. Empties when full.
2. Dome: The top of the bladder is the dome and is thin and collapsible.
   a. Extends, as the bladder fills much like a hot air balloon.
   b. Collapses when empty.
   c. Figure 25.1 shows the anatomy of the bladder.
3. Base: The base of the bladder is the thicker and less distensible portion.

        a. The trigone is the lower portion where the ureters enter the bladder.

        b. The bladder fills from the bottom and rises above the pubic bone when full.

        c. Bladder fills in 1cc per minute.

        d. Has an average capacity of 400–500 cc's.

B. The bladder wall consists of three layers.

    1. Outer: Adventitial layer of connective tissue.

    2. Middle: Contains the main muscle of the detrusor.

    3. Inner: Mucous membrane.

C. Urethral sphincter.

    1. Passes through the urogenital diaphragm and acts as a purse string to tighten the sphincter.

    2. Muscles provides passive compression to keep the urethra closed during filling.

D. Pelvic Floor Muscle. The levator ani is an internal diaphragm, which supports and stabilizes the pelvic organs.

    1. Acts as a voluntary sphincter for the urethra.

    2. Forms an occlusive layer which closes the lower pelvic floor to resist the down thrust of an increase in intra-abdominal pressure.

    3. Consists of a strong striated long muscle.

E. Neurophysiology.

    1. Distension of the bladder activates stretch receptors at approximately 200 cc's of urine.

    2. Sympathetic response facilitates urine storage by inhibiting the bladder contractions and stimulating the urethra to contract.

    3. Afferent impulses travel to the sacral spinal cord and the urge to urinate is felt.

    4. Efferent impulses return via the parasympathetic system.

        a. Detrusor contracts and the bladder empties.

        b. The urethral sphincter at the bladder neck simultaneously relaxes to allow the urine to escape.

    5. Pudendal nerve causes voluntary relaxation of the external sphincter and levator ani.

    6. Figure 25.2 provides a schematic diagram of the neurologic innervation of the bladder.

III. Urinary incontinence explained.

    A. Functional classification.

        1. Failure to store.

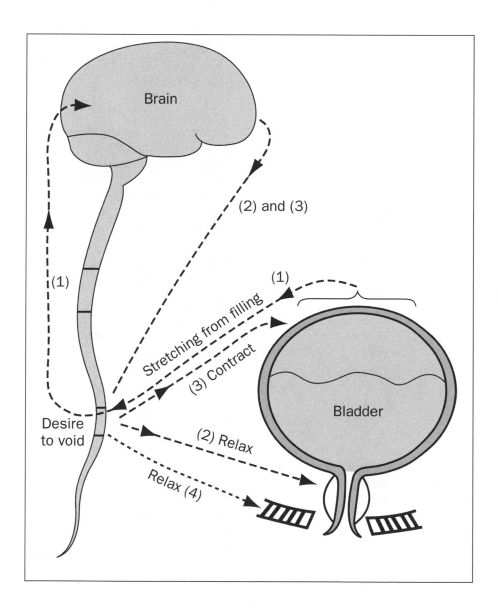

Figure 25.2 Schematic of neurologic innervation of the bladder.

        a. Bladder.
           (1) Involuntary muscle contractions.
           (2) Low compliance or stretchability.
           (3) Hypersensitivity to filling pressures.
      2. Failure to empty.
        a. Bladder does not contract efficiently.
        b. Outlet obstruction due to a stricture or kink in the urethra (cystocele) or the pressure of an enlarged prostate.
      3. Incontinence is the ultimate sign of storage failure.
    B. Requirements for urinary continence.
      1. Intact intrinsic urethral sphincteric mechanism.
      2. Well supported bladder neck and urethra.
      3. Normal bladder storage capacity at low pressure.
      4. Good compliance.
      5. Competent pelvic floor muscle.

IV. Types of urinary incontinence.
    A. Stress urinary incontinence (SUI).
      1. Involuntary loss of urine due to increased abdominal pressure on the bladder which exceeds maximal urethral pressure (the ability of the urethra to hold the urine in).
      2. Symptoms.
        a. Urine loss, usually occurring at unexpected or inappropriate times.
        b. Volume varies and is often described as occurring in spurts or drops.
        c. Precipitated by cough, sneeze, change in position, or other types of exertional activities often related to sports.
        d. Rare nighttime occurrence.
      3. Cause.
        a. Pelvic muscles act as a backboard or spring to absorb any increases in abdominal pressure and prevent overwhelming the urethral sphincter.
        b. When backboard becomes weakened or damaged, the bladder neck becomes displaced and opens the urethra to allow leaking.
        c. Abdominal forces generated to the bladder overcome the closing ability of the urethra and leaking occurs.
    B. Overactive bladder.
      1. Symptom.
        a. Symptom complex consisting of urgency, frequency, and urge incontinence. May not always be incontinent.

Table 25.1   **Comparison of Presenting Symptoms**

	OAB	Stress Incontinence	IC
Urgency	X		X
Frequency	X		X
Leaking with physical activity		X	
Leakage volume	Large	Drops to small amounts	Variable
Nighttime urination	X	Rare	X
Inability to reach toilet in time with urgency	X		X
Pelvic pain			X

Mixed is a combination of the symptoms of urge and stress incontinence.
OAB = overactive bladder; IC = interstitial cystitis.

    b. Characterized by sudden, strong feeling of urgency caused by uncontrolled (overactive) contractions of the detrusor during filling.

    c. The urgency may be very strong or very subtle.

    d. The urge a woman experiences is actually a bladder contraction that creates a false need to empty the bladder before it is full.

    e. If the force of the contractions is too strong or the seal of the urethra is weak, uncontrollable urine leakage can occur.

C. Urge incontinence.

    1. The involuntary leakage of urine that is often immediately preceded by an urge to urinate in the absence of physical activity.

    2. Frequency associated with "triggers" such as running water, or placing the house key in the front door.

    3. Urine loss may be substantial since contractions may continue until the bladder is empty.

    4. Must distinguish from a normal strong urge to void which can be controlled.

D. Mixed incontinence.

    1. A combination of stress and urge incontinence (see Table 25.1, which compares the symptoms of both).

    2. Probability increases with age.

    3. Usually described as being "stress dominant" or "urge domi-

Table 25.2   **Comparison of the Causes of Incontinence**

Causes of Stress Incontinence	Causes of Urge Incontinence/OAB
Pregnancy	Urinary tract infection
Genetic factors	Bladder stones or tumor
Vaginal delivery, particularly if multiple	Lack of vaginal estrogen
Mild to moderate cystocele	Urethritis/urethral diverticulum
Inadequate estrogen levels	Cystocele
Previous pelvic surgeries/radiation	Neurological problems associated
Obesity, particularly a high waist-to-hip ratio	with stroke, Parkinson's disease, multiple sclerosis, or spinal cord
High impact sports	problems
Medications (ACE inhibitors, Alpha-adrenergic blockers)	Habitual frequent voiding
Long-term heavy lifting	Diabetes
Chronic constipation	Incomplete emptying of the bladder
Elevated body mass index (BMI)	Smoking
Chronic cough, often related to smoking	
Vascular changes associated with aging	

nant" depending on which type of symptoms is more prevalent.

4. It is a combination of symptoms in which each requires special consideration.

5. Table 25.2 compares the causes of stress and urge incontinence.

E. Transient incontinence. Causes of incontinence that are usually caused by outside forces, which can be controlled or reversed (see list in Box 25.2).

F. Interstitial cystitis.

1. Symptoms.

a. Complex of symptoms characterized by urinary urgency and frequency, pelvic pain, dysuria, dyspareunia, and nocturia.

b. Bladder is tender and pain increases with filling and is relieved with emptying.

c. Is often misdiagnosed in the early phases of the condition as overactive bladder or urge incontinence.

Causes of Transient Incontinence   BOX 25.2

- Delirium/dementia
- Bladder infection
- Atrophic vaginitis/urethritis
- Medications
- Endocrine causes
- Restricted mobility
- Stool impaction/constipation
- Polyuria

    d. Pelvic pain increases over the years and is often diagnosed as endometriosis.

    e. Symptoms worsen with intercourse (12–24 hours), menstrual cycle changes, seasonal allergies, and stress.

    f. No underlying cause has been identified.

    g. Diagnosis is difficult and may take up to seven years of seeing various providers. It is usually made by exclusion.

V. Diagnostic testing and differential diagnosis.

  A. The health history.

    1. Begin by reassuring the woman that incontinence is a relatively common problem and that effective treatment is available.

    2. History includes the patient's perception of her symptoms, which helps determine the type and extent of urinary incontinence.

    3. Urinary symptoms of frequency, urgency, and incontinence mimic other bladder disorders and require special evaluation.

    4. Assess bowel function and type.

    5. Address the impact that incontinence has on the patient's life, self-esteem, and activities of daily living.

    6. Inquire about prior pelvic surgeries, number of vaginal deliveries, patient motility, medications, and history of urinary tract infection.

    7. Review use and extent of "self help" measures such as pad use and fluid reduction.

  B. Bladder Voiding Diary.

    1. Obtain a 3-day recorded history of the woman's day-to-day bladder habits and patterns.

2. Objectively document intake and output and extent of the problem.
3. Diary allows the woman to focus on her behavior and how it relates to symptoms.
4. The mere keeping of the diary can be therapeutic and continence may improve once a causal relationship is established and documented.
5. See Box 25.3 for a sample recording of the bladder diary.
6. Review the use of any bladder irritants.
   a. The lining of the bladder is sensitive to certain types of foods and fluids, particularly those with high caffeine and acid content.
   b. It can cause "irritative symptoms" such as urgency and frequency.
   c. Box 25.4 lists the worse offenders in the Carcio "C" List.

C. The physical examination is outlined in Table 25.3.
1. Urinalysis (see chapter 11).
   a. Rule out infection. Elderly women may not have the characteristic symptoms of a urinary tract infection (UTI), such as burning urination, and may only have frequency and incontinence.
   b. The presence of leukocytes and nitrates on a Multistix Reagent strip is a sensitive and inexpensive indicator.
   c. The presence of glucosuria or proteinuria require further investigation.
   d. Hematuria may be indicative of bladder cancer and may require referral for cystoscopy.
2. Postvoid residual.
   a. It is the integral result of bladder contractility and urethral resistance.
   b. A high residual may indicate an inability of the bladder to contract against an increase in urethral pressure or a hypotonic bladder.
   c. A measurement of a residual that is 25% or less of the voided volume is acceptable.
3. Vaginal cultures should be obtained (see chapter 10).
   a. Urinary frequency may be a symptom of genital herpes.
      (1) Rule out genital herpes with herpes select serology type 2 testing. HSV 2 may be latent and/or asymptomatic for decades, activating in perimenopause or menopause. Presentations are atypical, further evading easy diagnosis.

Bladder Diary

BOX 25.3

BLADDER DIARY DATE _____ **NAME** _____

Complete one page for each of the next 3 days.
In order to keep the most accurate diary possible, try
to write down events as they happen.

Day: M___ T___ W___
TH ___ F___ Sat___ Sun___

TIME	FLUIDS	DID YOU URINATE?					ACCIDENTS		
	What did you drink? How much? (in ounces) 1 cup = 8 oz	Did you feel a strong, sudden urge to urinate?	What amount each time? (small, moderate, large)	Did you feel any pelvic dis-comfort?	What activity did this interrupt?	Circle if urine; square if stool	How much urine did you leak? Small: drops; Med: < 1/4 cup; Lge: > 1/4 cup	What were you doing at the time?
8:45	Coffee 6 oz	Yes No	S M L	Yes No	Walking	Yes No	Drops	Coughing
		Yes No	S M L	Yes No		Yes No		
		Yes No	S M L	Yes No		Yes No		
		Yes No	S M L	Yes No		Yes No		
		Yes No	S M L	Yes No		Yes No		
		Yes No	S M L	Yes No		Yes No		
		Yes No	S M L	Yes No		Yes No		
		Yes No	S M L	Yes No		Yes No		
		Yes No	S M L	Yes No		Yes No		
		Yes No	S M L	Yes No		Yes No		
		Yes No	S M L	Yes No		Yes No		

Common Bladder Irritants	**BOX 25.4**

Coffee and tea (sometimes even decaffeinated)

Chocolate

Carbonation

Coke and colas (Pepsi)

Citrus (whether juice or fresh)

Cranberry juice or pills

C vitamin

Cocktails

Crystal light

Candy and other sugars

Chili and other tomato-based products

Chinese food (spicy or with MSG)

Cigarette smoking

Condiments such as honey and artificial

   sweeteners—Aspartame (NutraSweet, Equal)

Cold remedies

---

    4. Assess for atrophic vaginitis (see chapter 23).
       a. The "Maturation Index" should be assessed in order to determine the presence and extent of atrophic vaginitis.
       b. The presence of any parabasal cells on a wet mount may be considered documentation of atrophic vaginitis.
       c. Observe for the presence of a urinary caruncle which can cause symptoms of urgency, frequency, and bleeding.
  D. Assess pelvic muscle tone (see chapter 24).
    1. Ask patient to squeeze around your two examining fingers while palpating the levator ani muscle.
    2. Note the patient's ability to sustain constriction and deflection of finger or fingers upward with a good squeeze. No deflection indicates weaker muscles.
    3. Constriction lasting a few seconds indicates weakening.

Table 25.3   **The Focused Physical Examination in the Evaluation of Incontinence**

Abdominal	Abdominal skin condition
	Bowel sounds
	Masses
	Suprapubic tenderness
	Bladder distention
Pelvic examination	Perineal skin condition
	Urethral characteristics
	Atrophism
	Vaginal infection
	Pelvic floor deficits such as cystocele or rectocele
	Palpation of the strength and symmetry of the levator ani muscle
	Bladder base tenderness in the anterior vagina
	Pelvic muscle laxity
	Pelvic mass
	Provocative stress test with direct observation of urine loss
Rectal examination	Skin irritation
	Perineal sensation
	Sphincter tone
	Presence and consistency of stool
	Masses or fecal impaction
Neurological examination	Gait
	Mental status
	Knee and ankle reflexes
	Perineal sensation of S2–S4 dermatones
	Anal reflex or "wink" (S2–S5)
	Bulbocavernosus reflex (S2–S4)
Laboratory assessment	Urinalysis for infection, blood, glucose, protein
	Urine culture for infection
	Cytology for atypical or malignant cells

    4. A weakness may be indicative as the cause of SUI.

  E. Provocative stress test.

    1. Stress testing has a sensitivity and specificity of > 90%.

    2. Ask the patient to stand and cough with a moderately full bladder (150 cc's).

3. Observe for small spurts of urine that escape simultaneously with each cough. (May place pad between legs to catch and observe any urine released.)
4. Delayed or persistant leakage suggest detrusor overactivity (triggered by coughing) rather than outlet incompetence.
5. If urine escapes, place one finger on either side of the urethra to compress it.
6. Ask the patient to cough again.
7. If there is no loss of urine during the cough, the test is considered positive for stress urinary incontinence.

F. Assess the neuronal support to the sacral dermatone, S2, S3, and S4. These dermatones innervate the micturation reflex (Figure 25.3).
1. Lightly stroke the skin area innervated by the dermatones in the inner thighs (Figure 25.3).
Note response to light touch. Compare contralateral sides.
2. Bulbocavernosus reflex.
   a. Stroke or gently squeeze the clitoris.
   b. Note contraction of the bulbocavernous muscle around the clitoris.
3. Anal reflex (so-called anal wink).
   a. Lightly stroke the skin lateral to the anus.
   b. Note contraction of the anal sphincter.

G. The cotton-tipped swab (Q-tip) test.
1. Determines the degree of the detachment of the proximal urethra (Figure 25.4).
2. Place cotton-tipped swab through the urethra to the midurethral area.
3. Ask patient to perform a Valsalva maneuver (hold breath while bearing down).
4. Note change in the angle of the cotton-tipped swab.
   a. Normally, 10 to 15 degrees from the horizontal position.
   b. If there is significant urethral detachment and loss of urethral sphincter muscle, the angle will exceed 30 degrees (Figure 25.4).

H. Perform a simple CMG (see chapter 37).

VI. **Follow-up.**
A. Follow-up visits may range from 2 weeks to 3 months based on the patient's problems, response to therapy, and clinician/patient preference.
B. Once the diagnosis is established an individualized plan of care is developed with the patient. Options include:
1. Pelvic floor muscle strengthening.
   a. Kegel exercises, which include a rectal tightening and

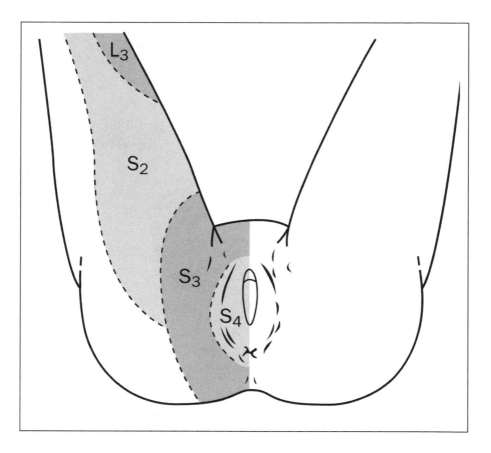

Figure 25.3 Sacral neuronal dermatones S2, S3, and S4 that innervate micturition reflex.

hold for 10 seconds followed by an equal period of relaxation.
   b. Exercises should be repeated 30 times a day, 10 reps three times a day.
2. Biofeedback training.
   a. Uses computerized technology to isolate the pelvic floor muscles.
   b. Monitors the electrical activity of the muscles through a vaginal or anal sensor and records any unwanted contraction of the accessory muscles using a sensor.
   c. Can cure 30 to 70% of motivated patients over a series of 6 visits.
3. Vaginal support pessary (see chapter 24).

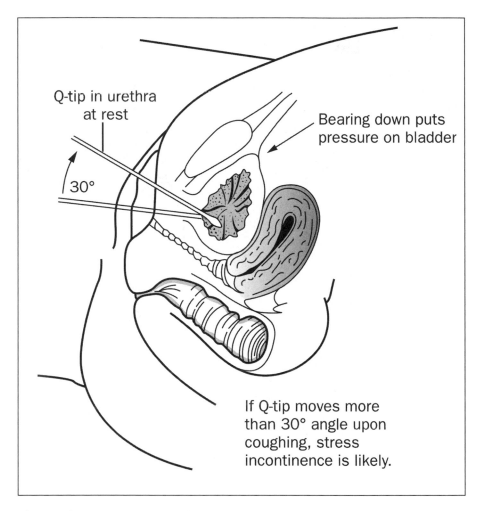

Q-tip in urethra
at rest

Bearing down puts
pressure on bladder

30°

If Q-tip moves more
than 30° angle upon
coughing, stress
incontinence is likely.

Figure 25.4 Cotton-tipped (Q-tip) swab test is used to determine the degree of detachment of the proximal urethra.

        a. Vaginal device that elevates and stabilizes the bladder neck and increases urethral resistance.

        b. Takes up redundant vaginal tissue, forming a sling that will support and elevate the uterus, and flatten and support a cystocele.

    4. Electrical stimulation.

        a. Delivers a weak, painless electrical current to the pelvic floor muscles.

Urge Suppression

**BOX
25.5**

PATIENT EDUCATION: Urge Suppression
In the following exercises you will learn to decrease frequency and urgency by calming the bladder.
The urgency curve is similar to a labor contraction, you simply have to mentally and physically suppress the urge and ride through the contraction. It is a matter of "mind over bladder." Follow these simple steps: (You may leak a little during this training period.)

The urge strikes!

- Avoid rushing to the toilet. It will make matters worse.
- Sit down and try to relax.
- Do 5 "quick flicks." This is done by tightening your rectal sphincter for a couple seconds, and releasing for another few seconds. Quickly repeat this sequence 5 times in a row.
- Next, relax your body totally—try imagery—think of something pleasant and unrelated. (Preferably not the running water of a peaceful waterfall!) The urge should be decreasing by now.
- Do another set of 5 "quick flicks."
- This may completely make the urge go away, or at least suppress the urge long enough to allow you to squeeze and calmly walk to the bathroom.

        b. Inhibits bladder spasm by affecting the neural pathways between the pudendal nerve and the bladder.
    5. Urge suppression.
        a. Contracting the muscle of the pelvic floor reflexively causes the muscles of the bladder to relax.
        b. Box 25.5 lists the steps to use when teaching urge suppression.
    6. Table 25.4 summarizes the treatment options in the treatment of urinary incontinence.
  C. Certain clinical conditions should be referred to a specialist.
    1. Uncertain diagnosis.
    2. Hematuria without urinary tract infection.
    3. Urinary retention with persistent symptoms of inadequate bladder emptying.
    4. History of previous incontinence surgery, radical pelvic surgery, or pelvic irradiation.
    5. Neurological conditions such as MS (muscular sclerosis), spinal cord injury, or neuropathy.
    6. Suspicion of fistula or suburethral diverticula.

VII. There are valuable resources for information on urinary incontinence.

Table 25.4   **Options in the Treatment of Incontinence**

Continence Treatment Options	Stress	Urge	Mixed	IC
Pelvic muscle exercises	X	X	X	X
Biofeedback/EMG	X	X	X	X
Reduction in use of bladder irritants		X	X	X
Treatment of vaginal atrophism	X	X	X	X
Pessary use	X	X	X	
Anticholinergics	sometimes	X	X	X
Bladder retraining	sometimes	X	X	X
Urge suppression		X	X	
Weight reduction	X		X	
Vaginal weights	X		X	
Smoking cessation	X	X	X	X

Note how mixed incontinence requires a combination of treatment options for stress and urge incontinence.

A. National Association for Continence (NAFC) Web site: www.nafc.org
B. Society for Urologic Nurses and Associates (SUNA).

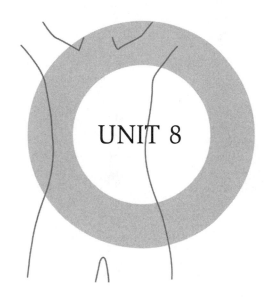

UNIT 8

Assessment of the Infertile Woman

CHAPTER 26

Initial Evaluation of Infertility

Helen A. Carcio

I. Infertility explained.

  A. Infertility is a major health care concern.

  1. Nearly 5.3 million American women are infertile.

  2. Twenty-five percent of all women in America will have a concern related to their fertility at some point during their reproductive years.

  3. The number of infertility clinics for assisted reproductive techniques has increased tenfold in the past 10 years.

  4. Contemporary therapy in the treatment of infertility is progressing faster than in any other field of medicine.

  5. Advanced practice clinicians can play a key role in the assessment and management of the infertile woman (see Box 26.1).

  B. More women than ever before are seeking diagnosis and treatment of fertility. There are many factors that have caused this increase.

  1. Couples are putting off starting their families until later in their reproductive lives.

  2. Many women today are older than 35 years of age—when reproductive potential begins to decline—before they even begin to attempt pregnancy.

Responsibilities of Midlevel Practitioner by Office Setting

BOX
26.1

Primary Care Setting	Initial workup to include:
	History and physical
	Ovulation assessment (BBT or OPK)
	Semen analysis
	HSG, if indicated
	Laboratory testing as indicated
	Emotional support
Specialty Setting	The above, plus:
	Endometrial biopsy
	Ovulation induction with clomiphene citrate
	Intrauterine insemination Sperm washing

3. The number of women in the United States between 35 and 44 years of age is increasing and will continue to do so.
4. More couples are aware of aspects surrounding infertility and the availability of new techniques.
5. Couples without male partners are taking advantage of various options available to them.
6. The number of adoptable babies has decreased, probably because of improved contraceptive methods.
C. Causes of infertility.
   1. Infertility affects 15 to 20% of all couples trying to conceive.
   2. The cause may be due to a female factor, a male factor, or both (see Table 26.1).
   3. Female factors involve various organs.
      a. Hypothalamus.
         (1) Weight changes may cause the hypothalamus to decrease levels of sex hormone-binding globulin. (SHBG). Weight loss or gain on either side of ideal body weight can greatly affect fertility.
         (2) Exercise decreases gonadotropin levels and increases prolactin levels.
         (3) Polycystic ovarian syndrome increases luteinizing hormone.

Table 26.1   **Etiologic Causes of Infertility**

Male Factor	35–40%
Female Factor	40%
Ovulatory	20–40%
Tubal	20–40%
Endometriosis	10%
Advanced age	18–50%
Luteal phase defect	< 10%
Uterine factors	10%
Fibroids	2–3%
Unexplained	10–15 %
Combination	10–20 %

       (4) Systemic disease such as liver and kidney disorders.
  b. Pituitary gland.
       (1) Hyperprolactinemia, causing anovulation.
       (2) Hyperthyroidism, which may cause menstrual ir-
           regularities.
       (3) Sheehan's syndrome, causing hypopituitarism.
  c. Ovary.
       (1) Premature ovarian failure where estrogen declines
           prior to menopause.
       (2) Polycystic ovarian syndrome causing an increase in
           ovarian cysts.
       (3) Luteal phase defect (low production of progesterone).
  d. Cervix.
       (1) Stenosis, which inhibits sperm motility through the
           os. Poor cervical mucus during midcycle, creating a
           barrier to sperm.
  e. Fallopian tubes.
       (1) Infection with chlamydia, gonorrhea, or mycoplasma,
           especially if pelvic inflammatory disease has
           occurred.
       (2) Narrowing of the tubes in the presence of en-
           dometriosis.
  f. Uterus.
       (1) Asherman's syndrome, due to scarring of the uterine
           lining from a traumatic dilatation and curettage (D &
           C).

       (2) Fibroids may distort the shape and size of the uterus.
  4. Male factors ultimately mainly affect the quality of the sperm. These factors include:
    a. Anatomic factors.
       (1) Varicocele.
       (2) Cryptorchidism.
       (3) Congenital anomalies, such as hypospadias or epispadias.
    b. Endocrine factors.
       (1) Cushing's disease.
       (2) Acromegaly.
       (3) Pituitary tumor.
    c. Genetic factors.
    d. Previous or current infection.
       (1) Gonorrhea and chlamydia.
       (2) Prostatitis.
       (3) Epididymitis.
    e. Idiopathic factors.
    f. Prescription medications.
    g. Toxins and environmental factors.
       (1) Radiation, including X-rays and isotopes.
       (2) Heavy marijuana use; cocaine and alcohol consumption.
       (3) More than three to five cups of caffeinated beverage per day.
       (4) Frequent use of hot tubs or saunas.
    h. Mechanical damage.
       (1) Trauma and torsion of testes.
       (2) Prolonged or competitive bicycling.
    i. Ejaculatory dysfunction.
       (1) Retrograde ejaculation.
       (2) Ejaculatory failure.
       (3) Neurologic impairment.
    j. Neurologic dysfunction.

II. Health assessment of the infertile woman.
  A. Important to develop a trusting, long-term clinical relationship with both partners.
  B. Unique in that it involves the collective history of two individuals who may have separate issues of confidentiality.
  C. Recognize the underlying issues.
    1. Stress placed on the intimate relationship.

2. Conflicts with friends and family members.
3. Religious or moral concerns.
D. Understand the range of emotions that the couple may experience including:
   1. Denial.
   2. Anger.
   3. Confusion.
   4. Disappointment.
   5. Frustration.
   6. Anxiety.
   7. Depression.
E. A thorough health history is the first piece of the puzzle and involves attention to detail as well as an investment of time.
F. See Appendix 26.1 for assessment forms for both the male and female partner.

III. **Physical examination of the infertile woman.**
   A. A complete physical is recommended as an integral part of the initial infertility workup.
   B. The approach should be systematic, thorough, calm, and relaxed.
   C. Particular emphasis is placed on:
      1. Body habitus.
      2. Hair distribution.
      3. The presence of thyroid enlargement.
      4. Breast discharge.
   D. See chapter 4 for techniques of the physical examination.

IV. **The initial workup.**
   A. An infertility evaluation should proceed in a systematic manner beginning with the consultation visit.
      1. Acknowledge the couple's frustrations and fears in their zeal to have a child.
      2. Set realistic goals.
      3. Discuss overall direction of the impending evaluation (see Table 26.2).
      4. Although it is demanding, the workup can usually be accomplished in the first 2 to 3 months.
      5. Most of the tests are noninvasive, straightforward, and relatively cost effective.
      6. The couple must realistically accept that the workup can be invasive—temporarily affecting work schedules, relationships, and sexual patterns.

Table 26.2 **Initial Interview and Evaluation of the Infertile Couple**

History	Physical Examination	Laboratory Screening	Education
Genetic screening	Thyroid/breast	HIV encouraged	Expected workup
Reproductive history	Abdomen/pelvic	Rubella	Review of procedures
Ovulation assessment	Wet mount cultures if indicated	Semen analysis	Realistic outcomes
Identification of risk factors for uterotubal dysfunction or hormonal disorders	Pap (< 1 year)	Hormonal assays as indicated	Preconception counseling
Previous infertility treatments		FSH if over age 35 Varicella	

FSH, follicle-stimulating hormone; HIV, human immunodeficiency virus.

7. As the evaluation proceeds, keep the couple informed, interpreting each finding's relevancy to fertility.
8. Long-term goals should be set rather than monthly goals.

B. Concerns of the infertile couple are often related to:
1. The reasons they are not conceiving.
2. Types of treatments available.
3. Their chances of conceiving.
4. The costs.
5. The timeline.
6. Any long-term health consequences of the treatments.

C. After the plan has been identified, the couple should be educated regarding:
1. The necessity for the test.
2. The rationale for its use.
3. Necessary preparation.
4. Special timing.
5. Possible discomfort.
6. Time the procedure may take.
7. Anticipated recovery time.
8. Expected outcomes.

  D. An evaluation is warranted for couples who are:
   1. Younger than age 35: Have not been able to conceive after 12 months of unprotected intercourse.
   2. Older than age 35: Have not been able to conceive after 6 months of unprotected intercourse.
   3. Lesbian couples: Have made insemination attempts per the above-mentioned age criteria.
  E. The investigation attempts to answer the following four questions:
   1. Is the woman ovulating?
   2. Are there adequate motile sperm?
   3. Can the egg and sperm meet?
   4. Can implantation occur and be maintained?

V. **Ovulatory assessment.**
  A. Ten to 15% of infertile women have a problem related to ovulation.
   1. Ovulation is usually easy to determine.
   2. There are many tests available to predict ovulation.
      a. For women with regular cycles: An inexpensive initial screen for ovulation is the basal body temperature (BBT) chart.
      b. Ovulation predictor kits (OPK) or luteinizing hormone (LH) surge kits are more expensive, but can predict ovulatory cycles more accurately.
  B. A health history helps provide documentation of ovulatory cycles. The presence of moliminia predicts ovulatory cycles 95% of the time (see Box 26.2).
  C. The health history also documents the woman's anovulatory cycle. Anovulation should be suspected when history reveals:
   1. A history of amenorrhea.
   2. Long periods of oligomenorrhea (skipped menses).
   3. Irregular cycles (shorter than 26 days or longer than 35 days).
   4. No further assessment of ovulation is necessary if the history clearly indicates anovulatory cycles.
  D. Some comments related to the BBT.
   1. It is easy to record, inexpensive, and noninvasive.
   2. It is a useful indicator of ovulation, providing graphic documentation of the temperature rise and fall throughout a menstrual cycle.
   3. Can be used as a visual guide for the scheduling of tests and procedures.

Presumptive Signs That Ovulation Is Occurring (Moliminia)

BOX 26.2

Menstrual characteristics

- Premenstrual breast tenderness
- A predictable bleeding pattern lasting from 3–5 days
- Monthly menses occurring between 21 and 35 days
- Mild to moderate menstrual cramps

Periovulatory period

- Vaginal "wetness" (like that of the white of an egg)
- Slight cramping (Mittelschmerz)
- Spotting (Hartman's sign)
- Increase in sexual arousal

---

    4. Can be used to document menstrual cycle symptoms and co-ital events.

    5. Recording the BBT is considered a necessary adjunct to the menstrual history to confirm the presence or absence of ovulatory cycles.

    6. The woman's temperature should be monitored until a pattern can be determined, usually for at least two to three menstrual cycles.

    7. Use of the BBT chart is not necessary for a woman who, by history, is anovulatory.

E. The temperature.

    1. Normally considered to be 98.6°F, but it actually fluctuates around 98°F during rest (at least 6 hours).

    2. During the first half of the menstrual cycle, before ovulation, the BBT can range from 97.2° to 97.4°F.

    3. It will rise 0.4° to 0.8°F, to above 98°F with ovulation.

    4. It may drop slightly before ovulation (the nadir), but this drop is often difficult to capture on the BBT chart.

    5. It will remain elevated for the rest of the cycle.

    6. This temperature change from low to high at midcycle produces the classic *biphasic* pattern, which is characteristic of an ovulatory BBT recording. A monophasic chart usually indicates an anovulatory cycle.

F. The role of progesterone in relation to BBT.

    1. Progesterone acts on the hypothalamus, the thermoregulatory center of the brain.

2. Progesterone is prevalent in the second half of the menstrual cycle.
3. The rise in BBT is probably the result of progesterone levels because these two curves plotted on a graph are the same.
4. The temperature usually remains elevated for 10 to 14 days and then drops 1 to 2 days before menses, as progesterone levels fall.

G. Pregnancy.
1. The BBT will remain elevated beyond expected menses if a woman is pregnant, as a result of the continuing influence of progesterone. This prolonged temperature elevation can be used as an indicator of a possible pregnancy.

H. Use of BBT in the timing of intercourse.
1. Not routinely recommended for the timing of coitus to achieve pregnancy. Documents ovulation after it occurs.
2. If the couple is unable to afford commercial ovulation kits, the BBT may be used instead.
   a. Intercourse should occur every 36 to 48 hours during a 5- to 7-day period around the time of suspected ovulation (averaging previous recordings), usually from 3 to 4 days before, to 2 to 3 days after the temperature shift.
   b. Other sources recommend intercourse for 3 days in a row at the time of expected ovulation.

I. Advantages.
1. Inexpensively predicts the presence of ovulatory cycles.
2. Helps document the presence of a luteal phase defect (a luteal phase more than 11 days as counted during the temperature rise indicates the presence of ovulatory cycles).

J. Disadvantages.
1. Considered to be very bothersome and time consuming.
2. It dictates that the woman wake each morning, think of her fertility status, and plop a thermometer into her mouth.
3. The woman is constantly concerned over the adequacy of a temperature that she has no control over.
4. It is a daily reminder of her infertility problem.
5. It is imprecise as to the exact day of ovulation. Temperature rise occurs after ovulation.
6. There is considerable variation in BBT from cycle to cycle and from woman to woman.
7. Ten to twenty percent of monophasic charts (the temperature graph maintaining a relatively straight line because the temperature did not rise) occur in ovulatory cycles; the pres-

ence of a biphasic chart may not always indicate that ovulation has occurred.

K. Education.
   1. An accurate understanding of how to use the chart is imperative.
   2. A special form to record the BBT is available (http://www.babycenter.com/0_sample-basal-body-temperature-cervical-mucus-chart_7252.bc)
   3. Instructions for use: See Appendix 26.2.
      a. Begin a new chart on the first day of every monthly cycle and bring completed forms to subsequent appointments.
      b. Use a standard oral or rectal thermometer, calibrated in tenths of degrees.
      c. Place a dot on a temperature grid representing the temperature each cycle day, and then connect the dots when complete.
      d. Record menses and frequency of intercourse in the space provided.
      e. Note any observable signs of ovulation such as mittelschmerz or the presence of wet, watery vaginal discharge.
      f. Record any factors that can alter the BBT:
         (1) Inadequate sleep (less than 6 hours).
         (2) Travel.
         (3) Alcohol consumption the evening before.
         (4) Use of electric blanket or heated water bed.
         (5) Emotional upset.
         (6) Illness such as a cold or infection.
         (7) Voiding during early morning hours before taking the BBT.

VI. Ovulation predictor kits (OPK).
   A. Key concepts.
      1. The OPK monitors the level of LH in the urine.
      2. The peak of LH is called the LH surge.
      3. During a regular menstrual cycle, the LH surges just before ovulation.
      4. This surge stimulates the mature egg to be released from the follicle.
      5. Commercially available kits are relatively inexpensive and are accurate predictors of ovulation.
   B. The commercially available kit.

1. Contains five to nine sticks or wands.
2. This number usually lasts for one to two cycles, depending on the number of sticks used before the surge.
3. Once the surge occurs, testing should cease.
4. Kits are available at most pharmacies and supermarkets.
5. It is convenient for the patient to have them available for sale through the office or clinic. A reduced cost may be negotiable with the manufacturer.

C. The procedure and education.
1. Proper use of the OPK is essential.
2. Written instructions help ensure proper timing (see Appendix 26.3).
3. The LH surge is assessed by the daily testing of the urine at midcycle.
4. The second morning urine should be used. It is best to test within an hour of the first voiding (only a few drops are needed).
5. The LH surge tends to occur between midnight and 7 a.m. in two thirds of women. The physiologic basis is not understood.
6. Ovulation occurs in 24 to 48 hours, plus or minus 6 hours, following a positive test result.
7. The LH surge has occurred when the urine test shows an equal or darker color than the control.
8. The menstrual cycles are averaged. (See the chart supplied by the manufacturer, which pinpoints the day to begin testing.)
9. Single, daily testing is adequate.

D. Advantages.
1. LH testing is reliable in documenting that a woman's cycle is ovulatory.
2. It accurately predicts ovulation.
3. It is easy to use following simple directions.
4. It is convenient, only requiring a few minutes' time for each test.
5. It does not have to be performed on a daily basis but often only a few days a month.
6. It can be used to time other procedures related to the infertility workup such as:
   a. Inseminations.
   b. Hormonal assays.
   c. Postcoital tests.

  d. Follicular sizing.

  e. Embryo transfer.

  f. It can be used during hyperstimulated cycles to document that ovulation is occurring.

  7. More convenient (no daily temps).

  8. Can be purchased online less expensively.

  9. The most commonly used kits are Clearplan Easy and Ovu Quick.

  10. The cost is between $3 and $7 a kit or $15–70 a month.

E. Disadvantages.

  1. The OPK does not always indicate that ovulation has occurred.

  2. Although OPKs are comparatively inexpensive, at a cost of $20 to $50 per cycle, the money spent may add up if the test is used for many months.

  3. Interpreting the color of the two lines is very subjective and may be difficult to interpret.

F. Timing in the infertility workup.

  1. Should be used as an adjunct (along with the BBT) in documenting the presence of ovulatory cycles during the first 2 to 3 months of the infertility workup.

VII. Other comments.

A. Additional testing.

  1. Many other hormones and procedures may be ordered as indicated as part of the infertility evaluation.

  2. Table 26.3 lists those tests and clinical indications for ordering them.

B. Indications for referral.

  1. No pregnancy after three to six cycles of therapeutic management.

  2. Severe sperm factor for possible intracytoplasmic sperm injection (ICSI).

  3. Complex hormonal picture requires referral to an endocrinologist.

  4. Surgical management of any assessed condition.

  5. Box 26.3 lists a sample referral form for use in standardizing care.

Table 26.3   Summary of Tests

Test	Indications for Ordering	When to Test	Normal Findings
Progesterone	Shortened luteal phase (< 11 days), monophasic BBT, unexplained infertility	Midluteal Day 21 or 7 days after BBT rise or LH surge	10–15 ng/dL
Endometrial biopsy	Shortened luteal phase (< 11 days), unexplained infertility	11–13 days after BBT rise or LH surge or 1–3 days before next expected menses	Endometrium within 2 days of cycle day
Prolactin	Irregular menses, luteal phase defect, headache/blurred vision, galactorrhea, unexplained infertility	Luteal phase (around day 20)	< 20 ng/mL Values > 25 ng/dL indicate need for a CT scan
TSH	Manifestations that may suggest hyperthyroidism or hypothyroidism Hyperprolactinemia	Any point during menstrual cycle	
LH/FSH ratios	Indicators of PCOD present such as hirsutism, oligoamenorrhea, acne, obesity	Secretory phase Day 3–5	< 3:1
FSH	History suggestive of premature ovarian failure or menopause such as hot flashes, irritability, or irregular menses	Secretory phase Day 3, also day 10, if clomiphene citrate is used	< 15–20

BBT, basal body temperature; CT, computed tomography; FSH, follicle-stimulating hormone; LH, luteinizing hormone; PCOD, polycystic ovary disease; TSH, thyroid-stimulating hormone.

Sample Referral Form: Summary of Infertility Evaluation and Treatments

BOX
26.3

Member: _____ P_____ G_____ Ab_____(S, T)
DOB: _____ Insurance# _____
Partner: _____ DOB _____
Fertility Diagnosis: _____
General medical problems: _____
Surgical history: _____
Medications: _____ Allergies: _____
❒ rubella immune   ❒ folic acid supplements
❒ genetic history complete   ❒ HIV risk assessment complete
Pertinent Female History or CPE Findings:
❒ negative   ❒ hirsutism
❒ previous infertility   ❒ habitual abortion
❒ obstetrical complications (bleeding,   ❒ cervical cultures if indicated.
   infection)
❒ risk for tubo-peritoneal disease   Results: _____
   ❒ history STDs or PID   ❒ contraception: _____
   ❒ previous ectopic   ❒ galactorrhea
❒ family history of congenital   ❒ smoking/alcohol use
   anomalies

Menstrual History
Cycle length _____ Regularity: _____ Duration of flow _____ days.

   ❒ dysmenorrheal
   ❒ dyspareunia

❒ Other
_____
Description of any abnormal responses _____
_____

Male Evaluation
❒ negative   ❒ undescended testicle
❒ testicular surgery   ❒ varicocele/repair
❒ genital infection   ❒ environmental/heat exposure/
❒ medical problems   smoking/alcohol use
❒ other: _____   ❒ medications: _____
                                    ❒ sports/bicyclist
Fathered child: ❒ yes ❒ no
Semen analysis: Date: _____   Results _____

Description of any abnormal responses _____
_____

Documentation of Ovulation:
❒ Ovulatory   ❒ Anovulatory
   ❒ molinimia present
   ❒ OPK # months _____   Response _____
   ❒ BBT # months _____   Curve _____
❒ Progesterone level (if indicated) _____ Day_____ of_____ day cycle.

APPENDIX (26.1)

Health History

FEMALE FERTILITY EVALUATION
Please complete the following:
Name: _____
Member #: _____
Date of birth: _____ Age: _____
Partner's name: _____ Member #: _____
Date of birth: _____ Age: _____
Primary care provider: _____
OB/GYN provider: _____
How long have you been trying to get pregnant? _____
Weight: _____ Height: _____ Current medications: _____
Allergies: _____ Reaction: _____
Menstrual History:
a) Date of last menses:
b) Age at onset of your menstrual period:
c) Average length between cycles:
d) Any history of irregular menses, spotting, or missed menses?
If yes, please explain (include dates):
e) Painful menses?
List any medications you take for cramps.
Ovulation: Do you experience?
Premenstrual cramps?   Yes ☐   No ☐
Clear discharge midcycle?   Yes ☐   No ☐
Monthly cycles?   Yes ☐   No ☐
Pain at midcycle?   Yes ☐   No ☐
Have you ever used the following?:
• Basal body temperature: _____ months. Temperature shift: _____
• Day of shift: _____
• Ovulation predictor kit:
• Name of kit: _____
• # of cycles: _____ LH surge seen? Yes _____ No _____
• Day of surge: _____

Birth Control: Have you ever used any of the following?
Birth control pills, IUD, diaphragm, condoms, Norplant, Depo-Provera, foam, sponge, other
(please describe)

Method	Dates	How long	Why stopped	Complications

Obstetric History:

Preg. #	Year	Time to conceive	Type of fertility treatment? (if any) Weeks carried	Outcome	Type of delivery (vaginal/c-sect)	Complications	Current partner

Gynecologic History: Please include dates and treatment if you ever had:

Mother who took diethylstilbestrol (DES)

Pelvic infection

Chlamydia/gonorrhea

Herpes

Vaginitis

Endometriosis

Ovarian cysts

Genital warts

Ectopic pregnancy

Miscarriage

Abortion

List date and nature of any pelvic surgery: Have you had a tubal ligation? If so, when was it reversed? Were you ever treated for an abnormal Pap smear? If yes, list date and nature of treatment.

Sexual History: Please describe any positive responses.

Do you have painful intercourse?

Do you use vaginal lubricants or douches?

Hormonal Assessment: Have you experienced any of the following:

Weight gain /loss of 10 + lb

Discharge from nipples

Change in vision

Unusual sensitivity to hot or cold

Excessive change in hair growth/loss

Thyroid disease, diabetes, or other hormonal abnormalities

Medical History: Please list any medical or psychiatric conditions that you have or had in the past and any medications used in treatment. List dates.

Surgical/Hospitalization History: Please list any surgeries or hospitalizations you have had. List dates.

Family History
Please list any family history of infertility, genetic problems, thyroid disease, diabetes, cancer, or any other major medical problems.

Social History
Occupation: Travel for work?   Frequency?
Caffeine intake:
Do you smoke cigarettes?   _____ Packs per day
Alcohol consumption: _____ Drinks/week   Type:
Medications:
  Prescription:
  Over the counter:
  Recreational (marijuana, hallucinogens, crack/cocaine, other addictive drugs; if yes, explain):
List the form and frequency of any regular exercise:
Have you ever been told you have or suspected you have an eating disorder?

Previous Infertility Treatment: Describe results. Include dates.
Name of physician/practice:
Has your partner ever had a semen analysis?

Have you had any hormonal blood tests?
Have you ever had an endometrial biopsy?
Have you ever had an X-ray of your tubes and uterus (HSG)?
Have you ever had a laparoscopy?
Have you ever taken medications to stimulate ovulation?
Have you ever had intrauterine inseminations?
Have you ever had advanced reproductive technology procedures performed (IVF,
GIFT, ICSI)?
Why do you think you are not getting pregnant?

FEMALE PARTNER FERTILITY EVALUATION
Please complete the following:
Name: _____ Member #: _____
Date of birth: _____ Age: _____
Partner's name: _____ Member #: _____

Gynecologic History: Please include dates and treatment if you ever had:

Pelvic infection
Chlamydia/gonorrhea
Herpes
Vaginitis
Genital warts
Were you ever treated for an abnormal Pap smear? If yes, list date and nature of
treatment.

MALE FERTILITY EVALUATION
Please complete the following:
Name: _____ Member #: _____
Date of birth: _____ Age: _____
Partner's name: _____ Member #: _____
Date of birth: _____ Age: _____
Primary care provider: _____
Weight: _____ Height: _____
Current medications: _____
Allergies: _____ Reaction: _____

Male Medical History: Please explain any positive answers.

History of mumps? Complications?

History of undescended testicles?

Any illness and/or high fever in last 6 months?

Have you ever had any injury, cancer, tumor of testicles?

Have you ever had x-rays to your groin area?

Have you ever been treated for a genital infection (i.e., chlamydia, gonorrhea, syphilis, herpes, prostate)?

Other medical problems, past and present. List treatment.

History of Any Operations: (Give data and surgeon.)
Hernia repair
Testicular surgery
Pelvic surgery
Varicocele repair
Vasectomy/reversal

Sexual History
Describe any difficulty having or maintaining an erection.
Describe any premature ejaculations.
Any other sexual difficulties? Explain.

Social History
Occupation: Travel for work?   Frequency?
Caffeine intake:
Do you smoke cigarettes?   _____ Packs per day
Alcohol consumption? _____ Drinks/week   Type: _____
Medications: _____
_____

Educational Series

Basal Body Temperature Chart

Evaluation of the basal body temperature (BBT) curve is one of the indicators that helps document that ovulation is occurring monthly. Ovulation is important to assess because 10 to 15% of women unable to conceive do not ovulate. However, other signs are also reliable. If you have a history of regular menstrual cycles, varying from within 2 to 4 days per month, you probably ovulate. Cycles shorter than 21 days or longer than 35 days may indicate a problem with ovulation. Other symptoms such as premenstrual breast tenderness, lower abdominal discomfort at midcycle, with or without spotting, painful menstruation (dysmenorrhea), and an increase in vaginal moisture or "wetness" are additional signs that ovulation is occurring.

The temperature of humans is usually 98.6°F, but it fluctuates to around 98° during rest. In the first part of the menstrual cycle, before ovulation, the temperature can range even lower, from 97.2° to 97.4°. When ovulation occurs, it rises to over 98°F, with a temperature increase varying from 0.4° to 1.0°. This temperature shift produces what is called a "biphasic" chart, in which the second half of the chart contains a higher curve than the first half. It is estimated that the ovary probably releases the egg or ovum the day before the first temperature elevation.

The temperature rise is probably the result of the hormone progesterone, which is prevalent in the second half of the menstrual cycle. It acts on the thermoregulatory centers of the brain. It usually remains elevated for 10 to 14 days and then drops 1 to 2 days before menses. There may be a concurrent dip in the temperature preceding the rise, although this is usually difficult to detect on the chart. BBT will remain slightly elevated if you are pregnant, so it will help you diagnose pregnancy should it occur.

The BBT should be taken daily when you first wake up before any type of activity, even brushing your teeth. Your temperature should be timed for a full 5 minutes. A regular oral or rectal thermometer can be used, or you may purchase a special thermometer that shows a range of only a few degrees and is easier to read.

There are special charts on which to record your BBT. Days of intercourse or inseminations should be recorded on the chart to review appropriateness of timing with your provider. Record any medications taken. Start a new chart when menstrual bleeding begins.

The BBT chart is useful in providing graphic documentation of ovulatory cycles but is not as useful in predicting the exact timing of ovulation. It can be used to time intercourse, although it is not as accurate as the urinary ovulation predictor kit. It is less expensive, however. You should time intercourse every 1 to 2 days in the 5- to 7-day period around ovulation, usually 3 to 4 days before expected temperature rise to 2 to 3 days after. It is unclear how long the sperm can actually survive, but it is estimated that sperm can retain their ability to fertilize an ovum for 24 to 48 hours. The human egg is probably able to be fertilized for 12 to 24 hours following its release from the ovary. For fertilization to occur, it is best that the sperm be present in the area when the egg is released. The transportation of sperm to the ovary occurs from 5 minutes to more than a day after intercourse.

It is important to understand that there is only about a 20% to 25% chance of conceiving during each ovulatory cycle, even if optimally timed.

Once ovulation has been well documented, usually after 2 to 3 months of BBT, and if your cycles are fairly regular, it is usually not necessary to continue taking your temperature unless you are using the BBT to time intercourse.

Educational Series: Ovulation Predictor Kit

The ovulation predictor kit (OPK) is an accurate test used to establish the presence of ovulatory cycles for diagnostic purposes or to predict ovulation for timing of intrauterine insemination. The kits are easy to use, requiring only a few minutes of time. OPK testing is a reliable method of predicting ovulation. Ninety-five percent of the time, ovulation occurs within 24 to 48 hours following a positive test result.

The OPK documents the rise of luteinizing hormone (LH) in the urine. LH is a hormone secreted by the pituitary gland. During a regular menstrual cycle, the LH level will peak before ovulation. This is called the *LH surge*. This surge stimulates the egg to be released from the follicle 1 to 2 days later. When timing inseminations, the OPK is used as an adjunct to other indicators such as vaginal wetness and cycle averaging.

The LH surge is assessed by testing the urine daily during the days before expected ovulation. You first need to determine the average length of your menstrual cycle by averaging the length of the cycles during the past 6 months. Next, count the first day of bleeding as day 1. Start testing your urine on the appropriate cycle day. If your cycles are irregular, use the shortest cycle that occurred during the 6-month period.

The LH surge occurs between midnight and 7 a.m. in two thirds of the female population. Test your urine each morning using the second morning urine. It should be done as the bladder begins to fill, usually within an hour after the first voiding. Only a few drops are needed. If you have risen during the night to empty your bladder, the first morning urine may be used if it was only 3 hours since you last voided. Do not force fluids to fill your bladder more quickly because it may only dilute the urine. Because of various schedules, you may prefer to test your urine at night. This is okay. Regardless of when you test, it is important to test your urine at approximately the same time each day. Daily testing is adequate. Testing every 12 hours rather than every 24 hours may more closely pinpoint the exact time of the LH surge, but this is usually not necessary.

CHAPTER 27

The Postcoital Test

Helen A. Carcio

I. **The postcoital test or PCT explained: PCT evaluates the cervical mucus following intercourse. It is also called Sims-Huhner test after its original developers.**
   A. The cervical mucus is important to assess because it potentially acts as the first barrier to the union of the egg and sperm, addressing the question of whether the egg and sperm can meet. Actions of the cervix include the following:
      1. It serves as a conduit for sperm transport through the cervical os during the ovulatory period.
      2. It stores sperm in the cervical folds.
      3. It acts as a biologic filter for bacteria and poor sperm.
      4. It is believed to serve as a source of nutrients necessary for capacitation.
   B. The PCT determines the adequacy of many reproductive functions (see Box 27.1).
   C. Prognostic value. Sources vary.
      1. Seventy-eight percent of reproductive endocrinologists still include the PCT as part of their initial workup.
      2. Additionally, there are many tangential benefits to the PCT.
         a. Provides a time for trust building between the couple and the clinician early in the relationship.
         b. If the office or clinic setup allows, the clinician should permit the couple to view the microscopic findings.

Purpose of the Postcoital Test   **BOX 27.1**

The postcoital test determines:
- If the ejaculate is appropriately delivered during the act of coitus
- The quantity and quality of preovulatory cervical mucus
- The character of the cervical os
- The ability of the sperm to survive in that mucus
- The adequacy of the number of sperm
- The presence of any immunologic incompatibility

Future Treatments:
- Determine if cervical mucus is hostile to the sperm

---

      c. Gives a realistic perspective to the many unknowns of the infertility workup.

      d. In a normal PCT, the couple is reassured by the results.

      e. If the test in abnormal, it provides an opportunity to educate the couple in sperm transport mechanisms and to discuss strategies to overcome the observed problem.

   3. It helps the couple time intercourse during the cycle, which could result in a pregnancy early in the infertility workup.

   4. Despite the above-mentioned benefits, the clinician must be aware that some couples may view the PCT as just one more intrusive step in their evaluation.

   5. They are asked to have "sex on demand," which interferes with the privacy of the sexual relationship of the couple.

   6. Some women feel unclean being seen by a clinician so soon after intercourse.

   7. The clinician must weigh the risks versus the benefits in relation to prognostic value.

II. **Timing. Proper timing of the test is crucial.**

  A. There is lack of standardization as to when to perform the PCT.

    1. It must be performed during late follicular phase or early ovulatory phase, when the highly estrogenized cervical glands secret mucus that is most receptive to sperm.

    2. Improper timing will result in inaccurate abnormal results.

  B. The practice of arbitrarily scheduling the PCT around cycle day 14 should be discouraged.

    1. Scheduling is imprecise because ovulation can occur at any point in any given cycle.

  C. Most agree the PCT should be scheduled before ovulation.

    1. One to three days before the expected rise in BBT *or*:

    2. The day of, or the day following the luteinizing hormone (LH) surge.

D. The ovulation predictor kit (OPK) is more accurate than the basal body temperature (BBT) chart for the timing of the PCT.

E. The PCT should be performed at least 3 hours, but no more than 12 hours, after intercourse.

    1. Some couples prefer to have intercourse the night before, which is okay, but they must arrive the next morning within the designated time frame.

    2. It is important to keep the routine sexual practices of the couple as normal as possible.

F. The woman is allowed to shower following intercourse, but she should not bathe.

G. In certain practices where there is not a large infertility program, the appropriate day may not coincide with the availability of a provider.

    1. Unfortunately, the test will then have to be rescheduled during a subsequent menstrual cycle.

    2. The timing of the test is not lost; intercourse should still occur, which may potentially result in a pregnancy.

H. An instruction sheet that clearly describes the expected procedure should be reviewed with the woman and her partner (see Appendix 27.1).

III. The procedure.

A. Before the test, record:

    1. Day of the woman's menstrual cycle.

    2. Hours since intercourse.

    3. Days of abstinence before.

    4. Method of ovulation determination.

    5. Confirm that no lubricants were used.

B. The technique. Carefully explain each step.

    1. The woman assumes the dorsal lithotomy position, and a speculum is inserted into the vagina.

    2. Insert an endometrial biopsy pipelle 2 to 3 mm into the cervix.

    3. Pull back on the suction applicator, and withdraw a drop of cervical mucus.

    4. Prepare two slides.

        a. Slide #1. Place drop of cervical mucus on a glass slide, and immediately cover with a coverslip and view under microscope. (Evaluate number of sperm.)

      b. Slide #2. Spread the residual mucus on the pipelle tip uniformly across the slide. Allow to air dry while viewing the first slide (Grade ferning).

  5. View both slides under high power.

  6. Many fields are evaluated.

  7. When the mucus is dried on slide #2, evaluate and grade ferning.

C. The following are important to assess:

  1. The cervical os.

    a. Size and shape. Should be open, even gaping.

    b. Color. Should be hyperemic.

    c. Determine if any unusual discharge is present, which might indicate the presence of a vaginal or cervical infection. If an unusual discharge is present, a wet mount of the vaginal secretions should be performed (see chapter 10).

  2. Mucus quality and quantity.

    a. Cervical mucus is produced by the mucus-secreting cells of the endocervix.

    b. As ovulation approaches, ovarian secretion of estrogen rises, increasing the volume and water content of the mucus.

    c. Just before ovulation, the cervical discharge changes from thick, scant mucus to become acellular, nonviscous, watery, and abundant, providing an environment that is conducive to sperm transport.

    d. At ovulation, nearly 98% of the mucosal volume is water.

    e. Suboptimal mucus may simply indicate poor timing rather than an anomaly of mucus production.

    f. The mucus may be so thick that it tends to plug the cervical os.

    g. Poor mucus in not an absolute barrier to fertility but may lower the possibility of conception.

    h. If the mucus is poor, 0.625 mg of conjugated estrogen (Premarin) could be given daily for 8 to 9 days before expected ovulation (between days 5 and 13 in a 28 day cycle). The dose can be doubled in the subsequent cycle if the mucus does not improve. A mucolytic agent, guaifenesin, which is usually used as a cough syrup, has anecdotally been used successfully to thin the cervical mucus.

  3. Spinnbarkeit explained.

    a. The mucus usually remains clear for 2 to 3 days during ovulation.

    b. It should resemble the white of an egg (uncooked of course).

    c. The mucus actually develops the ability to stretch as estrogen levels rise before ovulation.

    d. Spinnbarkeit can be evaluated in a variety of ways.

        (1) A small sample of mucus can be grasped between thumb and forefinger, and the stretchability can be measured in centimeters.

        (2) The mucus can be pulled away from the os with nasal polyp forceps.

        (3) Place a coverslip over the discharge that has been placed on a slide and lift it, noting the distance it stretches.

    e. A stretch of 6 to 10 cm is indicative of adequate ovulatory mucus.

4. Arborization or ferning.

    a. This characteristic ferning is seen microscopically when the cervical mucus is allowed to dry on a slide (without a coverslip; Slide #2).

    b. Ferning is due to the crystallization of the mucus from electrolytes, mainly sodium chloride, interacting with glycoproteins in the mucus.

    c. The presence of ferning indicates adequate estrogen production.

    d. It is interesting to note that some sources suggest that the fernlike channels may actually provide a passageway for sperm transport.

5. Sperm.

    a. Slide #1 is viewed, and the presence of motile sperm is evaluated.

    b. A good PCT is one in which at least 5 to 15 motile sperm with good linear progressive movement are visualized.

    c. Visualization of 20 or more sperm is almost always associated with a sperm count above 20 million/mL.

    d. Fewer than five may affect fertility.

    e. If clumping or shaking of the sperm is noted, further immunologic testing for antisperm antibodies may be indicated.

    f. Results in which there are progressively motile sperm in the PCT indicate significantly higher pregnancy rates.

6. Cellularity.
   a. The presence of white blood cells might indicate infection.
   b. Because the mucus is a combination of a woman's cervical mucus and sperm, it is not possible to ascertain the source of the white blood cells.
   c. Each partner needs to be evaluated separately.
   d. A wet mount can easily be scheduled for the woman a few days after the PCT.
   e. An infection needs to be diagnosed accurately and treated.

7. pH.
   a. pH of the cervical mucus at midcycle should be determined.
   b. If the pH is below 7, a precoital douche of 1 tablespoon of sodium bicarbonate (baking soda) or an over-the-counter baking soda douche should be used.

IV. **Following the procedure.**
   A. Findings from the PCT should be recorded in the patient's chart. See Table 27.1 for a sample recording.
   B. Results are known at the time of the test and have the following indications:
      1. Good result.
         a. Presence of 10 motile sperm moving in a forward direction.
         b. Full, branching fern pattern.
         c. Open, gaping cervical os with abundant mucus that stretches 8 to 10 cm.
      2. Poor result. Table 27.2 presents a summary of poor result parameters.
         a. Fewer than 5 motile sperm, or no motile sperm.
         b. Shaking movement indicative of antisperm antibodies.
         c. Lack of cervical mucus.
   C. The PCT should be repeated if results are poor, if the timing is not right, or if a vaginal infection is present—all of which may alter the results.
      1. The test may be repeated in 1 to 2 days if the timing occurred before the preovulatory period.
      2. If ovulation has already occurred, it should be rescheduled during the next cycle at an earlier cycle day.

Table 27.1   Postcoital Test Evaluation

Patient name: _____ Date of birth: _____
Partner name: _____ Date of birth: _____
Time of coitus _____ Date: _____

Timing of ovulation: ❐ Natural
                      ❐ Serophene Day: _____
                      ❐ BBT Results: _____
                      ❐ Ovulation predictor kit
  Brand name: _____ Day of cycle for color change: _____
Day of menstrual cycle: _____
Circle Results:

Mucus Score	0	1	2	3
Quantity	None present	Scant	Pooled on cervix	Abundant
Quality	None	Clear	Clear, thick	Clear, watery
Spinnbarkeit	None	Slight—a short (2 cm) stretch	Moderate length string (2–6 cm)	Long (6–8 cm) string
Ferning	None, amorphous	Fine lines, no branching	Fine lines with side branches present	Full ferning with multiple side branches
Cervical os	Closed, pale pink	Partially open, Pink	Open, fully hyperemic	Gaping, hyperemic
Add columns: _____				
Total score	0–6	6–10	10–12	12–15
Results (circle)	Negative	Fair, early ovulation	Good	Excellent
Sperm/high power field (circle):	None present	Sperm present, all immobile	4–10 present 2–6 forward progression	> 8 present 8–10 forward progression

    3. If any infection was noted, it should be treated and the test repeated.

  D. Two abnormal PCTs are indicative of a cervical problem or the presence of antisperm antibodies.

V. Advantages.
  A. The test is relatively inexpensive.
  B. It provides the clinician with additional data with which to proceed during the infertility investigation.

Table 27.2   **Causes of Poor Postcoital Test**

Finding	Cause
Immobile Sperm	
Poor cervical mucus production	Inappropriate timing
	Diethylstilbestrol (DES) exposure
	Cervical cautery/conization
	Low estrogen levels
Agglutination/Shaking	Antisperm antibodies
No Sperm	Poor coital practice
	Retrograde ejaculation
	Hostile mucus
	Azoospermia

    C. The clinician is able to view the interaction of the sperm with the cervical mucus, as well as the abundance of the mucus.

    D. Motile sperm found in the mucus documents the adequacy of coital technique.

    E. The test provides useful information concerning the presence of a cervical factor as a cause of infertility, with the presence of immobile or absent sperm indicating the need for intrauterine insemination (IUI).

  VI. Disadvantages.

    A. Subjective nature of the test in grading the various parameters, which is thought to decrease the test's validity.

    B. Lack of strong evidence that links the predictive value of the test to successful pregnancy. (Although a normal PCT is a good sign, a poor result does not preclude conception.)

    C. Considered by some couples to be invasive, which may further burden the couple and increase their frustration.

    D. Considered obsolete by some because the results usually do not alter the treatment of the infertile couple because most couples quickly progress to IUI, superovulation, or both, fairly early in the investigation.

  VII. Infertility time line.

    A. The PCT should be scheduled during the first 1 to 2 months of the initial evaluation, after it has been determined that the woman is ovulatory and that the male partner has adequate sperm.

B. If a serum progesterone measurement or endometrial biopsy is indicated, it may be scheduled during the concurrent cycle.

C. If the PCT is abnormal, it should be rescheduled during the next cycle, with timing and any use of lubricants reviewed.

D. At this point in the workup, any identified problems should be treated.

E. If the PCT shows good mucus and adequate actively motile sperm, it does not need to be repeated.

F. If no cause for infertility has been found, and if the history and physical do not indicate other potential causes, the couple should be treated at this point with clomiphene citrate (Serophene), IUI, or combined regimens for the next three to four cycles.

G. The couple needs to be involved in this decision. An HSG should be considered.

H. If a cervical factor is suspected, IUI is recommended. See Figure 27.1 for a summary of the PCT workup.

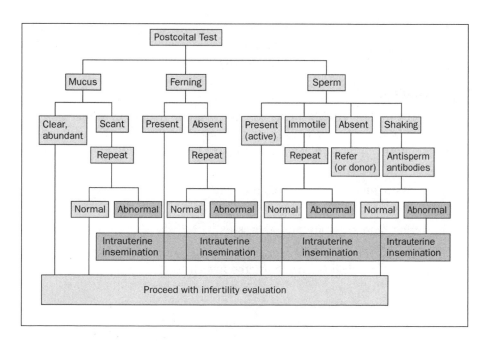

Figure 27.1 Summary of postcoital test workup.

APPENDIX 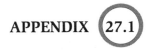 27.1

Educational Series

Instructions for Postcoital Test (Sims-Huhner Test)

Purpose:

To examine the quality and amount of the cervical mucus at midcycle and to evaluate the sperm's ability to survive in that mucus.

The mucus is most conducive to sperm movement just before ovulation.

The mucus is assessed for clarity, amount, and its ability to stretch (spinnbarkeit).

The presence of any motile sperm and the development of a fernlike pattern are viewed microscopically.

Ferning is due to high estrogen levels in the mucus and becomes visible as the mucus dries on the slide. Mucus is examined for the presence of any white blood cells, which may indicate infection.

Preparation:

The test should be performed 1 to 2 days before ovulation (expected basal body temperature rise) or on the day of or the morning after the urine luteinizing hormone (LH) surge, as indicated by the ovulation predictor kit.

The woman should have intercourse 4 to 12 hours before the appointment.

Showering before the appointment is okay, but she should not douche or take a tub bath.

Avoid use of lubricants during intercourse. If lubricants must be used, use vegetable oil.

The Test:

The test is painless and takes approximately 15 minutes.

A pelvic examination will be performed, as with a Pap smear.

A speculum is inserted into the vagina, and the opening to the cervix is visualized.

A narrow pipelle is inserted just inside the opening, and a small amount of cervical mucus is withdrawn.

The mucus is placed on a slide and examined under the microscope.

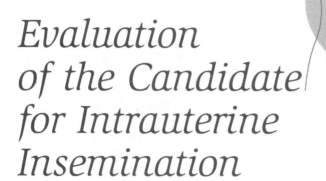

CHAPTER 28

Evaluation of the Candidate for Intrauterine Insemination

Helen A. Carcio

I. **Intrauterine insemination (IUI) explained.**
   A. IUI is the direct placement of processed, highly motile, concentrated sperm, washed free of seminal plasma and other cells, into the uterus.
      1. Washing the specimen before IUI refines and concentrates the sperm, thus enhancing the fertility potential of the ejaculate.
      2. The specimen, which contains a high proportion of morphologically normal cells, is placed high in the uterine cavity, adjacent to the medial ends of the fallopian tubes, as close to the ovulated oocyte as possible.
      3. This procedure greatly reduces the distance that the sperm have to travel, eliminating the necessity of the spermatozoa traveling from the vagina, through the cervix, and into the uterus.
      4. The sperm leave the uterus, migrate to the ampullary portion of the fallopian tube, and attach to the zonapellucida of the oocyte in order for fertilization to occur.

>   **5.** The number of sperm to reach the fallopian tubes is increased as much as 25% with IUI.
> **B.** Some comments.
>>   **1.** IUI is one of the oldest treatments of infertility, and it is still an integral part of the management of the infertile couple.
>>   **2.** IUI has consistently been shown to be a safe method with minimal complications related to the procedure itself or any increase in the number of congenital abnormalities.
>>   **3.** IUI is appropriate to use in the office with adequate quality control, but requires a significant commitment of time and resources.
>>   **4.** The procedure is within the scope of practice for midlevel practitioners who have been specially trained and educated.
>>   **5.** IUI may be an appropriate first step in the infertility management continuum for women with patent tubes.
>>   **6.** It is cost-effective and appropriate to continue IUI for three to six cycles before considering assisted reproductive technologies (ART) because it may maximize fertility while minimizing patient risk and expense.
>>   **7.** IUI has many indications (see Box 28.1).
> **C.** Before beginning IUI, the couple should be informed of the following:
>>   **1.** Expected course of treatment.
>>   **2.** The technical aspect of the procedures.
>>   **3.** The risks of any complications.
>>   **4.** Expected outcomes.

> **II. During the initial workup, the following items should be discussed.**
> **A.** Number of expected inseminations per cycle.
>>   **1.** Current recommendation is that only one, well-timed insemination is necessary.
>>>   **a.** A recent study showed little difference in the pregnancy rate in 4,935 cycles in which IUI was performed on 1, 2, or 3 days (11.9%, 11.5%, and 9.9%, respectively).
>>>   **b.** A decrease in semen volume and sperm motility has been seen on the second consecutive day of ejaculation.
>>>   **c.** Some studies demonstrate an increase in pregnancy rates with two consecutive inseminations, but this finding may be explained by poor timing of insemination involving the single day.
> **B.** Total number of cycles of IUI.

Intrauterine Insemination Indications   **BOX 28.1**

Cervical factors

Poor sperm–mucus interaction/failed postcoital test (poor spinnbarkeit or ferning)

Cervical stenosis

Destruction of endocervical glands as a result of cone, laser, or cryosurgery

Ovulation induction with Serophene (tends to thicken cervical mucus)

Male factor—mild to moderate oligospermia or asthenospermia (count below 20 million)

Poor sperm motility or volume (either seen in semen analysis or postcoital test)

Sperm antibodies in seminal plasma

Retrograde ejaculation

Minimal endometriosis

Antisperm antibodies

Unexplained infertility, pregnancy is not achieved with other medical interventions

Donor insemination

Table 28.1   **Cumulative Pregnancy Rates With IUI**

Month of Insemination	Pregnancy Rate
First	9%
Sixth	38%
Ninth	48%
Eighteenth	56%

1. Most clinicians agree that six cycles represent an adequate trial in women younger than 35 years of age. Some believe that three or four cycles are adequate.
2. Up to 9 or 10 cycles may be warranted for the older woman.
3. The fecundity rates (number of pregnancies per cycle) plateau or decline after 4 to 6 insemination attempts (see Table 28.1).

4. A good guideline is that there should be some results after 6 months of IUI. If no results are seen, then the plan needs to be changed.
   a. The sperm washing technique may be changed.
   b. Controlled ovarian hyperstimulation may be added.
   c. Further testing may be performed (hysterosalpingogram [HSG] or hysterogram, if not previously done).
1. The chances of enhanced success with in vitro fertilization (IVF) must be explained while discussing realistic outcomes.
2. The couple needs to be made aware that the option to return to IUI after failed ART is usually available. A forward step does not preclude reverting back to a previous step.
3. Every time a new technique is added, the clinician must be careful not to give rise to any false hopes that the chances of pregnancy will be substantially increased.
4. An information sheet explaining IUI is helpful (see Appendix 28.1).

C. Use of superovulation (medication to induce ovulation). Superovulation combined with IUI serves many purposes.
   1. Superovulation increases the number of sperm and oocytes available in the upper genital tract, resulting in an increased chance of fertilization and embryo development.
   2. Helps regulate any subtle luteal phase defects.
   3. Pregnancy rates improve with stimulated cycles.
      a. One study demonstrated an increase in fecundity to 9.5%, versus 3.3% in cycles using clomiphene citrate (Serophene).
      b. A recent study at California Fertility Associates in California documented that fewer women conceived following IUI during natural cycles (9.1%) compared with those who had stimulated cycles (13.3%).
   1. Superovulation induces ovulatory cycles in most women who were previously anovulatory.
   2. Parameters for the use of clomiphene citrate.
      a. Begin with 50 mg per day for 5 days, either days 4 to 8, or 5 to 9 of the menstrual cycle.
      b. Increase by 50-mg increments if ovulation is not achieved, but not more than 150 mg.
      c. Refer to an infertility specialist if ovulation does not occur.
      d. Monitor the woman for signs of ovarian hyperstimulation such as lower pelvic pain.

Table 28.2   **Conception Rate by Age With IUI**

Age, Years	Conception Rates With Intrauterine Insemination
< 31	15.1%
31–35	12.9%
36–40	14.6%
41–45	6%
> 45	0%

       e. Inform the woman that her chances of twins increases 5% to 8%. The chance for triplets is rare.

  D. Relationship of age to fertility. Age also affects the outcome of IUI.

    1. Research of thousands of IUI cycles showed the chances of pregnancy were fairly stable through age 40, after which it decreases 2.5-fold (see Table 28.2).

    2. No patient older than 45 years of age conceived in 126 patient cycles.

  E. Use of IUI versus intracervical insemination (ICI).

    1. The pregnancy rate is considerably higher using IUI than ICI because the cervical mucus is bypassed and sperm are placed closer to the site of ovulation.

    2. Statistics document that IUI increases cycle fecundity fourfold compared with ICI.

    3. Studies have shown that ICI leads to sperm recovery in the cul-de-sac 50% of the time, whereas IUI led to recovery in 85% of the cases.

    4. Considering the difference between these two routes, IUI is the treatment of choice.

    5. ICI has advantages.

      a. It is considered less invasive to the woman, both physically and mentally.

      b. There is less risk for complications during the procedure itself than with IUI.

      c. It could actually be performed by the woman herself or her partner in the privacy of their home.

III. Clinical evaluation before IUI.

  A. A complete evaluation should include:

1. A comprehensive history and physical examination including:
   a. A Papanicolaou (Pap) smear if less than a year has passed since the previous smear.
   b. A wet mount to evaluate for any signs of genital infection.
2. Functionally patent fallopian tubes documented by HSG, sonohysterogram, or hysteroscopy.
   a. Recommended within 12 months of anticipated IUI, particularly if factors are present that would put the woman at risk for tubal disease such as:
      (1) A history of sexually transmitted infection (STI), chlamydia, or gonorrhea.
      (2) A history of pelvic inflammatory disease (PID).
      (3) A history of infection following:
         • Abortion.
         • Delivery.
         • Pelvic surgery.
      (1) Documented endometriosis (implants may obstruct the tubes).
      (2) Past or present use of an intrauterine device (IUD).
   b. Some studies indicate an increase in the pregnancy rate following HSG.
3. Tubal evaluation may not be initially performed under the following circumstances:
   a. In the clear case of poor cervical mucus and semen parameters as possible causes of infertility.
   b. Prior anovulatory cycles, which are treated with superovulation.
   c. In the absence of any risk factors for endometriosis, some clinicians proceed to IUI for three cycles. If no pregnancy occurs, recommend to progress to tubal evaluation.
4. Semen analysis should always be performed and kept current (within 6 months of first IUI).

APPENDIX **28.1**

Patient Education: Intrauterine Insemination

Intrauterine insemination (IUI) is the direct placement of highly motile concentrated sperm, washed free of seminal fluid and other cells, into the uterus. Washing the specimen before IUI refines and concentrates sperm, thus enhancing their ability to fertilize the egg.

Intrauterine insemination has consistently been shown to be a safe method to increase a woman's chances of becoming pregnant. There has been no increase in the number of congenital abnormalities when IUI is used. It is usually indicated when the sperm count is low or if the postcoital test shows poor sperm interaction in the cervical mucus. It is sometimes used for unexplained infertility.

In women with open tubes, IUI is an appropriate step. It should definitely be considered as a treatment before referral for assisted reproductive technologies (ART) because it may maximize a woman's chance of conceiving, while minimizing exposure to more complex invasive procedures that are more costly in both time and money. Pregnancy rates in infertile couples who have been trying to get pregnant for a period of 1 year are 10 to 30% higher with IUI when compared with natural intercourse.

Before beginning IUI, you and your partner should be informed of the expected course, the technical aspects of the procedures, the risks of complications (which are very rare), and the chances of getting pregnant. The emotional impact must be addressed. A medication to stimulate follicular development in the ovary may also be recommended.

Timing is very important. You will be given separate instructions on how to use the ovulation predictor kit. A mature egg is able to be fertilized for approximately 12 to 18 hours following ovulation, and fresh sperm have the ability to fertilize for up to 48 hours. A single, well-timed insemination at the time of ovulation is performed each cycle. Call the health center the day of the color change. IUI will be performed on the day after the luteinizing hormone (LH) surge, which is the day of expected ovulation. IUI will be performed for four to six well-timed cycles.

Your treatment plan will be continuously reevaluated as the treatment progresses. The overall pregnancy rate is about 8% per cycle.

Contact your provider if your period is in any way different from your usual flow or if any pelvic pain or unusual discharge develops. IUI cannot be performed if an infection is present.

The procedure is simple. You may bring your partner with you. A pelvic examination is performed, and a speculum is inserted into your vagina. Once the opening to the cervix is visualized, a small catheter is inserted through the cervix and into your uterus. The procedure takes only a few minutes and is rarely uncomfortable. The specimen is placed high in the uterine cavity, adjacent to the area where the ends of the fallopian tubes leave the uterus, as close to the ovulated egg as possible. Simply put, this procedure greatly reduces the distance that the sperm must travel, eliminating the necessity of the spermatozoa traveling from the vagina, through the cervix, and into the uterus. The washed sperm sample is slowly injected. You should remain on the table for an additional 15 minutes, after which you may leave the office and resume normal activities.

The risk of developing any complications following the procedure is very low but call the office if any abdominal pain, cramping, bleeding, or abnormal vaginal discharge occurs after the procedure. Call in 2 weeks should menses occur, or if menses does not occur in 16 days, return for a pregnancy test.

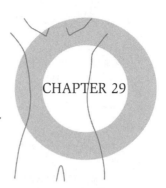

CHAPTER 29

Sperm-Washing Technique

Helen A. Carcio

I. **The gradient technique of sperm preparation explained.**
   A. Some comments.
   1. Sperm are not sterile but need to be carefully washed before direct placement into the uterus. There are many purposes served by sperm washing (Box 29.1).
   2. Semen contains nonmotile, morphologically abnormal sperm and nonsperm cells that need to be separated from the normal motile sperm.
   3. Sperm that are placed directly into the uterus bypass the protective effects of the cervical mucus.
   4. While washing, sperm selection, hyperactivation, and partial capacitation occur—a process that usually occurs in the cervical mucus.
   5. The washing separates the seminal plasma from the spermatozoa, which is important because the seminal plasma contains prostaglandins, which in turn can cause intrauterine contractions.
   6. The advantages of intrauterine insemination (IUI) and sperm washing:
      a. They are inexpensive techniques and therefore cost-effective as an office practice.
      b. They are relatively simple procedures that involve little risk.

| *Purpose of Sperm Washing* | **BOX 29.1** |

1. Removes the seminal plasma, which contains prostaglandins.
2. Removes contaminated cell debris and immobile or morphologic abnormal sperm.
3. Concentrates and hyperactivates the normal sperm.

    c. IUI places the sperm directly into the uterus, which is much closer to the ovulated egg, bypassing the vagina and cervix.

  7. The final sperm count should have at least 1 million motile sperm for IUI to be effective. If there are fewer than 1 million sperm, the couple should be referred for assisted reproductive technologies (ART).

  8. The gradient technique is fairly easy and straightforward, but does require careful adherence to the various steps involved in the procedure.

  9. The gradient technique is effective in separating motile sperm.

    a. Cellular debris, abnormal and immobile defective spermatozoa, seminal fluid debris, and white blood cells are removed from the ejaculate when it is filtered through a concentration gradient during spinning in a centrifuge.

    b. The gradient technique is cost-effective and requires minimal equipment and expertise to perform.

    c. For the concentration gradient to work correctly, extreme care must be taken to keep the two layers separate.

  10. In performing IUI, the spermatozoa can be prepared for insemination in numerous ways. The method explained here is the most reliable technique employed at this time. Many principles must be followed (Box 29.2).

B. Gradient technique: The preparation.

  1. Liquefaction. Liquefaction, or thinning, of the semen normally occurs 20 to 60 minutes following ejaculation. The semen must be liquefied before washing.

    a. Once the sample is collected, it may be left for at least 30 minutes and up to 1 hour at 37°C or room temperature to liquefy.

    b. Determine gross estimate of viscosity (Box 29.3).

    c. Liquefaction is considered normal if it has occurred within 60 minutes.

Important Principles for the Washing of the Ejaculate

BOX 29.2

Laboratory must have Clinical Laboratory Improvement Act (CLIA) approval under the moderate complexity license.

Protective eyewear and gloves should be used when handling the specimen. The same pipette should not be used to enter more than one bottle.

A semen analysis for count and motility is performed and recorded before and after the sperm-washing procedure. This is an important part of quality assurance.

If many white blood cells (WBCs) are present in the ejaculate, intrauterine insemination should not be performed. The partner should be appropriately diagnosed and treated. Remember that immature sperm can look very similar to WBCs.

The total volume of the nongravid uterus is 0.5 mL. If more than 0.5 mL of fluid is instilled, the specimen will flow back out the os.

Properly label all tubes and syringes containing the specimen.

Although the semen is not sterile, sterility should be maintained through the sperm-washing procedure.

Grading of Liquefaction

BOX 29.3

0 Freely drips off end of pipette
1 Forms drop that sticks briefly to pipette before it drops off
2 Forms drop that is delayed in dropping off
3 Forms string as it leaves pipette
4 Thick, syrupy in consistency—may not even form an individual drop (in some cases may not be able to pipette at all)

If viscosity is 3 or 4, the clinician may want to dilute with medium.

    2. Transfer the liquefied semen to a sterile conical tube.
       a. Label with the patient's name and date of collection.
       b. Record volume.
       c. There should be a maximum volume of 2 mL. If volume is over 2 mL, additional tubes need to be used (Table 29.1).

Table 29.1   **Guidelines for Number of Tubes to Centrifuge Based on Volume of Sperm**

Volume	Centrifuge Tube(s) (No.)
1–2 mL	1
3 mL	2
4 mL	3

    3. A small amount of sperm should be left in the original container so a sperm count can be performed on it.

    4. The identity of the donor must be checked by a valid driver's license (explain that it is for the donor's protection), and his Social Security number should be recorded.

C. Equipment.

    1. Makler containing chamber.

    2. Centrifuge capable of operating at 300x *g*.

    3. Incubator or water bath at 37°C.

    4. Sterile plastic graduated 15-mL conical tubes with screw caps

    5. Sterile plastic graduated transfer pipettes (15–20).

    6. Sterile specimen container.

    7. One-mL insulin syringe.

    8. Insemination catheter.

    9. Isolate sperm-washing kit containing upper phase, lower phase, and sperm-washing medium.

    10. Microscope with 20X objective.

D. Technique. Extreme care must be taken to keep the layers of isolate separate.

    1. Warm all medium to room temperature or 37°C.

    2. Using a bulb pipette, transfer 1.5 mL of lower phase medium to the bottom of the centrifuge tube.

    3. Carefully layer 1.5 mL of upper phase medium over lower phase medium.

        a. Allow the pipette tip to contact the surface of the lower phase medium and slide back to allow a wet channel for the solution to slide along.

        b. Hold the tube at an angle, and slowly dispense the upper phase solution along the side of the tube, drawing back the tip as the level of the upper phase medium rises.

    c. A visible line should be seen.

    d. The tube should be filled to the 3.0-mL mark.

4. Gently mix the liquefied semen sample, being careful to avoid bubbles. If a frozen specimen is used, it should be thoroughly warmed to 37°C to maximize sperm motility.

5. Pipette up to 2 mL of liquefied semen, and layer over the upper phase medium.

6. The total volume should not exceed 5 mL.

7. Cap the tube, and centrifuge for 20 minutes at 300x *g*.

    a. Be sure that the centrifuge is balanced with a tube filled with the same volume of water.

    b. After the 20 minutes has elapsed, the normal sperm, by action of their tails, migrate to the bottom of the tube, forming a pellet.

    c. Debris, leukocytes, and sperm with abnormal forms remain in the middle or top layers.

    d. Do not centrifuge for more than 20 minutes, after which the dead sperm may also be forced down to the pellet.

8. Using the bulb pipette, remove the medium until it is within the 0.5-mL mark.

    a. Do not disturb the pellet.

    b. If the pellet is disturbed, recentrifuge for a few minutes longer until another pellet is formed.

    c. Sometimes, there may not be a clearly defined sperm pellet.

9. Combine pellets (if more than one tube was used).

10. Next, the pellet is washed and nourished with a special wash medium.

    a. Add sperm-washing medium up to the 5-mL mark, and mix well to resuspend the pellet.

    b. Tap against the palm of hand to resuspend sperm cells into the medium, or slowly invert the capped tube three to four times.

11. Centrifuge for an additional 10 minutes.

12. Again, carefully remove supernatant as described earlier, leaving 0.5 mL above the pellet.

13. Repeat the washing procedure by resuspending the sperm pellet into the new medium.

14. Add medium as needed to the 5-mL mark.

15. Centrifuge for another 10 minutes.

16. Remove medium to pellet.

Documentation Required for Intrauterine Insemination

BOX 29.4

- Document the pre- and postsperm count and motility of the specimen
- Any degree of trauma associated with the IUI procedure, especially any bleeding
- Date of LH surge in relation to IUI procedure
- Day of menstrual cycle
- The number of IUI procedures per cycle (one is recommended)
- The number of the insemination cycle
- Character of cervical mucus and cervical os
- Any use of ovulation induction
- Results of previous evaluation of fallopian tube adequacy

IUI, Intrauterine insemination; LH, luteinizing hormone.

---

17. Add sperm-washing medium to 0.5-mL mark.
18. Place one to two drops on Makler counting chamber. Analyze and record.
    a. Movement of the sperm will look very different.
    b. Motility increases as hyperactivation occurs.
    c. Washed sperm undergo a transition from a forward progression (a linear swimming motion) when they are in the semen, to a shaking dance, or "thrash" trajectory.
    d. The sperm are capacitated at this point.
19. Load remaining medium into 1-mL syringe (tuberculin) attached to a catheter for insemination.
20. Leave a bolus of air in the syringe or have washing medium available to flush the catheter of any sperm.
21. Labeling the container, or paper wrapper, is critical. Record:
    a. Patient's name
    b. Partner's name or number of donor sperm.
    c. Replace the catheter with syringe attached into the sterile paper wrapper and store at room temperature until ready to use.
22. The washed sample should be used within a half hour.
23. Review the final sperm count with the patient, and show the patient the donor number on vial, if donor sperm is used.
24. Documentation is vital (Box 29.4).
25. The solution should be used within 2 hours when it is stored at room temperature.
26. See Box 29.5 for a quick reference to the above-mentioned procedure; Figure 29.1 depicts the process.

Quick Reference: Sperm Preparation
for Intrauterine Insemination

BOX 29.5

1. Warm all media to room temperature or 37°C.
2. Allow time for liquefaction of semen (20 minutes).
3. Transfer 1.5 mL of lower phase to centrifuge tube.
4. Carefully layer 1.5 mL of upper phase over lower phase.
5. Add semen on top of upper layer (no more than 2 mL). Total volume should not exceed 5 mL.
6. Prepare a second tube as above if volume of sperm is more than 2 mL.
7. Centrifuge for 20 minutes.
8. Perform semen analysis on unwashed specimen for number and motility. Record.
9. Remove and discard layers down to the pellet (0.5 mL).
10. Combine pellets (if more than one tube).
11. Add sperm-washing medium to 5 mL and mix well to resuspend the pellet.
12. Centrifuge for 10 minutes.
13. Again, remove old medium and resuspend pellet in new medium as above.
14. Centrifuge for 10 more minutes.
15. Remove old medium and add new medium to 0.5-mL mark. Mix well.
16. Perform semen analysis on washed specimen for number and motility. Record.
17. Load specimen into 1-mL syringe (tuberculin) and catheter for insemination. Label.

II. Swim-up technique.

A. Some comments.

1. The *swim-up technique* involves the washing of the liquefied semen with an isosmotic solution and centrifugation.

2. If either a low number of sperm or poor motility is the major factor that may be contributing to infertility, the swim-up method may not yield enough sperm.

3. Longer incubation times may be necessary to allow for more sperm to swim up.

4. The more highly mobile sperm are harvested, and the morphologically abnormal sperm are left behind.

5. It is not known if the presence of these abnormal forms has any effect on conception.

B. Equipment: As in Section I.C.

C. Technique.

1. Allow the specimen to liquefy at room temperature for 30 minutes.

2. Estimate count and motility of the semen sample. Record.

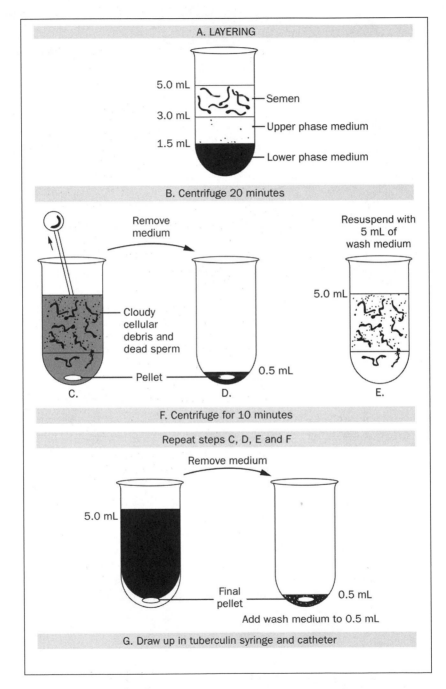

Figure 29.1 Steps in sperm-washing procedure in preparation for intrauterine insemination.

3. Using a pipette, place the semen into a sterile, 15-mL centrifuge tube with a conical bottom.
4. Should the volume be greater than 5 mL, divide into two sterile tubes.
5. Add 3 mL of medium and mix with semen by gentle pipetting. (Do not use a needle because it may damage the sperm.)
6. Centrifuge for 10 minutes.
7. Carefully remove medium to just above the sperm pellet and discard.
8. If more than one tube is used, combine several suspensions into one tube.
9. Add fresh medium and resuspend.
10. Again, carefully remove supernatant, and gently add 0.5 mL of medium.
11. Hold the tube at an angle so that the medium runs down the side of the tube with minimal disturbance of the sperm pellet.
12. Tap the tube gently to loosen the sperm pellet. Be careful not to mix the pellet with the medium.
13. Next the sperm pellet is overlaid with a culture medium solution and incubated at 37°C for 60 minutes.
14. During that time, the more mobile spermatozoa swim out of the pellet up to the overlying medium, which becomes cloudy with the increasing concentration of sperm. This process is termed *sperm migration.*
15. The top 0.5 to 0.8 mL of the upper cloudy layer contains the motile sperm immediately above the pellet.
16. Using a syringe attached to a catheter, carefully remove a portion of the upper, cloudy layer.
17. Estimate and record count and motility from a small drop (aliquot).

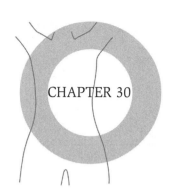

CHAPTER 30

Intrauterine Insemination Procedure

Helen A. Carcio

I. The procedure explained.
  A. Obtaining the specimen.
    1. The semen specimen is obtained by masturbation into a sterile container.
    2. It can either be collected at home or produced in a nearby bathroom.
    3. If it is collected at home, it must be brought to the laboratory or office within 1 hour.
    4. The container should be one supplied by the office and is usually a green-capped sterile urine container. (Use of a container sterilized at home is usually discouraged.)
    5. The semen must be kept at body temperature. It should be transported inside the clothing, with the container in direct skin contact. The warmth of the body can help maintain the quality of the specimen as much as possible.
    6. Avoid excessive heat. Do not place in front of the car heater because this may damage the sperm.
    7. It is essential to establish the identity of the partner. A driver's license is an excellent form of identification. Record driver's license (or Social Security) number.

Documentation of Intrauterine Insemination   **BOX 30.1**

Record:
The name and Social Security number of husband or intimate partner
The number of days of abstinence prior to today's ejaculate
Collection problems
Any transportation problems
Time of specimen collection
Any medications the donor is taking

8. Once the semen is left at the center, the patient and her partner can leave and return in 1 hour. It should be suggested that they go someplace to relax and have a light snack.
9. There may be a time when the man is unable to "perform on demand." Be as supportive as possible and try to schedule the insemination for later that day, schedule permitting.
10. Documentation is important (Box 30.1).

B. Preparing the woman.
  1. When the woman returns, she should empty her bladder.
  2. Inquire as to whether there has been any significant change in her menses in any way during the intrauterine insemination (IUI) cycle. (Any change should be carefully explored before IUI can proceed.)
  3. Elicit whether there has been any change in the character of the vaginal discharge, which may indicate an infection.
    a. IUI should not be performed if any infection is present.
    b. A wet mount can be performed before IUI to observe for any white blood cells or vaginitis.
    c. If an infection is present, the infection should be identified and treated, and the IUI rescheduled for the next month.
  4. It is a nice idea to have the room be as relaxing as possible. Never forget that a new life may be created here.
    a. Dim the lights or have a lamp on the counter, which can be used rather than bright overhead lights.
    b. Silk flowers on the counter lend to a more informal atmosphere.

C. Insemination technique.
  1. Bring the prepared specimen into the room in the syringe with catheter attached. It should be replaced in the sterile wrapper. The name should be on the wrapper.

Table 30.1   Timing of Insemination

Method	Timing of Insemination
Urinary LH kit	Day after the color change
Clomiphene d5-9	Day 16 or 17
Ultrasound	18-mm diameter: 24–36 hours later

2. The partner may be present in the room and is encouraged to remain for the insemination procedure.
3. Review the expected procedure with the patient and her partner.
4. Reassure her that the procedure takes only a few minutes and is usually painless.
5. Verify that ovulation has occurred (using luteinizing hormone [LH] predictor kit and ultrasound).
6. Document the method, timing, and use of any superovulation technique, and day of menses (Table 30.1).
7. Review any potential complications.
8. Obtain written consent (Box 30.2).
    a. Many states require written consent from both partners.
    b. The consent form needs to be completed only for the first insemination.
    c. Consent is also required for any donor sperm; either both husband and wife or a single woman must sign. Note: This is separate from the form required by the cryobank.
9. Record sperm count and number of donor specimen (Box 30.3).
10. Ask the woman to assume a lithotomy position (perhaps to a slight degree of Trendelenburg's position).
11. Perform a bimanual examination to assess uterine size and positioning. Explain the procedure.
12. Insert bivalvular speculum into the vagina to visualize the cervix.
    a. Note and record the appearance of the cervical os and the character of ovulatory discharge.
    b. A mirror may be used to show the cervix to the patient and her partner.

Consent for Intrauterine Insemination   BOX 30.2

I, _____ and my partner, _____,
understand that intrauterine insemination (IUI) has been recommended for
me for the purpose of achieving pregnancy. The purpose of the procedure,
the technique itself, and potential complications have been fully explained
and I/we have been provided with the opportunity to ask questions
regarding this procedure that have been answered to my/our satisfaction.

I understand that IUI will be performed once per cycle and that several
attempts at IUI may be necessary over a course of four to six cycles.

I understand that the procedure involves the use of washed sperm from
my husband or intimate partner, which will be placed directly into my
uterus.

I understand that there is a possibility that complications may occur
during childbearing and delivery separate from the IUI.

I understand that the risk of fetal abnormalities and miscarriage are the
same as for other pregnancies achieved by natural sexual intercourse.

I understand that other unexpected risks or complications not discussed
may occur.

I understand that a pregnancy may not result and that no promises or
guarantees have been made concerning the results of the IUI.

I am not allergic to penicillin or streptomycin.

By signing this consent form I hereby accept the risks inherent in an IUI
procedure, including, but not limited to, the risks set forth in this informed
consent form.

I hereby authorize _____ to perform IUI.

Patient: _____ Witness: _____

Date: _____ Date: _____

Clinician Certification

I certify the above procedure and its complications/risks have been
explained to the patient and her partner.

Clinician signature/date: _____

---

13. The cervix may be cleansed with a dry rectal swab or a
    swab dipped in normal saline.
14. Thread the preloaded catheter through the cervix.
    a. Do not force.
    b. Once the fundus is felt, pull catheter back a few centime-
       ters to allow the sperm to flow unobstructed through the
       tip.
    c. This approach places the sperm close to the opening of
       the tubes.
15. Usually, a tenaculum does not need to be used, except with
    patients who have a marked degree of uterine anteversion or
    retroflexion.

Microscopic Analysis Technique   **BOX 30.3**

The semen analysis is performed twice during the intrauterine insemination procedure. The original count is performed before washing; the second is a postwash analysis. A Makler counting chamber is recommended. This device has a base with a flat disc over which a nondisposable cover is placed.

- The specimen should be mixed well once liquefaction has occurred.
- A drop of the specimen is placed in the center of the disc with a sterile pipette. Holding the cover next to the two dots, the cover is placed over the disc. The drop should spread over the entire surface of the disc.
- Rotate the coverslip to evenly spread the specimen over the entire field.
- Place the chamber under the microscope.
- Using the 20x objective, scan the chamber to find the grid and focus on the sperm.
- The sperm should be evenly distributed over the disc.
- Count and record the number of *all* sperm in 10 squares.
- Next, count and record the number of actively motile sperm in 10 squares. This represents the number of total motile sperm in millions per milliliter. Record in medical record.
- Divide the total motile sperm by the total sperm count to calculate the percentage of actively motile sperm.
- Record in medical record.

16. If cervical stenosis is present, a stiffer catheter should be used, or the catheter can be placed in the freezer and frozen.
17. The new catheters are very narrow, making it possible to deposit the spermatozoa atraumatically and accurately high in the uterine cavity.
18. Ask the partner if he or she would like to inject the sperm.
    a. Some partners are very pleased with being offered this opportunity, whereas others are simply appalled.
    b. Be open to either response.
19. Slowly inject the specimen over 30 to 60 seconds to avoid flushing the uterus too fast and causing retrograde flow.
    a. Be careful that the catheter does not act as an outflow wick.
    b. Injecting the solution too rapidly can force semen through the tubes into the peritoneum, causing considerable pain.
    c. Any excess semen should be allowed to flow out of the uterus.
    d. Some sources suggest leaving the catheter in the cervix for another minute.

e. If the catheter has traumatized the lining of the uterus and bleeding occurs, the chance of fertilization is reduced because immunoglobulins may be secreted from the endometrium, immobilizing the sperm.

f. Slight bleeding from the cervix is acceptable as long as blood does not enter the uterus.

20. Remove the catheter with a slight twist to avoid any spillage.

21. Slowly inject 0.5 ml of air to clear the catheter of any remaining specimen. Be careful not to force any of the sperm from the uterus.

22. Remove the speculum.

23. Rotate the speculum sideways to dump any spilled sperm into the vagina.

24. Leave the woman in a reclining position for 5 to 20 minutes.

a. Remove her legs from the stirrups, and pull out the drawer to support her legs.

b. Dim the lights, if possible.

c. It is controversial whether elevating the hips is of any benefit.

25. As the woman is leaving, it is sometimes a nice idea to allow her and her partner to view the sperm under the microscope. It somehow helps validate the process.

26. Instruct the woman to call:

a. To report the development of abdominal pain, cramping, or fever (Box 30.4).

b. To report the onset of menses and to discuss the next steps.

c. If menses are 2 or 3 days late, or for pregnancy test and further instructions.

Complications of Intrauterine Insemination   **BOX 30.4**

Complications: The complication rate of IUI is extremely low but not totally absent.

Cramping: Occurs in approximately 5% of all patients. Usually the cramping subsides within the hour. Although the majority of the prostaglandins have been washed away, it may be possible for some residual prostaglandins to remain. Additionally, the introduction of the catheter through the cervical os may set up a cramping reflex. The endometrium may become disrupted by the insemination catheter, causing a prostaglandin cascade, leading to cramping.

Mild spotting: Spotting is rarer than cramping, occurring in 1% of patients. It is probably caused by the minor irritation of the catheter as it penetrates the outer cervical os. Spotting usually subsides within a few hours after the procedure.

GI upset: Gastrointestinal upset and nausea occur in 0.05% of women. This is probably caused by the disruption of the endometrium, leading to the eventual production of intrauterine prostaglandins. It also will subside in a few hours.

Infection: Occurs in fewer than 0.2% of patients. Antibiotics are not necessary for either the woman or her partner before or after the procedure.

Donor Insemination

CHAPTER 31

Helen A. Carcio

I. **Donor insemination explained.**
   A. More than 30,000 babies are conceived by donor insemination each year.
   B. There has also been an increase in the number of single women and lesbian couples who are interested in having a biologic child. It may be the only alternative for women without male partners who wish to conceive.
   C. The reduced availability of adoptable babies has greatly increased its use.
   D. Although donor insemination may be very appropriate for some couples, many psychological, social, and ethical questions remain (and are beyond the scope of this chapter).
   E. If pregnancy with a certain donor is requested, the patient can ask that the vials from the same donor be saved for future pregnancies at a fee. Through this method, offspring will have a father in common.
   F. There is no increase in pregnancy complications or fetal anomalies in babies born with donor sperm.

II. **Indications.**
   A. Donor inseminations are useful for couples in which the male partner has the following:
      1. Azoospermia.

       a. Previous vasectomy.

       b. Congenital or surgical absence of either the testes or the vas.

    2. Severe oligospermia.

    3. Poor sperm motility.

    4. Presence of antisperm antibodies in either partner.

    5. Male sexual dysfunction.

  B. Women without male partners.

    1. Lesbian couples.

    2. Single women.

  C. Genetic disorders.

    1. Autosomal dominant disorder in male.

    2. Recessive genetic trait in both partners.

       a. Tay-Sachs disease.

       b. Cystic fibrosis.

  D. Women who have a history of fetal loss caused by Rh sensitization. (These patients would be able to choose an Rh-negative donor.)

III. Success rates.

  A. The success rates with frozen semen are lower than with fresh semen.

  B. The chances of getting pregnant each cycle with frozen sperm is only 5%, compared with nearly 20% with fresh semen.

  C. It usually takes twice as many inseminated cycles to conceive.

  D. The effects are cumulative, whereas the success rates using fresh semen seem to plateau or drop.

IV. Source of donor.

  A. Some comments.

    1. When exploring the donor lists, an attempt should be made to match the physical characteristics with those of the husband or partner, if applicable.

    2. Some sources recommend mixing the donor sperm with the husband's in cases of a low sperm count.

    3. Counseling is often recommended.

  B. All donor sperm is frozen and used only after a 6-month quarantine period has passed, after which the donor has been tested and is determined to be free of human immunodeficiency virus (HIV) and other sexually transmitted diseases.

  C. Known donors.

    1. Donors may be a friend or the male partner's brother, father, or uncle.

  2. Patients desiring such services should be referred to area cry-obanks, where they can make arrangements for testing, collecting, freezing, quarantine, and storage of sperm. Use of untested sperm is not recommended.
  3. Raises legal and social issues for both the recipient and the donor, which they must both be made aware of. Use of a lawyer is strongly recommended.
  4. There are advantages.
     a. Enhances knowledge of the personal traits of the donor.
     b. Avoids impersonal nature of anonymous donors.
     c. If the donor is a relative, it ensures some continuity of family.
  D. Anonymous donor.
  1. Sperm banks do not reveal the identity of the donor.
  2. Some banks leave open the opportunity of the donor to contact the woman if she so desires at some future time.
  3. The donor is not usually informed whether a child results from insemination with his sperm.

V. Shipping of frozen specimens.
  A. Transportation tanks.
  1. Portable liquid nitrogen vapor tanks.
  2. Usually hold specimens frozen for 7 days.
  3. Do not open tank until ready to use.
  B. Cost. Cost varies among laboratories but generally:
  1. Local shipping by courier: $50.
  2. Federal Express: $150.
  C. It is often up to the patient to make her own payment and shipping arrangements.

VI. Preparation of donor sperm.
  A. The Centers for Disease Control and Prevention (CDC) and the Food and Drug Administration (FDA) have imposed restrictions on the use of donor specimens by mandating that only guaranteed frozen specimens be used, as described below.
  B. Testing.
  1. The donor is tested for HIV. The specimen is quarantined for 60 to 180 days and released only after a second HIV antibody titer is negative.
  C. Additional tests required of donors.
  1. Blood type and Rh.
  2. Complete blood count.
  3. Blood chemistry.

      4. Antihepatitis B surface antigen.

      5. Antihepatitis B core.

      6. Gonorrhea.

      7. Rapid plasma reagin (RPR) test for syphilis.

      8. Herpes simplex virus.

      9. Antihepatitis C.

     10. Hepatitis B surface antigen.

     11. Chlamydia.

     12. HIV-1 and HIV-2.

     13. Fluid culture on semen.

D. Unable to test for herpes.

E. Testing on donors from certain ethnic groups.

      1. α-thalassemia.

      2. Tay-Sachs carrier screen.

      3. Sickle cell carrier screen.

F. Performed on request.

      1. Ureaplasma.

      2. Mycoplasma.

      3. Karyotyping.

      4. Canavan, gaucher, or both.

G. Donors generally between 18 and 35 years of age.

H. Evaluation of candidate.

      1. Completes an extensive questionnaire.

      2. Health history spans three generations.

      3. Complete physical examination.

      4. Screens for history of genetic disease.

I. Description of donor usually includes:

      1. Ethnic origin.

      2. Blood type.

      3. Color of hair and eyes.

      4. Height and weight.

      5. Religion.

      6. Occupation, education, and interests are often included.

J. Matching can be done either by:

      1. Sperm bank.

      2. Recipient.

VII. Specimen quality.

   A. Vials prepared for intracervical insemination (ICI) are packaged in 0.8- to 1.0-mL volumes.

   B. Each vial is guaranteed to contain a minimum of 20 million motile sperm.

   C. The minimum postthaw motility of each vial prepared for ICI is 25 to 35%.

D. Vials for IUI are packaged in 0.5-mL volumes.

E. Most sperm banks grant full credit if the specimen is substandard.

F. The vials are guaranteed to be kept frozen for 7 to 10 calendar days from the shipping date.

VIII. The initial visit.

    A. Complete history and physical of the woman.

    B. If findings suggest normal fertility, may begin insemination process.

    C. If there are indicators of infertility, see chapter 26

    D. Perform routine prenatal tests.

        1. HIV.

        2. Hepatitis.

        3. Syphilis.

        4. Immunity to rubella and varicella.

    E. Begin the woman on prenatal vitamins.

    F. Provide the couple with a list of available cryobanks and potential donors. See http://www.ihr.com/infertility/provider/spermbank.html for a nationwide list of spem banks.

    G. Monitor for ovulation verification, and instruct in how to use ovulation predictor kits (see chapter 28).

    H. Discuss and review the consent form, and have the patient sign it.

        1. Donor insemination should involve the consent of both partners, male and female, or female and female.

        2. See Box 31.1.

IX. Home insemination using frozen sperm.

    A. After discussing the various alternatives, a woman may decide on home insemination.

    B. It is the clinician's responsibility to offer support, education, and guidance.

    C. Review timing of procedure.

        1. Using ovulation predictor kits:

            a. Day of color change or day after if using frozen sperm.

            b. Day after color change if using sperm from a known donor.

    D. Thawing of specimen (see Section X, D).

    E. Procedure for deposition of sperm in the vagina.

        1. Intravaginal. May use syringe and catheter to simply deposit sperm in the vagina.

        2. Purchase sperm cup.

Authorization for Artificial Insemination With Frozen Donor Sperm

BOX 31.1

Artificial insemination using donor sperm has been recommended for me/us.

I/We understand the nature and purpose of the procedure and its potential benefits and risks, and outcomes.

I/We understand that the purpose of this procedure is to induce pregnancy in a situation in which spontaneous conception is not possible.

I/We understand that during this procedure sperm is given by a donor to a commercially accredited sperm bank, frozen for storage, and thawed immediately before injection by syringe into my cervix.

I/We understand that pregnancy is not guaranteed and that the production of a child with undesirable traits, hereditary tendencies, disabilities, or abnormalities is possible as with any conception.

I/We understand that infection, including the possibility of venereal disease or AIDS, is possible, even though all donors are thoroughly screened and the frozen sperm is quarantined for 6 months while donors are tested.

I/We are aware that there is a possibility that complications may arise during childbearing or delivery. These have not been shown to be increased by the process of donor insemination.

I/We are aware of the possible side effects, including pain, infection, scarring, and uterine perforation.

I/We are aware that there may be other risks or complications not discussed that may occur. No guarantees or promises have been made to me/us concerning the outcome of this procedure.

I/We have been given the opportunity to ask questions about the procedure and expected outcomes and have received satisfactory answers.

I/We consent to the performance of artificial insemination with frozen donor sperm by the clinician named below or his/her designee.

Date: _____

Patient Name: _____

Medical Record Number: _____

(Please print)

Patient Signature: _____

Partner Signature: _____

Clinician Signature: _____

Date: _____

      a. The entire specimen of semen is placed in the cup and placed against the cervix, thus protecting the semen from a hostile vaginal environment.

      b. The sperm cup should be left in place for approximately 8 hours.

   3. The advantage of the home-insemination option is that it eliminates the necessity of transporting the specimen to the provider's office, electing for the quieter, more natural environment of the home. Seems to be less invasive.

   4. Disadvantage of home inseminations.

      a. Technique is not monitored.

      b. No check of adequacy of sperm specimen.

X. Preparation for the insemination procedure.

  A. Equipment.

    1. Vial containing specimen with donor number clearly visible.

    2. Paperwork validating donor number.

    3. Insemination syringe and catheter.

    4. Thermometer if using water bath.

  B. Verify with woman the correct donor number and number of vials received.

  C. Remove the vial from the shipping tank.

    1. Do not remove tank from box—save for return shipment.

    2. Carefully lift the cap off the tank by raising it straight up. *Do not twist it.*

    3. Lift the inner canister out by the handle, and remove the thin silver can that contains the vial.

    4. Gloves must be worn to eliminate freezer burn of the fingers and hands.

    5. Protective eyewear should be worn.

    6. Select the appropriate vial by checking the donor number.

    7. Note: Vials that have been thawed cannot be refrozen.

  D. Thawing of the specimen. Thawing varies with individual cryobanks. Vials must be removed from the tanks approximately 10 minutes before the insemination procedure.

    1. Thaw at room temperature for 5 minutes, then at 37°C for 5 minutes.

    2. If a 37°C plate or incubator is not available, hold the vial tightly for 5 minutes.

    3. Some sources recommend not placing vials in a water bath because this may increase the chances of contamination, should water seep in through the cap. (Vial may not be watertight.)

    4. Never heat specimens above 37°C.

    5. Best results are achieved when insemination takes place immediately after the completion of the thawing process.

    6. An alternate method is to place the frozen vial in a water bath of 38°C to 42°C for 3 minutes, shake, and replace in the water bath (should recheck the temperature) for an additional 3 minutes. Note: A temperature higher than 40°C will severely decrease sperm motility.

E. Gently agitate.

F. Perform a semen analysis for the number and motility of sperm. Most banks will not charge for an inadequate postthaw specimen.

G. Return tank by date indicated on packing slip.

H. Sperm washing.

    1. Many sperm banks offer specimens that are already washed.

    2. Controversy still exists as to whether or not frozen sperm for IUI need to be washed.

    3. Cryobanks do use synthetic cryoprotectants, which have the potential to cause cramping and inflammation. Infection is rare, however.

XI. The insemination.

A. Draw up the specimen into the syringe, and note the volume.

B. Attach insemination catheter.

C. Intravaginal.

    1. This procedure is usually not done in an office setting.

    2. It may be indicated in the woman who does not want the invasiveness of intracervical or intrauterine insemination but wants the specimen prepared and evaluated by a clinician.

D. Intracervical insemination (ICI).

    1. Some believe that the cervix acts as a time-release reservoir, releasing sperm over 24 to 48 hours, allowing the fertilization to occur even if the insemination has not been precisely timed.

    2. It is believed that with ICI, the timing is not as critical because the sperm retain their fertilizing capacity for a longer time in the reservoir of the endocervical mucus than in the endometrium.

    3. Explain the procedure for placement of sperm.

        a. The patient is placed in stirrups and draped appropriately.

        b. A speculum is inserted, and the cervical os is visualized.

        c. Thread the catheter, which is attached to the syringe containing the sperm, just inside the cervical os.

      d. Slowly instill the specimen into the lower part of the cervical canal or in the cervical os.

      e. With ICI, the woman should remain with her hips elevated.

      f. The clinician may allow the speculum to remain in place for 5 or 10 minutes to hold sperm in closer contact with the cervical os.

    4. Alternate method. The clinician may deposit sperm in cervical cup, which is then secured over the cervix.

      a. Fit the cup over the cervix, choosing from the nine available sizes. Should be self-retaining on the cervix, yet leave room for the semen to be injected into the cup.

      b. Aspirate semen from the vial into the syringe.

      c. Make sure the white ball in the stem is below the hole in the bottom of the stem.

      d. Push the polyethylene attachment tail on the syringe through the small hole in the bottom of the stem.

      e. Slowly inject the sperm directly into the cup

      f. Using the tamper rod supplied in the package, push the white ball up the stem as far as it will go. This acts as a plug to prevent the backflow of sperm from the cup.

      g. Fold the stem and put into loop provided.

      h. Have the woman remain on the exam table for 20 minutes. Elevate hips if possible.

      i. Woman may leave, with instructions to keep cup in place for 3 to 4 hours.

      j. Remove the cup by first breaking the seal on the cervix, then pull the device from the vagina using the stem attachment.

E. Intrauterine insemination (IUI) (see chapter 30).

    1. Disadvantages of IUI.

      a. More expensive than ICI.

      b. Must be performed in a health center.

      c. Must use washed specimens.

      d. Prostaglandins in the seminal fluid may cause severe cramping if the specimen is deposited directly into the uterus.

    2. The main advantage is an increase in pregnancy rate.

F. Number of inseminations. One to two inseminations are performed each month. Although recent studies indicate that only one insemination is necessary for cycles using fresh sperm, some research suggests that two inseminations should be performed with donor sperm.

G. Timing.
   1. Two-inseminations method. First is recommended on the day of the color change, and the second on the day after.
   2. One-insemination method. Done on the day following the color change, as with the fresh specimen.
H. If no pregnancy occurs after three cycles, some women elect to change the donor or switch to IUI if she has previously had ICI.
I. If no pregnancy occurs after four to six cycles of IUI, a more extensive infertility workup may be indicated, such as a hysterosalpingogram.

XII. Comparison of rate of pregnancy with fresh versus frozen sperm.
   A. Some comments.
      1. Pregnancy rates are lower for cervical inseminations.
      2. Frozen sperm tend to perform better when they are introduced directly into the uterus compared with being introduced at the cervix.
      3. It seems that with frozen sperm in particular, it is better to deposit as close to the site of fertilization as possible.
      4. Some sources believe that by using at least 20 million motile sperm, pregnancy rates with frozen sperm are comparable to those with fresh sperm. Sperm banks usually guarantee 20 to 25 million motile sperm.
      5. It seems that, in theory, the higher the number of sperm, the greater the chance of fertilization.
      6. Frozen sperm are usually washed before freezing, but probably should be washed afterward to remove the cryoprotectant. This is only necessary for IUI, not for ICI.

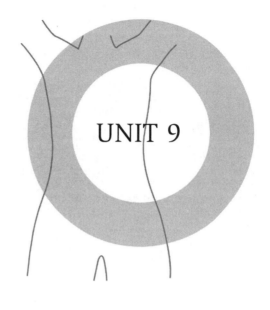

UNIT 9

Advanced Skills

CHAPTER 32

Vulvar Cancer and Biopsy

Helen A. Carcio

I. **Vulvar cancer explained.**
   A. Statistics.
      1. Accounts for 0.7% of all female cancers, occurring in 1.8 per 100,000 women.
      2. Is the fourth most common malignant tumor of the female genital tract.
      3. It causes 500 deaths annually in the United States.
   B. Occurrence.
      1. Occurs most frequently in women older than 65 years.
      2. Incidence is rising in younger women.
      3. Usually diagnosed in the localized stage (about 60%).
   C. Surgery is the usual treatment.
   D. Most tumors are squamous cell in origin.
   E. Long-standing pruritus is the most common complaint.
   F. The most frequent site is the labia minora, in the middle or anterior portion.
   G. Risk factors.
      1. History of herpes simplex virus type 2 (HSV2) or human papillomavirus (HPV).
      2. Multiple sexual partners.
      3. Smoking.

H. Early detection is key to reducing mortality rates.

I. Biopsy study.

  1. All white lesions of the vulva must undergo biopsy study if short-term medical treatment is unsuccessful. Two thirds of the lesions appear acetowhite (white when vinegar is applied).

  2. Any suspicious lesions of any color and persistent ulcerations should be excised.

II. Nonneoplastic epithelial disorders of the vulvar skin and mucosa.

  A. Squamous hyperplasia.

  1. Proliferative response to an irritant or allergen that has become chronic.

  2. The presenting symptom is pruritus, with or without vulvodynia.

  3. Suspect all substances that come in contact with the vulvar skin. (See Box 32.1 for a list of vulvar irritants.)

  4. Assessment includes:

  a. Thick white patches caused by localized thickening of the epidermis (lichenification).

  b. Raised lesions, often bilaterally symmetric.

  c. Vulva may appear dusky red in color.

  d. Vulvar skin thickened with prominent skin markings (Perdu's sign).

  5. Diagnosis.

  a. Punch biopsy.

  b. Histologic findings of acanthosis (irregular thickening of the malpighian layer), hyperkeratosis, and inflammatory infiltrate.

  B. Lichen sclerosis.

  1. Related to hormonal, genetic, and immunologic interactions.

  2. Usually seen after a long period of self-diagnosis and treatment.

  3. Symptoms include intractable itching, with or without vulvodynia.

  4. Assessment includes:

  a. Bluish-white papules, which progress to form thin white patches.

  b. Tissue is friable and may develop petechiae.

  c. Skin is thin and wrinkles like parchment paper.

Substances That May Cause Vulvar Irritation	BOX 32.1

Laundry detergents/fabric softeners

Chlorine bleach

Fiberglass particles (residue in washing machine after washing fiberglass materials such as curtains)

Propylene glycol in spermicides, lubricants, and vaginal medications

Formalin found in the wool of permanent press fabrics

Nylon (can give off formaldehyde vapors)

Deodorant substances on sanitary pads and liners

Vaginal sprays and douches

Creams in topical antifungal agents

Synthetic-fiber underwear

Fabric dyes, especially in colored underwear

Saliva

Semen

Bromine and chlorine compounds in hot tubs and swimming pools

Prescribed medications such as antifungals, antibacterials, crotamiton

Note: The distribution of lesions may provide a clue to which agent may be responsible for the allergic reaction.

　

5. Diagnosis.
　　a. Punch biopsy.
　　b. Histologic findings include loss of rete layers, homogenization, and inflammatory infiltrate.
C. Vulvar dermatologic manifestations that may be associated with systemic disease. May not need to be excised if the systemic condition is well documented.
　　1. Bechet's disease.
　　　a. Small vesicles that ulcerate.
　　　b. Systemic areas include oral ulcerations with uveitis and arthritis.
　　2. Pellagra.
　　　a. A history of anorexia or poor dietary intake.
　　　b. Hyperpigmentation and peeling of the vulva.
　　　c. Systemic areas include dry scaly body skin with erythema of the mucous membrane.

3. Diabetes.
   a. Chronic pruritus of vulva and erythema with a gray sheen.
   b. Systemic areas include dry body skin and changes related to the kidney, retina, and heart.
4. Crohn's disease.
   a. Knifelike slits in vulvar folds.
   b. Associated with gastrointestinal problems of varying degree.

III. **Differential diagnosis of other vulvar dermatoses.**
   A. Table 32.1 compares and contrasts other dermatoses.
   B. A biopsy may be indicated because symptoms vary and may be cancerous.

IV. **Vulvar biopsy.**
   A. Vulvar biopsy is a simple office procedure that is virtually free of complications and usually does not cause discomfort for the patient.
   B. It is appropriate to use on lesions smaller than 0.5 cm. Refer larger lesions to a gynecologist.
   C. The procedure takes approximately 15 minutes.
   D. Excising all lesions, particularly fissures, ulcerations, or thick plaques, is mandatory because of the risk of cancer, no matter how small (only 1–2% risk).
   E. Must be a full-thickness biopsy sample.
   F. Histologic findings are diagnostic.

V. **Assessment.**
   A. Ask about other dermatologic conditions on other parts of the body because a condition such as psoriasis can occur on the vulva.
   B. Carefully evaluate the vagina and cervix, remembering that discharge from these areas bathes the vulvar tissues.
   C. Perform a vaginal wet mount (see chapter 10) on any discharge.

VI. **Indications.**
   A. To differentiate between benign and malignant conditions: Women who smoke or who are infected with HPV 16 or HSV 2 are at higher risk for vulvar cancer.
      1. If the patient is seropositive, she is at even higher risk.
         a. Women with HPV seropositivity are 3.5 times more likely to develop in situ disease and more than 2.5 times more likely to develop invasive disease.

Table 32.1   **Differential Diagnosis of Other Vulvar Dermatoses**

Condition	Clinical Characteristics	Other Skin Areas Affected
Papulosquamous lesions		
Contact dermatitis	Pruritus, history of exposure to irritant or allergen, erythema and edema in contact areas	Other areas in contact with irritant/allergen, although vulvar skin more sensitive
Lichen Simplex Chronicus	Pruritus, history of chronic irritation, thickened, leathery skin with accentuated skin markings	Not common
Lichen planus	Pruritus, purplish plaques defined by cross-hatched skin lines	Flat-topped papules on wrist, lumbar back, thighs, lacey pattern on buccal mucosa
Seborrheic dermatitis	Usually pruritus, yellow or red lesions covered by greasy scales in areas of sebaceous glands	Face, scalp, particularly eyebrows and hairline
Psoriasis	Mild pruritus, red plaques or silvery scales with bleeding points beneath	Silvery plaques on scalp, knees, elbows, sacrum
Tinea curis	Variable, but usually dry, erythematous, annular lesions	May spread to buttocks and inner thighs
Vesiculobullous Lesions		
Erythema multiforme	History of recent genital herpes or drug allergy, "iris-shaped" lesions	Target lesions, especially on palms and soles
Pemphigus	Blisters and erosion	Any other skin areas on body
Infections		
Folliculitis	Tiny, red papules with white pustular center punctured by hair shaft	Any other skin in hairy areas
Impetigo	Superficial ulcer with yellow crust	Usually spread from infection of other body parts

    2. The more a woman smokes and the longer she smokes, the greater the risk.

        a. Current smokers are at almost 6.5 times the risk for in situ disease and at three times the risk for invasive disease.

  B. Confirm histologic characteristics.

VII. Patient preparation.

  A. Explain that discomfort during the procedure is usually minimal.

  B. The reasons for the biopsy study should be explained and the technique should be outlined.

VIII. The procedure.

  A. Some comments.

    1. It is important to have good lighting.

    2. Use of 5% acetic acid can greatly enhance identification of atypical areas such as intraepithelial neoplasia or HPV infection, which will often turn aceto-white a few minutes after application on the vulva.

    3. Toluidine blue dye is no longer used owing to the high rate of false-positive and false-negative results.

    4. A large magnifying lens is essential to highlight abnormal areas for biopsy study.

    5. Colposcopy may be used and is particularly helpful in diagnosing HPV infection. (Usually not available in primary care setting.)

  B. Equipment.

    1. Hand magnifying lens (or colposcope).

    2. Betadine swabs.

    3. Anesthetic agent.

    4. A 25-gauge needle.

    5. Syringe—0.3 mL.

    6. Two- to 4-mm Keyes' punch biopsy (disposable).

    7. Iris forceps.

    8. Fine scissors.

    9. Monsel's paste or silver nitrate sticks.

    10. Sterile gauze sponges.

    11. Labeled pathology container of formalin.

    12. Paperwork for lab requisition.

    13. Acetic acid (vinegar).

  C. Identify area to be biopsied. Multiple biopsy sites (2 to 3) may be indicated.

  D. Anesthesia.

    1. Local infiltration of 1% Xylocaine without epinephrine.

    2. Inject anesthetic solution subdermally with fine-gauge needle (0.5–1 mL per site).

3. A wheal (4–5 mm) is created, which facilitates the biopsy by raising the lesion above the dermas and promotes local vasoconstriction, minimizing blood loss.

E. The biopsy procedure.

1. Cleanse area using antiseptic solution or iodine-soaked swabs.
2. The dermal punch is like a corkborer.
3. Place the punch biopsy over the site, and rotate back and forth three or four times while holding the skin taut with the opposite hand (an assistant may be recruited to hold the skin).
4. The epithelium and dermis should be cut until the proper thickness is obtained.
5. Bore out in a circular manner.
   a. Depth comes with practice—too deep of a cut results in cutting large blood vessels, increasing bleeding.
   b. Too shallow a cut results in loss of an identifiable plug.
6. Once a plug is made, remove the cutter.
7. Grasp the plug with the forceps and separate from the skin. Snip dermal skin areas transversely to sever the base with scissors.
8. If the plug is lifted off and remains in the punch, dislodge the plug from the punch using a toothpick.

F. Control bleeding.

1. Bleeding is usually minimal because the dermis contains few blood vessels.
2. Pressure may be all that is required to stop any bleeding.
3. Use silver nitrate to cauterize area or put a drop of Monsel's solution over the site for hemostasis.
4. If bleeding persists, add a single suture using 4-0 Vicryl or Chromic.
5. A sanitary pad may be used for additional pressure.

G. Laboratory preparation.

1. Gently place the sample in formalin and properly label the container.
2. Complete required forms.
3. Document biopsy site(s) and the procedure itself, including the patient's response.
4. If biopsy samples from different sites are obtained, place in separate containers and label with the site.

IX. Follow-up.

A. Care of the biopsy site.

1. The patient is instructed to keep the incision clean and dry.
2. Baths should be taken daily until any soreness is gone.

     3. Blot dry. Be careful not to remove any healing scab.

     4. Reassure the patient that the biopsy site will become practically invisible in 1 to 2 weeks.

     5. Avoid intercourse for 2 or 3 days.

  B. The patient is instructed to call if any redness or increasing discomfort occurs or the signs of infection develop such as pus formation.

  C. Return to discuss results and recommendations for treatment.

  X. **Complications—rare bleeding or infection. Occasional oozing from the site may persist.**

  XI. **Teach vulvar self-examination.**

    A. Most vulvar malignancies are visible.

     1. Vulvar examination should be performed monthly by women who are sexually active or who are older than 18 years of age.

     2. The patient must recognize the importance of early detection of vulvar disease.

     3. Understand the basic vulvar anatomy and function.

     4. Learn the proper use of a hand-held mirror to optimize viewing the vulva.

     5. Perform the examination monthly between menses.

     6. Report any new growths or changes.

CHAPTER 33

Endometrial Biopsy

Helen A. Carcio

I. **Endometrial biopsy explained. Endometrial biopsy examination is used mainly to diagnose endometrial cancer and the presence of a luteal phase defect (LPD).**
   A. It is a method of removing a sample of representative tissue from the endometrium.
      1. It provides a histologic specimen of glandular epithelium from the uterine endometrial wall.
      2. It may be referred to as endometrial sampling because of the negative connotations that arise with the use of the word "biopsy."
      3. It is inexpensive and usually well tolerated by the woman.
      4. It is relatively easy to perform and can be performed appropriately by a trained nurse practitioner, midwife, or physician assistant.
      5. Advances in pipelles have made the procedure relatively simple to perform in the office, without the need for general anesthesia.
      6. Although the technique is relatively easy to perform by the clinician, it is often viewed as invasive by the patient.
      7. Although it is a blind procedure, its accuracy rate in identifying endometrial hyperplasia is greater than 90%.

II. **Some comments concerning endometrial cancer.**
   A. Incidence.

1. Endometrial cancer accounts for nearly 8% of all cancers in women.
2. Incidence is higher in Black and Hispanic women than in White and Asian women.
3. Most uterine cancers are adenocarcinoma of the endometrium.

B. Risk factors.
   1. Age. The incidence of endometrial cancer increases with age, particularly in those older than 65 years.
   2. Obesity causes an increase in the presence of exogenous estrogens from peripheral conversions of estrogen in the fat cells.
      a. No progesterone is present to counterbalance the excess estrogen (unless on hormone replacement therapy [HRT]).
      b. Uterine cancer develops in women who are more than 50 lb overweight 10 times more frequently than in women who are average weight.
   3. Hyperestrogenic state is possibly related to the following.
      a. Polycystic ovarian syndrome.
      b. Early menarche.
      c. Late menopause.
   4. Use of unopposed estrogen.
      a. During the 1950s and 1960s, estrogen was given as replacement therapy without progesterone.
      b. This practice caused a dramatic increase in the occurrence of endometrial cancer.
      c. Clinicians are now aware of the necessity to use progesterone supplementation with estrogen replacement therapy or to monitor the endometrium in a woman unwilling or unable to take progesterone.
   5. Use of tamoxifen therapy as treatment for women with breast cancer.
      a. It is antiestrogenic to breast tissue.
      b. It has an estrogenic effect on the lining of the uterus.
      c. It may contribute to endometrial stimulation, resulting in eventual hyperplasia and possible cancer.
      d. Its benefits in treating breast cancer probably outweigh the risk for development of endometrial cancer.
   6. Endometrial hyperplasia and endometrial polyps.
   7. Previous breast or ovarian cancer.
   8. Nulliparity.

    a. The risk for endometrial cancer is twice as high than in a woman who has one child.

    b. The risk is three times as high than in a woman who has five children.

   9. A personal history of hypertension or diabetes.

C. Protective factors. Progesterone use greatly diminishes hyperplasia of the endometrium. Oral contraceptives, particularly if used during the later reproductive years.

D. Clinical features.

   1. Abnormal uterine bleeding, particularly in postmenopausal women, including

    a. Heavy menses.

    b. Intermenstrual bleeding.

    c. Frequent menstruation.

   2. The older the woman, the higher the level of suspicion should be.

   3. Endometrial cells found on a Papanicolaou (Pap) smear.

III. Some comments concerning LPD.

A. The condition exists when the corpus luteum secretes an inadequate amount of progesterone.

B. Three to four percent of infertile women have LPD.

C. LPD is suspected when the luteal phase (the interval between ovulation and menstruation) is less than 11 days.

D. Causes.

   1. Inadequate progesterone production by the granulosa cells of the ovary.

   2. Hyperprolactinemia, which can cause an abnormal luteal phase.

   3. Psychogenic stress, nutritional factors, and exercise can cause a deficiency in the luteinizing hormone (LH) pulse.

   4. Kidney, liver, and immunologic diseases affect the corpus luteum cells.

IV. Endometrial biopsy examination explained.

A. Historical perspective.

   1. Endometrial biopsy was first performed as early as the Ancient Greek era and was originally used as a treatment for abnormal uterine bleeding.

   2. In the 1950s, the normal characteristics of the endometrium were established, which led to the ability to apply endometrial dating to help diagnose LPDs.

B. Relationship to dilatation and curettage (D & C).

1. Use of endometrial biopsy as a screen has replaced the need for D&C, which was previously the gold standard in many cases.
2. Recent studies found results were histologically similar between specimens collected by D&C and those obtained by endometrial biopsy.
3. Endometrial biopsy is more cost-effective and less invasive.

V. **Indications for biopsy study.**
  A. Complaints of uterine bleeding in any postmenopausal woman: The level of concern should increase with the patient's advancing age, particularly if the woman
     1. Is obese.
     2. Is taking unopposed estrogen replacement therapy (ERT).
     3. Has had no spotting or bleeding for 12 months or longer.
     4. The bleeding is excessive, prolonged, or irregular.
     5. Is taking cyclic ERT with an increase in bleeding pattern.
  B. Postmenopausal women in whom bleeding begins or increases (if previously present) with the initiation of hormone replacement therapy that does not resolve after 3 to 6 months of therapy.
     1. Some providers perform endometrial biopsy before the initiation of ERT, but most do not consider it necessary.
  C. Monitoring endometrial response to hormonal influences of unopposed ERT in those women undergoing ERT who are unable or unwilling to take progesterone.
     1. Progesterone protects the endometrium from the effects of unopposed estrogen.
        a. Women who are not taking progesterone are at increased risk for hyperplasia, which may lead to adenocarcinoma.
        b. Must monitor the patient yearly and document that the woman is aware of the increased risk for development of endometrial cancer.
        c. Biopsy study is sufficient, but the woman may choose to undergo ultrsonography to measure the width of the endometrial stripe.
           (1) The uterine lining is seen as a thin line or stripe.
           (2) The width of the stripe determines whether the lining of the uterus has thickened due to hyperplasia.
              (a) Less than 5 mm: no hyperplasia.
              (b) Between 5 and 10 mm: gray zone.
              (c) Greater than 10: hyperplasia.

Indications for Biopsy Study Before Age 40   **BOX 33.1**

Biopsy study before age 40 is only indicated if the following factors are present:

- Obesity (may have higher levels of estrogen)
- Long-standing anovulation or irregular menstrual cycles
- History of other adenocarcinomas such as of the breast or colon
- Functional metrorrhagia with dysfunctional uterine bleeding

   D. Endometrial cells found on a routine Pap smear, especially
      1. If taken more than 10 days from the first day of the menstrual period.
      2. In any patient older than 40 years of age.
      3. In the presence of irregular bleeding.
   E. Infertile women with suspected LPD.
      1. Documents endometrial response to progesterone.
      2. Evaluates the luteal phase, for endometrial dating in an infertile woman suspected of having an LPD.
         a. A discrepancy of more than 2 days between the woman's endometrial histologic stage and menstrual dating is diagnostically significant.
      3. Also obtains valuable information about the patency of the cervical os.
   F. It is rarely performed before age 40 years because 95% of cancers occur in woman older than 40 years of age. Box 33.1 lists the exceptions.
   G. Women who are undergoing tamoxifen treatment for breast cancer.
   H. Follow-up of abnormal ultrasound if endometrial thickness (stripe) is greater than 5 mm.
   I. Women in whom pelvic inflammatory disease (PID) is suspected (controversial).
      1. Endometritis is a fairly frequent cause of irregular bleeding in young women.
      2. Endometritis often precedes and then accompanies salpingitis.
      3. Offers an objective test in the diagnosis of PID to improve diagnostic accuracy.
         a. Positive if histologic findings of plasma cell endometritis are found.

VI. Contraindications to biopsy study.

A. Pregnancy or poorly involuted postpartum uterus (a sensitive pregnancy test can be performed before).

B. Infection.

  1. Any infection can be passed into the uterine cavity and tubes as the pipelle passes through the cervical os.

  2. Active or chronic cervicitis: defer until treated.

  3. Active or chronic vaginitis: defer until treated.

C. Uterine abnormalities such as a large myoma displacing the uterus, making obtaining of sample impossible.

D. Blood dyscrasias or suspected bleeding disorder.

E. Woman is febrile. Note: If there is a history of valvular heart disease or rheumatic fever, bacterial endocarditis is a risk and antibiotic prophylaxis is appropriate.

VII. Examination of the woman.

  A. Subjective information must include

   1. Date of last menstrual period (LMP).

   2. Use of contraception; discuss compliance issues.

   3. Risk-evaluation for sexually transmitted diseases (STDs) and human immunodeficiency virus (HIV).

   4. History of any bleeding problems.

   5. Presence of symptoms of vaginal or cervical infections.

   6. History of heart disease, especially rheumatic heart disease or mitral valve prolapse.

   7. Allergies, especially to lidocaine (Xylocaine) or povidone-iodine (Betadine).

   8. Level of pain associated with previous Pap smears.

   9. History of vasovagal episode or hypoglycemia.

   10. Inquire about food eaten that day. Offer sweetened juice to prevent a vasovagal reaction.

  B. Objective findings.

   1. Obtain vital signs, including temperature.

   2. Perform pelvic examination to assess for any signs of infection.

   3. Perform laboratory tests, if indicated.

    a. Sensitive pregnancy test.

    b. Hematocrit.

    c. Wet mount examination (see chapter 10, Vaginal Miscroscopy).

VIII. The procedure.

  A. Supplies.

   1. Nonsterile gloves.

2. Vaginal speculum.
3. Tenaculum.
4. Aseptic solution (Betadine).
5. Cotton rectal swab.
6. Sterile Pipelle (two).
7. Biopsy sample container (10% formalin or other fixative).
8. Two percent to 10% viscous lidocaine gels and Hurricane gel.
9. Sterile lubricant.

B. Characteristics of the pipelle.
   1. Advances in the pipelle have made the procedure relatively simple to perform in the office without the need for general anesthesia.
   2. Single-use, disposable, clear instrument with colored, graduated markings graded from 4 to 10 cm.
   3. Flexible polypropylene.
   4. Size. Small caliber, 3.1 cm (outside diameter) and 2.6 cm (inner diameter); 23.5 cm in length.
   5. Use: Histologic biopsy of uterine mucosal lining or sample extraction of uterine menstrual content.
   6. Negative pressure. Rapid movement of the piston creates a negative pressure within the lumen of the sheath, allowing for aspiration of the mucosal tissue through the curette opening and into the lumen of the tube as the curette scrapes against the endometrial walls while being moved within the uterine cavity. The piston cannot be fully pulled out.

IX. **Preparation.**
   A. Timing in the evaluation of LPD.
      1. Performed 1 to 3 days before the expected onset of menses (take average of previous cycles).
      2. Menses may begin on the day of the scheduled biopsy procedure because the timing is close. If this occurs, the biopsy procedure must be rescheduled for the next cycle, but a day or two earlier.
   B. Can schedule evaluation of abnormal uterine bleeding or endometrial monitoring at any time.
   C. Analgesia.
      1. Many clinicians suggest the use of nonsteroidal antiinflammatory medication in the event that mild cramping occurs.
      2. Administer ibuprofen, 400 mg, 30 to 60 minutes before the scheduled visit.

D. Anesthesia: In patients who are very sensitive to pain, topical anesthesia such as 20% benzocaine (Hurricaine) can be applied to the cervix a few minutes before the procedure.

X. Informed consent and education.
A. The clinician must clearly explain
   1. How much pain to expect.
   2. Reasons for the procedure.
   3. Risks involved, including perforation of the uterus, failure to obtain tissue, and infection.
   4. Overall safety.
   5. Realistic expectation of what will occur during the procedure.
   6. What the results may indicate.

B. Verbal or written consent should be obtained and documented.

XI. The procedure.
A. Position: The woman is asked to assume a comfortable dorsal lithotomy position.

B. Bimanual examination.
   1. A bimanual pelvic examination is first performed to determine the position and size of the uterus and to assess for any pelvic tenderness.
   2. A rectal examination may be necessary if the uterus is retroverted.
   3. Helps determine the direction of insertion of the catheter.
   4. It is important to assess the size of the uterus so that its proper depth can be determined.

C. Use of lubricant: A lubricant should not be used because it may prevent proper interpretation of cervical cytology tests.

XII. Technique.
A. Put on gloves (sterile gloves are not necessary). Care should be taken not to touch the parts of the instruments that will come in contact with the cervix or the endometrial cavity.

B. The speculum is inserted into the vagina, and the cervical os is visualized.
   1. The cervix should be well positioned, facing directly outward, between the blades of the speculum. (This helps with the insertion technique.)

C. Inspection.
   1. The vagina and cervix are inspected for the presence of any usual discharge.

   2. If an infection is suspected, a wet mount examination should be performed.
      a. If white blood cells are present, the condition should be diagnosed and treated.
      b. Reschedule biopsy surgery for the next cycle.
D. Cleansing the area.
   1. Using a rectal swab, the cervix and upper vagina are next swabbed free of discharge and cleansed with an antiseptic such as Betadine.
   2. Any excess Betadine should be removed to prevent contamination of the specimen.
E. Use of a tenaculum for anteflexion or retroflexion.
   1. A tenaculum is usually not necessary.
   2. It is only used 15% of the time.
   3. If it is used, a lidocaine gel should be placed at the site the tenaculum will grasp for 5 minutes, or 1% lidocaine (0.5–1.0 ml) should be injected at the tenaculum site via a spinal needle. Either method will significantly reduce the pain of tenaculum application.
   4. The tenaculum may be necessary to stabilize the cervix and straighten the uterus to facilitate passage of the pipelle if there is a marked degree of anteflexion or retroflexion.
      a. Anteflexion.
         (1) Grasp the anterior upper lip of the cervix between 2 and 10 o'clock. (Warn the patient that she will feel a pinch.)
         (2) This technique should compress approximately 1 cm of cervical tissue. (The tissue immediately turns white.)
         (3) Gently pull the cervix forward to straighten the cervical canal.
         (4) Guide the curved tip along the anterior surface of the endocervical canal.
      b. Retroflexion.
         (1) Grasp the posterior lip of the cervix.
         (2) Guide the curved tip along the posterior surface of the endocervical canal.
      c. Remember that the uterine artery runs laterally at 3 and 9 o'clock.
   5. The clinician may manually curve the tip of the pipelle while it is in the sterile package to accommodate the curvature of the uterus.

      6. If the tip is not curved, the straight tip may become embedded into the posterior or anterior wall of the canal.

F. Pipelle insertion.

    1. If a topical anesthetic is being used, instill it into the cervical os using a swab.

    2. Once the position of the uterus has been assessed; the cervical os, positioned, a thin pipelle or catheter is passed through the cervix, into the uterus to the fundus.

    3. The tip of the catheter can be bent manually for easier insertion to accommodate for the natural curve of the endocervical canal.

    4. However, the clinician must be aware that the rigidness of the catheter may slightly increase chances of accidental perforation.

    5. It is usually not necessary to sound the uterus.

    6. Hold the pipelle lightly with a grip similar to holding a pencil.

    7. As the pipelle is inserted through the cervix, the resistance of the internal os is felt as the pipelle is passed through.

    8. Slowly and gently advance the catheter the full depth of the endometrial cavity, until the resistance of the fundus is felt.

    9. Never use force against digitally felt resistance.

    10. Assess the length of the uterus by noting the centimeters marked on the pipelle.

       a. In premenopausal women, 6 cm or more.

       b. Less than 6 cm in postmenopausal women.

       c. The cavity has probably not been entered if only the 3- to 4-cm mark has been reached.

       d. The woman may feel mild uterine cramps at this point.

       e. Once the pipelle is fully inserted and the tip is positioned properly, release traction of the tenaculum, if it is used.

G. Aspiration.

    1. The pipelle should be stabilized with the nondominant hand, using the dominant hand to pull the plunger fully back.

    2. Rapidly pull the piston firmly, using one full motion, as far toward the proximal end of the sheath as it will go. The piston cannot be pulled out completely.

    3. Slow, irregular pressure, or incomplete withdrawal of the plunger will not supply the suction required for an appropriate sample.

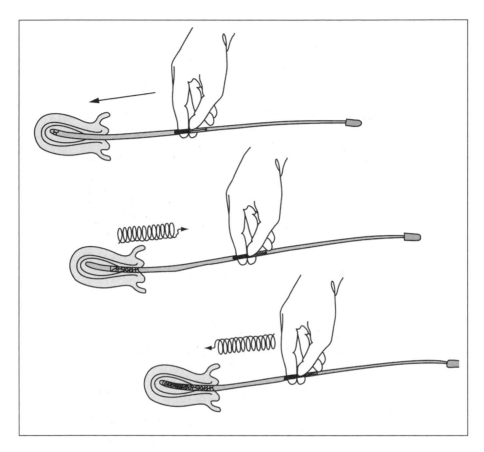

Figure 33.1 Simultaneously roll (twirl) sheath between fingers while moving sheath laterally and back and forth (in and out) between the fundus and internal os 3 or 4 times to obtain sample.

4. Correct technique creates negative pressure inside the pipelle, which allows for aspiration of the endometrial tissue into the open tip of the pipelle.
5. Next, the pipelle should be rotated continuously 360° by rolling or twisting it between thumb and index finger as it is rapidly, but gently, advanced and withdrawn between the fundus and internal os (Figure 33.1).
6. Withdraw and advance the pipelle three or four times (over 30 seconds).
7. As the tube is rotated, a column of tissue is seen as it is drawn into the tube, often filling it completely.

8. This suction from negative pressure generally yields an adequate sample.
9. If the pipelle is withdrawn from the os, the suction is lost.
10. If this occurs, the pipelle should be reinserted.
11. Once enough of a sample has been aspirated, the pipelle is slowly removed and the contents placed directly in preservative and sent to the pathology department for analysis.
12. If the instrument does not touch the container, it can be reinserted, if necessary.
13. Record the depth, ease of insertion, and patient response.
14. Any bleeding from the tenaculum site usually abates rapidly.
15. The patient should remain supine for a few minutes until any pain or dizziness passes.
16. Supply the woman with a perineal pad.

H. Sampling.
1. Recent studies suggest that the most representative samples are obtained from high in the corpus from both the anterior and posterior walls.
2. The samples should be superficial rather than deep because the deeper tissues often show less intense reactivity to progesterone.
3. If sufficient sample is not obtained, the procedure should be repeated at a later date.
4. The extent of the sample should correlate to the level of suspicion for malignancy.
5. For endometrial dating, only a single sample is necessary.

XIII. Common problems.

A. Difficulty entering the os due to cervical stenosis.
1. The cervix of a menopausal women is often tight. If this is the case, a smaller caliber (2 to 3 mm) pipelle should be used rather than the standard 4 mm.
2. If the flexible cannula bends in the middle with any pressure during attempts to pass through a tight cervical canal, grasp the cannula about 4 cm from its end with a ring or uterine dressing forceps. (This method minimizes the bending in the middle of the cannula as pressure is applied and eases its passage through the cervix.)
3. Additionally, the pipelle, with the tip curved, can be placed in a freezer to increase rigidity. Remember, this stiffness may slightly increase the risk of perforation.
4. A sterile lubricant can be placed on the pipelle to ease insertion in the elderly woman with a dry cervix.

5. Some clinicians recommend a 2-week course of vaginal estrogen before the biopsy sample is taken, to open the cervical os.

6. Refer if the os it still too tight or if the woman has severe atrophy, in which the external os may no longer be patent. The clinician should refer the patient to a gynecologist to open the os after the administration of paracervical anesthesia.

B. Minimal tissue obtained.
   1. Commonly seen in postmenopausal women evaluated for light spotting or bleeding.
   2. Consider the presence of a scant amount of tissue diagnostically sufficient if the following apply:
      a. The pipelle has passed at least 6 cm into the uterus.
      b. There is a clear sensation of having reached the fundus.
      c. The patient is not at high risk for endometrial cancer (due to factors other than age).

XIV. After biopsy procedure.
   A. Preparing the specimen for analysis.
      1. After the specimen has been obtained, clip off the tip of the cannula with scissors.
      2. Advance the piston so that the endometrial sample is expressed into a vial containing fixative.
      3. Fill out the paperwork and label the specimen, including information about the patient's clinical status.
      4. Indicate any hormone therapy the woman is receiving.
   B. Following the procedure observe the woman for
      1. Vasovagal response.
         a. The woman should be closely observed for a vasovagal response.
         b. She should remain supine for a few minutes and then slowly be assisted to a sitting position.
         c. She should remain sitting until equilibrium is restored and any discomfort passes.
      2. Cramping.
         a. Painful cramps usually subside rapidly and are well tolerated.
         b. If the cramps persist, an antiinflammatory agent can be used.
   C. Referral.
      1. Patient with contraindications.
      2. Patient with a severely stenotic os.

Table 33.1   **Complications Associated With Endometrial Biopsy**

Complication	Rate
Cervical stenosis	12/28
Excessive bleeding	5/28
Fever	4/28
Excessive pain	2/28
Vasovagal reaction	2/28
Uterine perforation	2/28
Interrupted pregnancy	1/28

3. Confer with supervising physician to discuss a patient at risk for bacterial endocarditis.

XV. Complications (see Table 33.1).

A. The client should be advised to monitor any bleeding and to return should any of the following develop:

1. Severe cramping or worsening discomfort or pain.

2. Heavy bleeding and clots or any bleeding lasting longer than 2 days.

3. Any foul-smelling discharge, with or without fever and chills.

4. Uterine perforation.

   a. Is very rare.

   b. Usually without serious sequelae.

   c. New catheters are very small and flexible, and carry little risk of perforation of the uterus.

   d. If perforation is suspected, the patient needs to be closely monitored for heavy bleeding.

5. Interruption of a pregnancy when evaluating LPD.

   a. There is a slight chance of disturbing an early pregnancy.

   b. Interruption of a pregnancy is rare, occurring in 1/1,500 biopsy procedures total, and in 1/500 biopsy studies for evaluating LPD. (The resulting miscarriage rate is 20%.)

   c. The woman may choose to use contraception during the cycle preceding surgery, or she may elect to continue trying to conceive because the risk is slight.

   d. Nothing is worse than disrupting an established pregnancy during an endometrial biopsy study in an infertile couple.

   e. A sensitive pregnancy test is recommended.

XVI. Follow-up.
   A. LPD evaluation.
   1. Ask the woman to call with the date that her next period begins.
   2. This information is essential for the accurate interpretation of results because they are based on the comparison of the histologic date to the day of menses.
   3. Normal results will confirm that ovulation has occurred and that there is adequate progesterone to support an early pregnancy.
   B. Results are usually available in 7 to 10 days.
   C. Have the client return in 2 weeks to discuss biopsy study results and any follow-up.

XVII. Diagnosis.
   A. LPD.
   1. LPD should be suspected if the endometrial tissue is "out of phase," demonstrating a lag of more than 2 days from the expected date of menses.
   2. The day of ovulation is counted forward to the date of the biopsy surgery.
   3. Additionally, the onset of the next menses is counted as day 28, counting back to the day of the biopsy surgery, and comparing it with the histologic date provided.
   4. A normal basal body temperature (BBT) or LH surge and an "in-phase" biopsy supports the adequacy of the hypothalamic-pituitary-ovarian axis.
   5. If the biopsy is out of phase, further hormonal assessment is warranted.
   B. The case against the use of endometrial biopsy study in diagnosing LPD.
   1. Endometrial biopsy examination is being used less and less because of the invasive nature of the test and the additional cost in both time and money.
   2. Some sources believe that there is a weak correlation between out-of-phase biopsy surgeries and infertility.
   3. Results are believed to be somewhat subjective, with different interpretations using the same sample.

    4. Other methods, such as the BBT, the over-the-counter ovulation predictor kit, and serum progesterone test, are accurate in documenting luteal function.

    5. Although a normal in-phase endometrial biopsy sample is strongly suggestive of an adequate luteal phase, an abnormal result does not always indicate LPD because 25 to 30% of abnormal biopsy samples are found in normally fertile women.

C. Adenocarcinoma.

    1. May note abundant friable fragments, which may appear as bits of rolled up tissue in the endometrial sample.

CHAPTER 34

Acrochordonectomy

Helen A. Carcio

I. **Acrochordonectomy (removal of skin tags) is a good technique for the advanced practice clinician to master.**
   A. Skin tags are commonly seen in the primary care setting.
   B. They are often bothersome to women because they appear around the neck and upper chest.
   C. The woman complains that her clothes and jewelry get caught on the tags, plus they are unattractive.
   D. The removal technique is easy and straightforward and can often be done during a routine physical examination.

II. **Acrochordonectomy explained.**
   A. Description: An acrochordon is a flesh-toned, papillomatous, cutaneous lesion.
      1. If they are pedunculated, they are called cutaneous papillomas and soft fibromas.
      2. Histologically: The lesion is hyperplastic epidermis enclosing a dermal connective tissue stalk.
      3. Loose, often edematous collagen fiber.
   B. They increase in number as one ages.

III. **Removal.**
   A. Technique 1.
      1. Identify the lesion to be removed.

        a. Cleanse the lesion and surrounding area with an iodine swab.

        b. Rinse with sterile saline.

    2. Apply a surgical clamp, such as a Kelly clamp, at the base of the acrochordon.

    3. Keep clamp in place for approximately 15 minutes.

    4. Remove the clamp.

    5. Grasp the lesions with a small clamp and lift away from the skin.

    6. Excise the lesions using fine-bladed scissors (iris scissors).

    7. Cut in the middle of the approximately 2-mm compressed area left by the surgical clamp.

    8. A small circular adhesive bandage may be applied or the area may be left open.

B. Technique 2.

    1. Identify the lesion to be removed.

    2. Apply petroleum jelly around the lesion, being careful not to cover the lesion itself with the petroleum jelly.

    3. Apply trichloroacetic acid (TCA) or bichloroacetic acid (BCA) to the lesion until it turns white, being careful not to get any chemical on the surrounding skin. (The immediate area around it will turn red and a slight burning may occur, which usually subsides in a few minutes.)

    4. Inform the patient that the lesion will turn black and eventually fall off.

    5. If the lesion is larger than 2 mm, the client may have to return for a second chemical application.

C. If the woman has many tags, only three or four should be removed at one time.

IV. Follow-up.

A. The patient is advised to call should burning increase or signs of infection occur.

B. Return for removal of other lesions.

Polypectomy

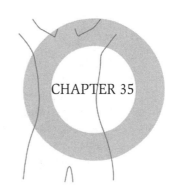

CHAPTER 35

Helen A. Carcio

I. **Polyps explained.**
   A. Description.
      1. Polyps are the most common tumors of the cervix.
      2. They are found most often during the menstruating years. (Parous women in 5th decade.)
      3. They are soft, pear-shaped, red to purple lesions and are usually pedunculated growths from the surface of the cervical canal.
      4. They contain a large number of blood vessels, particularly near the surface.
      5. Diameter varies from several millimeters to 2 cm.
      6. They occur with overgrowth of one of the cervical folds.
      7. They are usually asymptomatic but may bleed with intercourse.
   B. Microscopic analysis.
      1. Loose vascular connective tissue covered by endocervical epithelium.
      2. Stroma may be inflamed and edematous.
   C. Location.
      1. Usually found in the lower endocervix; may protrude from the cervical os.
      2. May be found at the squamocolumnar junction or portio vaginalis.
   D. Incidence: 6%.

II. **Removal.**
   A. Technique 1.

  1. Determine the site of origin.
  2. Grasp polyp with clamp.
  3. Twist until the polyp separates from the stalk.
  4. Apply silver nitrate or Monsel's solution for hemostasis.
 B. Technique 2 (if polyp is large).
  1. Determine the site of origin.
  2. Clamp approximately 0.5 cm above the origin of the pedicle.
  3. A surgical ligature is next tied between the clamp and the cervix.
  4. Remove the clamp.
  5. Using a pair of scissors with a fine blade, cut along the suture line to remove the polyp.
   a. Send specimen to the pathology department.
  6. It may be left attached to undergo infarction and slough.

III. Recommendations.
 A. All polyps should be sent to the pathology department because malignancy can occur in benign-appearing structures (0.2–0.4% incidence).
 B. There is no need for special follow-up. Polyps seldom recur after removal. The woman should report any bleeding.

CHAPTER 36

Colposcopy

Helen A. Carcio

I. **The colposcope explained.**
   A. The colposcope consists of two parts:
   1. Stereoscope.
   2. Binocular microscope with built-in light source that magnifies the cervix 3 to 10 times.
   B. By varying magnifications, the examiner can identify abnormal tissue from surrounding normal tissue.
   C. It is equipped with a green filter to filter out red, thereby enhancing the vascular appearance of the cervix by making the vessels dark.
   D. Used to diagnose cervical cancer, usually after an abnormal Papanicolaou (Pap) smear.
   E. Cervical biopsy allows for histologic evaluation of any abnormal lesions visualized. (Box 36.1 lists indications.)
   F. Purpose of the examination.
   1. Grade the lesion.
   2. Determine its size and location.
   3. Exclude invasive cancer by fully visualizing the area at risk.
   4. Excise any suspicious lesions for biopsy.
   G. Advanced practice clinicians need advanced training in colposcopy. Many courses are available.

II. **The preparation for colposcopy.**
   A. A woman is probably very frightened of the possibility of finding cervical cancer. She should be reassured by commenting on the following realities:
   1. There is a low probability of finding an invasive cancer.
   2. It is likely that only dysplasia will be found.

Indications for Colposcopy   **BOX 36.1**

Abnormal Pap smear

Presence of apparent lesion with normal Pap smear cytology

Undiagnosed vaginal bleeding

---

3. Cervical intraepithelial neoplasia (CIN) is composed of abnormal cells but is not cancer.
4. If found, CIN can be treated by simple methods without the need for hospitalization or major surgery.

B. Positioning.
1. Patient comfortably positioned in stirrups and draped appropriately.
2. Cervix should be at the clinician's eye level.
3. Plane of the cervix should be at right angles to the beam of the colposcope.

C. Equipment: The following equipment should be gathered:
1. Variously sized speculums.
2. Endocervical speculum cytobrush.
3. Wooden spatulas.
4. Lugol's solution.
5. Acetic acid (vinegar).
6. Monsel's solution.
7. Tenaculum.
8. Biopsy surgery instruments.
9. Cytofixative (Formalin).
10. Endocervical curette.
11. Silver nitrate sticks.
12. Swabs (small and large).
13. Topical benzocaine (Hurricaine).
14. Equipment for Pap smear.
15. Colposcope.
16. Vaginal wall retractor, if necessary.

D. Preparation and timing.
1. The procedure is best performed during the late follicular phase, when estrogen levels are highest and mucus is clear and not tenacious.
2. If the os is atrophic, treat with estrogen for 1 to 2 weeks before the procedure to open the os more fully.

E. Obtain informed consent.

Components of an Adequate Examination	**BOX 36.2**

Visualization of the entire transformation zone

Lesion must be seen in its entirety with no lesions extending into the endocervical canal

---

F. Box 36.2 lists components of an adequate examination.

III. Technique.
   A. Bring colposcope into position.
      1. Use bright light on vulva and perianal area to observe for signs of infection, inflammation, or ulceration.
   B. Insert speculum, and position to allow for complete visualization of the cervix.
      1. If lateral walls collapse in a patient who is pregnant, obese, or with poor pelvic muscle tone, two suggestions may help:
         a. Use a lateral wall retractor.
         b. A speculum with a condom or finger from a rubber glove with both ends exposed can be placed over the blades of the speculum.
   C. Cleanse the cervix. If thick secretions are present, two methods are appropriate for removal:
      1. Grasp the secretions with a large forceps and remove, being careful not to damage any underlying epithelial tissue.
      2. Moisten a cotton swab, and wipe free of discharge.
   D. Repeat Pap smear, if necessary.
   E. Perform wet mount examination on any vaginal discharge (see chapter 10, Vaginal Microscopy).
   F. Liberally wash cervix with 2% acetic acid.
      1. Acetic acid dehydrates the cells by causing a transient coagulation of cytoplasmic proteins in the superficial cells.
      2. Allows for easier identification of epithelial and vascular abnormalities.
   G. Examine the cervix with the colposcope.
      1. Begin with low power to look at transformation zone and associated topography. The clinician must be able to view the entire transformation zone.
      2. The transformation zone corresponds to that area of the cervix first covered with columnar epithelia.
         a. The area undergoes a process of squamous metaplasia as a woman ages.

      b. Morphology of columnar cells changes to squamous cells.

  3. Outside margin: Bound by the original squamocolumnar junction.

  4. Inner margin: Active squamocolumnar junction filled with columnar epithelium.

  5. Characterized by a white sheen, minute blood vessels, and small openings to glands.

  6. Dysplasia is thought to start in this area.

  7. The squamocolumnar junction varies with the amount of estrogen present.

      a. High-estrogen, low-pH state: Zone lies outside of the cervical os, where it is well visualized.

      b. Low-estrogen, high-pH state: Zone lies hidden within the os and may not be visible with colposcopy.

H. Reapply acetic acid as needed to keep the cervix moist.

  1. CIN lesions will become more prominent the longer they are exposed to acetic acid.

  2. Acetic acid coagulates the proteins of nuclei and cytoplasm, making the proteins opaque and white.

  3. It does not affect mature epithelium because the acid does not penetrate below the outer one third of the epithelium.

  4. Dysplastic cells contain large amounts of protein.

I. Examine the columnar villi. Villi will swell, making them prominent initially, and then fade and become harder to identify with each application of acetic acid.

J. Observe for aceto-white staining of epithelium, noting external and internal border of any aceto-white lesions.

K. Look for punctation and mosaic patterns.

L. Use a green filter to highlight any vascular abnormalities.

M. Lugol's solution can be applied next.

  1. The solution stains the glycogenated vagina.

  2. Areas that are poor in glycogen (columnar epithelium or regenerative epithelium) will not stain.

N. If the os is stenotic, the clinician may use an endocervical speculum to open the os for better visualization of the squamocolumnar junction.

O. Under direct visualization, selectively excise any abnormal areas.

  1. Anesthesia is usually not necessary; however, benzocaine may be applied a few minutes before the biopsy sample is taken.

P. Bleeding after the biopsy sample is taken.

  1. Apply pressure with a large swab; remove slowly to uncover bleeding area.

Table 36.1   Characteristic Findings During Colposcopy

Finding	Definition
Normal squamous epithelium	Devoid of blood vessels
Abnormal vascular patterns	Neovascularization of surface epithelium
Neoplasia	New vessels develop and extend into the surface epithelium
Mosaic pattern (have the appearance of mosaic tile)	New vessels that run parallel to the surface of the aceto-white epithelium taking on a mosaic pattern (epithelium is the tiles and the blood vessels are the grout)
Punctation	New vessels run perpendicularly to the plane of the epithelium appearing as small dots Indicate an abnormal epithelium, usually CIN
Atypical vascularity	Haphazard vascular growth with multiple branches
Abnormal epithelium	White color due to a decrease in tissue translucency
Aceto-whitening	Changes in nuclear proteins producing a white appearance when dehydrated
Leukoplakia	Plaque of white epithelium visible before application of acetic acid Layer of keratin on the surface epithelium usually found on immature squamous cells

CIN, cervical intraepithelial neoplasia.

    2. Swab with silver nitrate or Monsel's solution for 1 to 2 minutes.

IV. Interpretation of results. (See Table 36.1 for characteristic findings.)
    A. Colposcopic study is used to recognize abnormal patterns. It is not diagnostic in itself. Formal diagnosis occurs when the biopsy specimen has been examined histologically.
    B. Ideally, colposcopic findings, cytology, and histologic results correlate.
    C. Colposcopy is relatively simple to perform; however, the examiner must be able to recognize normal versus abnormal patterns.
    D. There are few complications outside of patient discomfort during the procedure.

V. Contraindications.

A. Colposcopy is usually well tolerated by the patient. As the examiner becomes more experienced, the duration of the procedure should decrease.

B. Absolute contraindications include:

    1. The possibility of metastatic choriocarcinoma of the cervix and vagina.

    2. Hemangioma of the cervix.

    3. Placenta previa.

VI. Follow-up.

A. Patients whose colposcopic findings are normal after low-grade intraepithelial lesion (LSIL) cytology.

    1. Serial Pap smears at 4- to 6-month intervals.

    2. Resume yearly Pap testing after three normal results.

B. Normal colposcopic findings after high-grade intraepithelial lesion (HSIL) cytology.

    1. Reevaluate results of Pap smear to confirm initial reading.

    2. Repeat colposcopy examination, with special attention to the vagina and vulva.

    3. If second examination and Pap smear results are normal, perform serial Pap smears at 4- to 6-month intervals.

    4. Resume yearly Pap testing after three normal results.

    5. If second Pap smear reveals HSIL, perform excision at the squamocolumnar junction.

C. Abnormal colposcopic findings: Therapy may include observation, laser treatment, loop electrocautery excision procedure (LEEP), cone biopsy, or cryosurgery.

D. CIN-II, CIN-III, or CIN-IV: Refer patient for physician management.

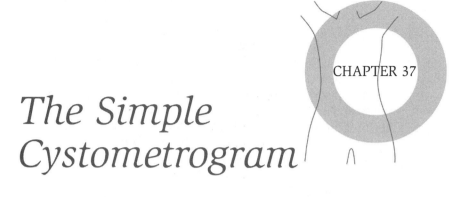

The Simple Cystometrogram

CHAPTER 37

Helen A. Carcio

I. **Simple cystometrography (CMG) explained.**
   A. Cystometrography is an important first step in the evaluation and management of bladder dysfunction.
   B. It is emerging as a reliable indicator to determine a diagnosis of overactive bladder, urinary incontinence, and interstitial cystitis.
   C. The patient must complete a 3-day voiding diary before the test (see chapter 25, Urinary Incontinence).
   D. Typical complaints that may lead to simple CMG testing include
      1. Incontinence, stress and urge
      2. Nocturia
      3. Frequency
      4. Pelvic pain
      5. Slow stream

II. **Patient assessment.**
   A. Assessment of strength of the pelvic floor muscles.
      1. Insert the index finger and middle fingers approximately 2 cm through the vaginal orifice (to the first knuckle).
      2. Palpate the band of muscle located just inside the vagina in the 5 and 7 o'clock positions.
      3. Ask the woman to squeeze and hold the contraction.
      4. Note the strength of the contraction and the number of seconds she is able to hold the contraction.

5. Ask the woman to squeeze her pelvic floor muscle tightly several times.
6. Note strength of the squeeze.
7. Compare the strength of contralateral sides.
8. The palpable contraction should be strong and sustained with fingers deflected upward and inward.
9. Decreased strength may signify weakened pelvic floor muscles and cause incontinence.

B. Measure postvoid residual (PVR).
   1. Have the woman void immediately before the test.
   2. The residual is the result of bladder contractility and urethral resistance.
   3. Should be obtained within 5 minutes of voiding.
   4. A high residual may indicate a hypotonic bladder or an inability to contract against an increase in urethral pressure.
   5. A PVR of 25% or less of voided volume is acceptable.

III. **The procedure.**
   A. Patient preparation.
      1. Patient should be mobile and alert.
         a. The bowel should be as empty as possible.
         b. An enema is not necessary.
      2. Explain the various phases of the testing procedure and show the equipment to be used to decrease any anxiety.
      3. Patient should not have taken any medications that may alter bladder function, such as an anticholinergic.
      4. It is imperative that measures be done to help patients relax because a tense patient is often unconsciously bracing against any leaking.
      5. Reassure the patient that every effort will be made to make her comfortable during the procedure.
         a. The procedure only takes 15 minutes.
         b. It is not uncomfortable.
      6. Ask client to respond to sensations during filling and to report any urgency or discomfort.
   B. Supplies.
      1. Twelve- to 14-French red rubber catheter.
      2. A 60-mL catheter-tipped syringe without piston.
      3. A liter bottle sterile water at room temperature.
         a. Cold water may stimulate the bladder to contract.
      4. Absorbent pads.
   C. The test.

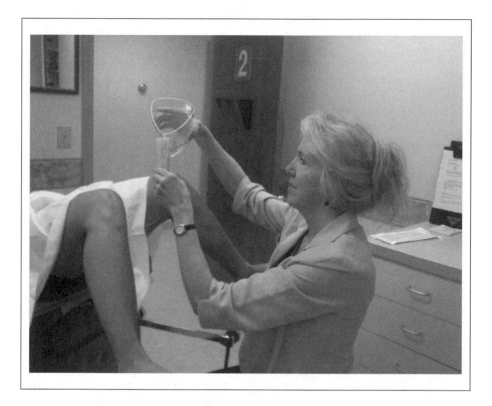

Figure 37.1 Performing a simple cystometrogram: After the patient is catheterized, the syringe acts as a funnel to fill the bladder.

1. Catheterize patient and measure and record the PVR.
2. Attach the 60-mL syringe (without the piston) to the red rubber catheter.
3. Hold the syringe 10 to 12 in. above the pubic bone (the syringe acts as a funnel to fill the bladder).
4. Slowly fill the bladder with warm, sterile water, 50 mL at a time (Figure 37.1).
5. Pinch the tube off between each aliquot to prevent putting air into the bladder.
6. Note the presence or absence of involuntary bladder contractions.
   a. Noted as an upward movement of the column of fluid in the syringe with each bladder contraction.

Table 37.1   Grading of Responses

Sensation	Observed Response	Normal Range (mL)
First sensation	First inclination to void	90–150
Second sensation	Normal desire to void Can be delayed	200–300

Third sensation	Strong and persistent desire to void
	Maximum capacity at which the patient
	  feels she can no longer hold her urine
	  or when the bladder spontaneously
	  empties
		400–550

7. Record fluid volume at which any contractions occur.
8. Perform provocative maneuvers to elicit potential leaking with each 100 mL of fluid instilled.
   a. Running water.
   b. Jingling of keys.
   c. Cough.
9. Record any leaking or contractions with these maneuvers and the volume at which they occur.
10. The contractions may be accompanied by leaking around the catheter or actual expulsion of catheter if the contractions are strong enough.
11. The examiner must also observe for the presence of any abdominal straining, which would alter the test results.
12. Sensation is the subjective response to bladder filling as communicated by the patient. The patient is asked to respond to three sensations:
   a. First sensation: the first indication of the need to urinate.
   b. Second sensation: a point in bladder filling when the patient would actually consider looking for a bathroom.
   c. Third sensation: a point where the patient can no longer hold the urine.
   d. Table 37.1 summarizes these responses.
13. Results.
   a. Contractions or severe urgency at relatively low bladder volumes (250 mL) suggest urge incontinence.
   b. Severe urgency at 150 mL and a volume less than 350 mL suggest interstitial cystitis.

    c. Provocative maneuvers may evoke a bladder contraction or an episode of leaking. Document which maneuver triggers leaking.

    d. Uninhibited detrusor contractions and urge incontinence may be stimulated by triggers.

    e. Leaking with straining or coughing suggests stress incontinence.

    f. Maximum bladder capacity is recorded at the end of the test. It measures the size of the bladder when full.

    g. Drain the bladder when test is complete.

IV. After the procedure.

    A. Results are immediate and can be explained to the patient.

    B. Inform the patient that she may note some burning with urination for the first 24 to 48 hours.

        1. This is normal and expected.

        2. The patient should call the physician if burning and frequency or blood in the urine occurs because this may indicate a urinary tract infection.

    C. Record findings (see Box 37.1 for a sample form).

    D. Reimbursement: The CPT code for a simple CMG is 57125 and is reimbursed between $175 and $325.

    E. Refer for complex CMG if findings are inconclusive.

Simple CMG Evaluation Form

BOX
37.1

Name _____ Date of birth _____ Age _____
Date of service _____ Urinalysis _____
Assessment summary _____
_____
_____
_____

Filling CMG
Capacity: Amount instilled _____ mL
Compliance
First sensation _____ mL (90–150 mL)
Second sensation _____ mL (200–300 mL)
Third sensation (max) _____ mL (400–550 mL)
Uninhibited contraction _____mL
Leaking _____ Provocative maneuver _____

PVR _____ (25% or less of voided volume)
❐ Bladder Diary completed
Clinical impression _____
Follow-up _____
_____

Provider _____

Bibliography

Chapter 1 Anatomy and Physiology of Female Reproduction
Chapter 2 The Reproductive Cycle
Chapter 3 The Health History
Chapter 4 The Physical Examination

Bates, B. (2008). *A guide to physical examination and history taking* (8th ed.). Philadelphia: J.B. Lippincott.

Carcio, H. A. (1985). *Manual of health assessment.* Boston: Little, Brown.

Carcio, H. A. (1998). *Management of the infertile woman.* Philadelphia: Lippincott-Raven.

Darney, P. D., Horbach, N. S., & Kom, A. P. (2005). *Protocols for office gynecologic surgery.* Cambridge: Blackwell Science.

Hogstel, M. O., & Curry, L. (2005). *Health assessment across the life span* (4th ed.). Philadelphia: FA Davis.

MacLaren, A. (1995). Primary care for women: Comprehensive sexual health assessment. *Journal of Nurse Midwifery, 40*(2), 104–119.

Scott, J. R., Gibbs, R. S. Karlan, B., & Haney, A. (Eds.). (2008). *Danforth's obstetrics and gynecology* (10th ed.). Philadelphia: Lippincott, Williams & Wilkins.

Williams, J. G., Paark, L. I., & Kline, J. (1992). Reducing distress associated with pelvic examination: A stimulus control intervention. *Women's Health, 18*(2), 41–45.

Chapter 5 Assessment of Vulvar Pain

Giglio, K., & Andrist, L. C. (2004). Understanding, diagnosing, and treating vulvodynia. *Women's Health Care: A Practical Journal for Nurse Practitioners, 3,* 24–30.

Glazer, H., Jantos, M., Martmann, E. H., & Swencionis, C. (1998). Electromyographic comparisons of the pelvic floor in women with dysesthetic vulvodynia and asymptomatic women. *Journal of Reproductive Medicine, 43,* 959–962.

Haefner, H. K., Collins, M. E., Davis, G. D., Edwards, L., Foster, D. C., Hartmann, E. D., et al. (2005).The vulvodynia guideline. *Journal of Lower Genital Tract Disea*se, *9,* 40–51.

Harlow, B. L., & Stewart, E. G. (2003). A population-based assessment of chronic unexplained vulvar pain: Have we underestimated the prevalence of vulvodynia? *Journal of the American Medical Women's Association, 58,* 82–88.

Jerzak, L. A., & Smith, S. K. (2006). Vulvodynia: Diagnosis and treatment of a chronic pain syndrome. *Women's Health Care: A Practical Journal for Nurse Practitioners, 5,* 29–32, 35–36, 41–42, 45–46.

Moyal-Barracco, M., & Lynch, P. J. (2004). 2003 ISSVD terminology and classification of vulvodynia: A historical perspective. *Journal of Reproductive Medicine, 49*(10), 772–777.

Oaklander, A. L. (1999). The pathology of pain. *Neuroscientist, 5,* 302–310.

Pascale, A. (2007). *The diagnosis and treatment of vulvovaginal complaints.* Presented at Nursing Conference at Harvard Vanguard Medical Associates, Boston.

Reed, B. D. (2006). Vulvodynia: Diagnosis and management. *American Family Physician, 73,* 1231–1239.

Reed, B. D., Gorenflo, D. W., & Haefner, H. K. (2003). Generalized vulvar dysesthesia vs. vestibulodynia. Are they distinct diagnoses? *Journal of Reproductive Medicine, 48,* 858–864.

Stewart, E. G. (2006, November). *Vulvar pain syndromes.* Presented at the New England Obstetric and Gynecology Society Annual Meeting, Boston.

Stewart, E. G., & Spencer, P. (2002). *The V book: A doctor's guide to complete vulvovaginal health.* New York: Bantam Books.

Zacur, H., Genadry, R., & Woodruff, J. D. (1980). The patient-at-risk for development of vulvar cancer. *Gynecology and Oncolology, 9,* 199.

Chapter 6 Assessment of the Female Breast

Bates, B. (2008). *A guide to physical examination and history taking* (8th ed.). Philadelphia: Lippincott.

Boyd, N. F., Guo, H., Martin, L. J., Sun, L., Stone, J., Fishell, E., et al. (2007). Mammographic density and the risk and detection of breast cancer. *New England Journal of Medicine, 356*(3), 227–236.

Casey, P. M., Cerhan, J. R., & Pruthi, S. (2008). Oral contraceptive use and risk of breast cancer. *Mayo Clinic Proceedings, 83*(1), 86–90.

Geiger, A. M., Thwin, S. S., Lash, T. L., Buist, D. S., Prout, M. N., Wei, F., et al. (2007). Recurrences and second primary breast cancers in older women with initial early-stage disease. *Cancer, 109*(5), 966–974.

Goldman, S. (1994). Evaluating breast masses. *Contemporary OB/GYN-NP, 1*(4), 76–94.

Mann, L. (1995). Physical examination of the augmented breast: Description of a displacement technique. *Obstetrics & Gynecology, 85*(2), 178–185.

Moss, S. M., Cuckle, H., Evans, A., Johns, L., Waller, M., & Bobrow, L. (2006). Effect of mammographic screening from age 40 years on breast cancer mortality at 10 years' follow-up: A randomised controlled trial. *Lancet, 368*(9552), 2053–2060.

Pennypacker, H. A. (1994). Achieving competence in clinical breast examination. *Nurse Practitioner Forum, 4*(2), 45–56.

Scott, J. R., Gibbs, R. S., Karlan, B., & Haney, A. (Eds.). (2008). *Danforth's obstetrics and gynecology* (10th ed., pp. 246–255, 291–292). Philadelphia: Lippincott, Williams & Wilkins.

Somkin, C. P. (1993). Improving the effectiveness of breast self-examination in the early detection of breast cancer: A selective review of the literature. *Nurse Practitioner Forum, 4*(2), 345–348.

Thompson, K. (2006). Evaluation and management of common breast complaints. *Female Patient, 31*, 28–38.

Chapter 7 Assessment of the Pregnant Woman

Centers for Disease Control and Prevention. (2006). *Sexually transmitted diseases treatment guidelines 2006.* Available at: www.cdc.gov/std/treatment/2006/toc

Gardiner, P. M. (2008). The clinical content of preconception care: Nutrition and dietary supplements. *American Journal of Obstetrics Gynecology, 199*(6 Suppl. 2), S345–S356.

Hobel, C. J. (1998, February). Routine antenatal laboratory tests and specific screening tests. *Contemporary OB/GYN,* pp. 25–34.

Klima, C., Norr, K., Vonderheid, S., & Handler, A. (2009). Introduction of centering pregnancy in a public health clinic. *Journal of Midwifery and Women's Health, 54*(1), 27–34.

Kriebs, J. (2009). Obesity as a complication of pregnancy and labor. *Journal of Perinatal and Neonatal Nursing, 23*(1), 15–22.

Parks, K., & Nouriani, M. (2006). *Frequently asked questions: Pregnancy tests.* Washington, DC: Office on Women's Health in the U.S. Department of Health and Human Services. Retrieved February 20, 2009, from http://www.4woman.gov/faq/pregnancy-tests.cfm#top

Schrag, et al. (2002). A population-based comparison of strategies to prevent early-onset Group B streptococcal disease in neonates. *New England Journal of Medicine, 347*(4), 233–239.

Scott, J. R., Gibbs, R. S., Karlan, B., & Haney, A. (Eds.). (2008). *Danforth's obstetrics and gynecology* (10th ed., pp. 246–255, 291–292). Philadelphia: Lippincott, Williams & Wilkins.

Chapter 8 Assessment and Clinical Evaluation of Obesity in Women

Center for Disease Control and Prevention. (n.d.). *National Health and Nutrition Examination Survey.* U.S. Department of Health and Human Services. Retrieved December 5, 2005, from http://www.cdc.gov/nchs/data/nhanes/databriefs/adultweight.pdf#search = 'National%20Health%20and%20Nutrition%20Examination%20Survey%20Weight%20gain'

Department of Health and Human Services. Center for Disease Control and Prevention. (n.d.). *Overweight and obesity: Defining overweight and obesity.* Re-

trieved December 5, 2005, from http://www.cdc.gov/nccdphp/dnpa/
    obesity/defining.htm
Hill, J. O., & Wyatt, H. (2002). Outpatient management of obesity: A primary
    care perspective. *Obesity Research, 10*(2), 124S–130S.
Jakicic, J. M. (2002). The role of physical activity in prevention and treatment of
    body weight gain in adults. *Journal of Nutrition* (Suppl.), 3826S–3829S.
Johnson, D. B., Gerstein, D. E., Evan, A. E., & Woodward-Lopez, G. (2002). Pre-
    venting obesity: A life cycle perspective. *Journal of the American Dietetic As-
    sociation, 106*(1), 97–102.
Klauer, J., & Aronne, L. (2002). Managing overweight and obesity in women.
    Clinical Obstetrics and Gynecology, 45, 1080–1088.
Kral, J. G. (2004). Preventing and treating obesity in girls and young women to
    curb the epidemic. *Obesity Research, 12*(10), 1539–1546.
Lyznicki, J. M., Young, D. C., Riggs, J. A., & Davis, R. M. (2001). Obesity: As-
    sessment and management in primary care. *American Family Physician, 63*,
    2185–2196.
National Center for Health Statistics. (2009). *Healthy People 2010 conference edi-
    tion.* Hyattsville, MD: Author. Available at: www.health.gov/healthypeople
National Research Council. (1989). *Recommended dietary allowances. Subcommit-
    tee on the Tenth Edition of the RDAs, Food Nutrition Board, Commission on
    Life Sciences* (10th ed.). Washington, DC: National Academy Press.
Ryan, D., & Stewart, T. (2004). Medical management of obesity in women: Of-
    fice-based approaches to weight mangement. *Clinical Obstetrics and Gynecol-
    ogy, 47*(4), 914–927.
WebMD. (n.d.). *Weight loss clinic, parenting & childhood obesity.* Retrieved De-
    cember 2, 2005, from http://www.weightlossmd.com/parenting_and_
    child_obesity.asp
Wing, R. R., & Hill, J. O. (2001). Successful weight loss maintenance. *Annual Re-
    view of Nutrition, 21*, 323–341.

Chapter 9 The Papanicolaou Smear

American Cancer Society. (2006). *Cancer facts and figures 2006.* Atlanta, GA:
    Author.
American Cancer Society. *Prevention and early detection. Pap test.* Retrieved
    March 24, 2009, from http://www.cancer.org/docroot/PED/content/
    PED_2_3X_Pap_Test.asp?sitearea = PED
American Cancer Society. (n.d.). Retrieved November, 12, 2009, from http://
    www.cancer.org/docroot/NWS/content/NWS_1_1x_Annual_Pap_Smears_
    May_Not_Be_Necessary.asp.
American Congress of Obstetricians and Gynecologists. (n.d.). Retrieved Novem-
    ber 12, 2009, from http://www.acog.org/
American Society for Colposcoy and Cervical Pathology (ASCCP). (n.d.). Re-
    trieved November 12, 2009 from http://www.ascccp.org
Castle, P. E. (2004). Beyond human papillomavirus: The cervix, exogeneous sec-
    ondary factors, and the development of cervical precancer and cancer. *Jour-
    nal of Lower Tract Genital Diseases, 8*, 224–230.

Center for Disease Control and Prevention. (n.d.). Retrieved November 12, 2009, from http://www.cdc.gov/cancer/hpv/

Fleischer, A. B., Parrish, C. A., Glenn, R., & Feldman, S. R. (2001). Condylomata acuminata (genital warts): Patient demographics and treating physicians. *Sexually Transmitted Diseases, 28*(11), 643–647.

Ho, G. F., Bierman, R., Beardsley, N. P., Chang, C. J., & Burk, R. D. (1998). Natural history of cervicovaginal papillomavirus infection in young women. *New England Journal of Medicine, 338*(7), 423–428.

Moscicki, A. B., Shiboski, S., Hills, N. K., Powell, K. J., Jay, N., Hanson, E. N., et al. (2004). Regression of low-grade squamous intraepithelial lesions in young women. *Lancet, 364,* 1678–1683.

National Cancer institute. (n.d.). Retrieved November 12, 2009 from http://seer.cancer.gov/statfacts/html/cervix.html.

Pinto, A. P., & Crum, C. P. (2000). Natural history of cervical neoplasia: Defining progression and its consequences. *Clinical Obstetrics and Gynecology, 43,* 352–362.

Thompson, D. W. (1993). *Adequate "Pap" smears: A guide for sampling techniques in screening for abnormalities.* Toronto, CAN: Laboratory Proficiency Testing Program.

Wartson, M., Saraiya, M., Bernard, V., Coughlin, S. S., Flowers, L. C., Collinides, V., et al. (2008). Burden of cervical cancer in the United States, 1998–2003. *Cancer, 113*(S10), 2855–2864.

Wright, T. C. (1995, March). Guidelines for colposcopic investigation of lower genital intraepithelial neoplasia. *Advances for Nurse Practitioners,* pp. 28–31.

Wright, T. C., Massad, S., Dunton, C. J., Spitzer, M., Wilkinson, E. J., & Solomon, D. (2007). 2006 consensus guidelines for the management of women with abnormal cervical cancer screening tests. *Journal of Lower Genital Tract Diseases, 11*(4), 2201–2222.

Chapter 10 Vaginal Microscopy

Agnew, K. J., & Hillier, S. L. (1995). The effect of treatment regimens for vaginitis and cervicitis on vaginal colonization by lactobacilli. *Sexually Transmitted Diseases, 22*(5), 269–273.

Centers for Disease Control and Prevention. (2008). *STD treatment guidelines.* Atlanta, GA: Author.

Cibley, L. J., & Cibley, L. J. (1991). Cytolytic vaginosis. *American Journal of Obstetrics and Gynecology, 165,* 1245–1249.

Horowitz, B. J. (2001). *Vaginitis and vaginosis: Recurrent and relapsing vaginitis.* New York: Wiley-Liss.

Horowitz, B. J., Mardh, P. E., & Nagy, E. (1994). Vaginal lactobacillosis. *American Journal of Obstetrics and Gynecology, 170,* 857–861.

Joesoef, M., & Schmid, G. (2003). Bacterial vaginosis. *Clinical Evidence, 10,* 1824–1833.

Kaufman, R. H., Frieddrich, E. G., & Gardner, H. L. (2004). *Benign diseases of the vulva and vagina* (5th ed.). Littleton, MA: Yearbook Medical Publishers.

Lowe, N. K., Neal, J. L., & Ryan-Wenger, N.A. (2009). Accuracy of the clinical diagnosis of vaginitis compared with a DNA probe laboratory standard. *Obstetrics & Gynecology, 113,* 89.

Raphaelidis, L., & Secor, R. M. (2006). Bacterial vaginosis update. *Women's Health Care, 5*(3), 21–29.

Secor, R. M. (Guest Editor). (1992). Vulvovaginitis: A comprehensive review (a series of articles). *Nurse Practitioner Forum, 3*(2).

Secor, R. M. (1994). Bacterial vaginosis: A common infection with serious sequelae. *Advances for Nurse Practitioner, 2*(4), 11–16.

Secor, R. M. (1997). Vaginal microscopy: Refining your technique. *Clinical Excellence for Nurse Practitioners, 1,* 29–34.

Sharp, H. C. (1993). Vulvovaginal conditions mimicking vaginitis. *Clinical Obstetrics and Gynecology, 36*(1), 129–135.

Sobel, J. D. (1994). Desquamative inflammatory vaginitis: A new subgroup of purulent vaginitis responsive to topical 2% clindamycin therapy. *American Journal of Obstetrics and Gynecology, 171,* 1215–1220.

STD/HIV Prevention Training Center of New England. (2002). *Online vaginal microscopy tutorial.* Jamaica Plane, MA: Available at: http://depts.washington. edu/nnptc/online_training/wet_preps_video.htm

Yudin, M. H. (2005). Bacterial vaginosis in pregnancy: Diagnosis, screening, and management. *Clinics in Perinatology, 32*(3), 617–627.

Chapter 11 Urinalysis

Darney, P. D., Horbach, N. S., & Kom, A. P. (2005). *Protocols for office gynecologic surgery* (pp. 245–263). Cambridge: Blackwell Science.

Scott, J. R., Gibbs, R. S., Karlan, B., & Haney, A. (Eds.). (2008). *Danforth's obstetrics and gynecology* (10th ed., pp. 334–339). Philadelphia: Lippincott, Williams & Wilkins.

Chapter 12 Sonohysteroscopy (Fluid Contrast Ultrasound)

Ashley, D. (1997). Sonohysterography in the office: Instruments and techniques. *Contemporary OB/GYN, 4,* 95–99.

Bradley, L. D., & Andrews, B. J. (1998). Saline infusion sonography for endometrial evaluation. *Female Patient, 123*(1), 12–25.

Breitkopf, D., Goldstein, S. R., & Seeds, J .W. (for the ACOG Committee on Gynecologic Practice). (2003). ACOG technology assessment in obstetrics and gynecology. Saline infusion sonohysterography. *Obstetrics & Gynecology, 102,* 659–662.

de Kroon, C. D., de Bock, G. H., Dieben, S. W., & Jansen, F. W. (2003). Saline contrast hysterosonography in abnormal uterine bleeding: A systematic review and meta-analysis. *British Journal of Obstetrics and Gynecology, 110,* 938–947.

Dijkhuizen, F. P., Mol, B.W., Bongers, M.Y., Brolmann, H. A., & Heintz, A, P. (2003). Cost-effectiveness of transvaginal sonography and saline infused sonography in the evaluation of menorrhagia. *International Journal of Gyneco-lology & Obstetrics, 83,* 45–52.

Mihm, L. M., Quick, V. A., Brumfield, J. A., Connors, A. F., Jr., & Finnerty, J. J. (2002). The accuracy of endometrial biopsy and saline sonohysterography in the determination of the cause of abnormal uterine bleeding. *American Journal of Obstetrics and Gynecology, 186,* 858–860.

Parsons, A. K., & Lense, J. J. (2003). Sonohysterography for endometrial abnormalities: Preliminary results. *Clinical Ultrasound, 21,* 87–95.

Rasmussen, F., Lindequiest, S., Larsen, C., & Justesen, P. (2001). Therapeutic effects of hysterosalpingograph: Oil versus water soluble contrast media—A randomized prospective study. *Radiology, 179,* 75–81.

Chapter 13 Bone Densitometry

"FRAX" Tool, Online tool to calculate risk of fracture. Available at: www.shef.ac.uk/frax/

National Osteoporosis Foundation. (2008). *Clinician's guide to prevention and treatment of osteoporosis* (p. 10). Washington, DC: Author.

North American Menopause Society. (2007). *Menopause practice: A clinician's guide* (3rd ed.). Philadelphia: Author.

Siris, E., & Delmas, P. (2008). Assessment of 10-year absolute fracture risk: A new paradigm with worldwide application. *Osteoporosis International, 19,* 383–384.

Szulc, P., & Delmas, P. (2008). Biochemical markers of bone turnover: Potential use in the investigation and management of postmenopausal osteoporosis. *Osteoporosis International, 19*(12), 1683–1704.

Wagner, E. H., Williams, C. A., Greenberg, R., Kleinbaum, D., Wolf, S. H., & Ibrahim, M. A. (2009). Simply ask them about their balance—Future fracture risk in a national cohort study of twins. *American Journal of Epidemiology, 169,* 143.

U.S. Department of Health and Human Services. (2004). *Bone health and osteoporosis: A report of the Surgeon General.* Rockville, MD: U.S. Department of Health and Human Services, Office of the Surgeon General,

Chapter 14 BRCA Testing

Goldman, S. (1994). Evaluating breast masses. *Contemporary OB/GYN-NP, 1*(4), 76–94.

Hall, J. M., Lee, M. K., & Newman, B. (2000). Linkage of early-onset familial breast cancer to chromosome 17q21. *Science, 250,* 1684–1689.

Hayes, D. (2007). Clinical practice. Follow-up of patients with early breast cancer. *New England Journal of Medicine, 356*(24), 2505–2513.

Ives, A., Saunders, C., Bulsara, M., & Semmens, J. (2007). Pregnancy after breast cancer: Population based study. *BMJ, 334*(7586), 194. Epub ahead of print, 2006 Dec 8.

Scott, R. J., Gibbs, R. S., Karlan, B., & Haney, A. (Eds.). (2008). *Danforth's obstetrics and gynecology* (10th ed., pp. 246–255, 291–292). Philadelphia: Lippincott, Williams & Wilkins.

Szabo, C. I., & King, M. C. (1995). Inherited breast and ovarian cancer. *Human Molecular Genetics, 4,* 1811–1817.

Wooster, R., Neuhausen, S. L., Mangion, J., Quick, Y., Ford, D., Collins, N., et al. (1994). Localization of a breast cancer susceptibility gene, BRCA-2, to chromosome 13ql2-13. *Science, 265,* 2088–2090.

Wooster, R., Bignell, G., Lancaster, J., Swit, S., Seal, S., Mangion, M. R., et al. (1995). Identification of the breast cancer susceptibility gene BRCA2. *Nature, 378*(6559), 789–792.

Zimmerman, V. L. (2002). BRCA gene mutations and cancer. *American Journal of Nursing, 102*(8), 28–36.

Chapter 15 The FemCap
Chapter 16 The Diaphragm

Archer, D. (2002). New contraceptive options. *Clinical Obstetrics and Gynecology, 44(*1), 122–126.

Cates, W. (1996). Contraceptive choice, sexually transmitted diseases, HIV infection and future fecundity. *Journal of the British Fertility Society, 1*(1), 18–22.

Chalker, R. (1987). *The complete cervical cap guide.* New York: Harper & Row.

FemCap prescribing information. FDA package insert is included with every device.

Gollub, E. L. (2000). The female condom: Tool for women's empowerment. *American Journal of Public Health, 90*(9), 1377–1381.

Hatcher, R. A., Trussell, J., Nelson, A. C., Cates, W., & Stewart, F. (2008). *Contraceptive technology* (19th ed.). New York: Ardent Media.

Mauck, C., Callahan, M., Weiner, D. H. & Dominik, R. (1999). A comparative study of the safety and efficacy of FemCap, a new vaginal barrier contraceptive, and the Ortho All-Flex diaphragm. The FemCap Investigators' Group. *Contraception, 60*(2), 71–80.

Moench, T. R., Chipato, T., & Padian, N. S. (2001). Preventing disease by protecting the cervix: The unexplored promise of internal vaginal barrier devices. *AIDS, 15*(13), 1595–1602.

Planned Parenthood Federation of America. (n.d.). *Diaphragms, caps, & shields.* Available at: http://www.plannedparenthood.org/pp2/portal/files/portal/medicalinfo/birthcontrol/pub-birth-control-13.xml

Shihata, A. (1998). The femcap: A new contraceptive choice. *European Journal of Contraceptive and Reproductive Health Care, 3,* 160–166.

Shihata, A. (2004). New FDA-approved woman-controlled, latex-free barrier contraceptive device: "FemCap." In D. Salim, D. R. Pierson, & J. Gumby (Eds.), *International Congress Series 12711* (pp. 303–306). Montreal, Quebec, Canada: Elsevier.

U.S. Food and Drug Administration. (n.d.). *Birth control guide.* Available at: http://www.fda.gov/fdac/features/1997/babyguide2.pdf

Chapter 17 The Intrauterine Contraception

American Heart Association. (n.d.). *New guidelines.* Available at http://circaha journals.org./cgi/reprint/CIRCULATIONAHA.106.183095

Bayer Healthcare. (2008). *Mirena product insert.* Bayer Healthcare.

Campbell, S., & Cropsey, K. (2007). Intrauterine device use in a high-risk population. *American Journal of Obstetrics, 197*(2), 193.

Grimes, D. A. (2000). Intrauterine device and upper-genital tract infection. *Lancet, 356*(9234), 1013–1019.

Inki, P. (2007). Long-term use of the levonorgestrel-releasing intrauterine device. *Contraception, 75*(6 Suppl.), S161–S166.

Peterson, H. B. (2005). Clinical practice. Long-acting methods of contraception. *New England Journal of Medi*cine, *353*(20), 2169–2175.

Shelton, J. D. (2001). Risk of clinical pelvic inflammatory disease attributable to an intrauterine device. *Lancet, 357*(9254), 443.

U.S. Food and Drug Administration. *New device approval: FemCap™-P020041.* Available at: http://www.fda.gov/MedicalDevices/ProductsandMedical Procedures/DeviceApprovalsandClearances/Recently-ApprovedDevices/ ucm082597.htm

Word Health Organization (WHO). (2009). *Medical eligibility criteria for contraceptive use, Update, 2009.* Available at: www.who.int/entity/reproductive health/topics/familyplanning/guidelines/en/ http://wnglibdoc.who.int/publications/2009/9789241563888

Chapter 18 Contraceptive Implants

Croxatto, H. B., & Minen, L. (1998). The pharmacodynamics and efficacy of Implanon. *Contraception, 58,* 91S–97S.

Croxatto, H. B., Urbancsek, J., Massai, R., Coelingh Bennink, H., & van Beek, A. (1998). A multicentre efficacy and safety study of the single contraceptive implant Implanon. Implanon Study Group. *Human Reproduction, 14,* 976–981.

Fu, H., Darroch, J. E., Haas, T., & Ranjit, N. (1998). Contraceptive failure rates: New estimates from the 1995 National Survey of Family Growth. *Family Planning Perspectives, 31,* 56–63.

Funk, S., Miller, M. M., Mishell, D. R., Jr., Archer, D. F., Poindexter, A., Schmidt, J., et al. (2005). Safety and efficacy of Implanon: A single-rod implantable contraceptive containing etonogestrel. *Contraception, 71,* 319–326.

Meckstroth, K., & Darney, P. D. (2002). Implantable contraception. *Obstetrics & Gynecology Clinics of North America, 27,* 781–815.

Organon. (2006). *Implanon* [package insert]. Roseland, NJ: Organon.

Sivin, I., Mishell, D. R., Jr., Darney, P., Wan, L., & Christ, M. (1998). Levonorgestrel capsule implants in the United States: A 5-year study. *Obstetrics & Gynecology, 92,* 337–344.

Chapter 19 The Sexual-Assault Victim

Mohler-Kuo, M., Dowdall, G. W., Koss, M. P., & Weshsler, H. (2004). Correlates of rape while intoxicated in a national sample of college women. *Journal of Studies on Alcohol, 65*(1), 37.

Resnick, H. S., Holmes, M. M., Kilpatrick, D. G., Clum, G., Acierno, R., Best, C. L., et al. (2000). Predictors of post rape medical care in a national sample of women. *American Journal of Preventative Medicine, 19*(4), 214–219.

Tjaden, P., & Thoennes, N. (2006). *Extent, nature, and consequences of rape victimization: Findings from the National Violence Against Women Survey.* Retrieved from www.ojp.usdoj.gov/nij

U.S. Department of Justice. (2004*). Bureau of Justice Statistics.* Retrieved May 7, 2005, from www.ojp.usdoj.gov/bjs

Workowski, K. A., & Berman, S. M. (2006). Sexually transmitted diseases guidelines, 2006. *Morbidity and Mortality Weekly Report.* Retrieved March 24, 2009, from http://www.cdc.gov/mmwr/preview/mmwrhtml/rr5511a1.htm

Chapter 20 Domestic Violence

Centers for Disease Control and Prevention. (2006). *Costs of intimate partner violence against women in the United States.* Atlanta, GA: CDC.

Family Violence Prevention Fund. (2004). *National Consensus Guidelines on identifying and responding to domestic violence victimization in health care settings.* Available at: http://endabuse.org/programs/healthcare/files/Consensus.pdf

Gerber, M. R., Lichter, E., Williams, C. M., McCloskey, L. A., et al. (2005). Adverse health behaviors and the detection of partner violence by clinicians. *Archives of Internal Medicine, 165*(9), 1016–1021.

Janssen, P. A. Holt, V. L., Sugg, N. K., Emanuel, I., Critchlow, C. M., & Henderson, A. D. (2003). Intimate partner violence and adverse pregnancy outcomes: A population-based study. *American Journal of Obstetrics and Gynecology, 188*(5), 1341–1347.

King, M. C., & Ryan, J. (1989). Abused women: Dispelling myths and encouraging intervention. *Nurse Practitioner, 14*(5), 47–58.

Lawson, D. M. (2003). Incidence, explanations, and treatment of partner violence. *Journal of Counseling and Development, 81*(1), 19–32.

National Center for Injury Prevention and Control. Retrieved May 22, 2006, from http://www.cdc.gov/violenceprevention/pdf/IPV-factsheet.pdf

Ryan, J., & King, M. C. (1997). Child witnesses of domestic violence. *Clinical Excellence for Nurse Practitioners, 1*(1), 47–57.

Chapter 22 Assessment of Menopausal Status

Bachmann, G. A., & Nevadunsky, N. S. (2000). Diagnosis and treatment of atrophic vaginitis. *American Family Physician, 61,* 3090–3096.

Carcio, H. A. (2009). Urogenital atrophy: A new approach to vaginitis diagnosis. *Advance for Nurse Practitioners, 10*(10), 40–47.

Cardozo, L., Bachmann, G., McClish, D., Fonda, D., & Birgerson, L. (1998). Meta-analysis of estrogen therapy in the management of urogenital atrophy in postmenopausal women: Second report of the hormones and urogenital therapy committee. *Obstetrics and Gynecology, 92,* 722–777.

Notelovitz, M. (2000). Urogenital atrophy and low-dose vaginal estrogen therapy (editorial). *Menopause, 7*, 140–142.
Pandit, L., & Ouslander, J. G. (1997). Postmenopausal vaginal atrophy and atrophic vaginitis. *American Journal of Medical Science, 314*, 228–231.

Chapter 23 Atrophic Vaginitis

Bachmann, G. A., & Nevadunsky, N. S. (2000). Diagnosis and treatment of atrophic vaginitis. *American Family Physician, 61*, 3090–3096.
Carcio, H . A. (1999). The maturation index. In *Advanced health assessment of women* (Vol. 12, pp. 226–228). Baltimore, MD: Lippincott.
Carcio, H. A. (2009). Urogenital atrophy: A new approach to vaginitis diagnosis. *Advance for Nurse Practitioners, 10*(10), 40–47.
Cardozo, L., Bachmann, G., McClish, D., Fonda, D., & Birgerson, L. (1998). Meta-analysis of estrogen therapy in the management of urogenital atrophy in postmenopausal women: Second report of the hormones and urogenital therapy committee. *Obstetrics and Gynecology, 92*, 722–777.
Notelovitz, M. (2000). Urogenital atrophy and low-dose vaginal estrogen therapy (editorial). *Menopause, 7*, 140–142.
Pandit, L., & Ouslander, J. G. (1997). Postmenopausal vaginal atrophy and atrophic vaginitis. *American Journal of Medical Science, 314*, 228–231.

Chapter 24 Pelvic Organ Prolapse

Carcio, H. A. (2008). Detour around surgery: Tuck and tone to treat pelvic organ prolapse. *ADVANCE for Nurse Practitioners, 12*(10), 61–64.
Davila, G. W. (1996). Vaginal prolapse: Management with nonsurgical techniques. *Postgraduate Medicine, 99*(4), 171–185.
Garely, A. (2001). Managing urinary incontinence: An expanding role for Ob/Gyns. *OBG Management, 13*(12), 26–33.
McIntosh, L. (2005). The role of the nurse in the use of the vaginal pessaries to treat pelvic organ prolapse and urinary incontinence: A literature review. *Urological Nursing, 25*(1), 41–48.
Poma, P. A. (2000). Nonsurgical management of genital prolapse: A review and recommendations for clinical practice. *Journal of Reproductive Medicine, 45*(10), 789–797.
Prietto, N. M., Luber, K., & Nager, C. W. (2003). Simple yet thorough office evaluation of pelvic floor disorders. *OBG Management, 15*(5), 80–95.
Schulz, J. A. (2001). Assessing and treating pelvic organ prolapse. *Ostomy/Wound Management, 47*(5), 54–59.

Chapter 25 Urinary Incontinence

Abrams, P., Cardozo, L., Fall, M., Griffiths, D., Rosier, P., Ulmsten, U., et al. (2003). The standardization of terminology in lower urinary tract function: Report from the standardization subcommittee of the International Continence Society. *Urology, 61*(1), 37–49.

Burgio, K. L. (2004). Behavioral treatment options for urinary incontinence. *Gastroenterology, 126*(1, Suppl. 1), 82S–89S.

Burgio, K. L., & Locher, J. L. (1998). Behavioral vs drug treatment for urge urinary incontinence in older women: A randomized controlled trial. *Journal of the American Medical Association, 280*(23), 1995–2000.

Carcio, H. A. (2003). Comprehensive continence care. *ADVANCE for Nurse Practitioners, 12*(10), 26–35.

Carcio, H. A. (2004). The vaginal pessary. An effective yet underused tool for incontinence and prolapse. *ADVANCE for Nurse Practitioners, 12*(10), 47–48, 50, 52–54, 56.

Carcio, H. A. (2004). Mixed signals: Treating overlapping symptoms of urinary incontinence. *ADVANCE for Nurse Practitioners, 12*(10), 32–36.

Carcio, H. A. (2005). Urodynamic testing: A reliable indocator of urinary dysfunction. *ADVANCE for Nurse Practitioners, 13*(10), 45–49.

Kegel, A. H. (1948). Progressive resistance exercise in the functional restoration of the perineal muscle. *American Journal of Obstetrics and Gynecology, 56,* 238–249.

Lukban, J., & Whitmore, K. (2002). Pelvic floor muscle re-education treatment of the overactive bladder and painful bladder syndrome, *Clinics in Obstetrics and Gynecology, 45*(1), 273–285.

Mahoney, C. (2002). Estrogen and recurrent UTI in postmenopausal women. *American Journal of Nursing, 102*(8), 44–52.

Ouslander, J. G. (2004). Management of overactive bladder. *New England Journal of Medicine, 35*(8), 786–799.

Parsons, C. L. (2002). Interstitial cystitis: Epidemiology and clinical presentation. *Clinical Obstetrics and Gynecology, 45*(1), 242–249.

Resnick, N. M., & Griffiths, D. J. E. (2003). Expanding treatment options for stress urinary incontinence in women. *Journal of the American Medical Association, 290*(3), 395–397.

Samselle, C. M. (2000). Behavioral interventions for urinary incontinence in women: Evidence for practice. *Journal of Midwifery and Women's Health, 45*(2), 94–103.

Chapter 26 Initial Evaluation of Infertility

American College of Obstetricians and Gynecologists. (2002). ACOG Practice Bulletin. Clinical management guidelines for obstetrician-gynecologists, number 34, February 2002. Management of infertility caused by ovulatory dysfunction. *Obstetrics & Gynecology, 99*(2), 347–358.

American Society for Reproductive Medicine and Society for Reproductive Endocrinology and Infertility. (2002). *Information on commonly asked questions about genetic evaluation and counseling for infertile couples. Practice Committee Report.* Birmingham, AL: Author.

Carcio, H. A. (1998). *Management of the infertile woman.* Philadelphia: Lippincott-Raven.

Miller, P. B., & Soules, M. R. (1996). The usefulness of LH kit for ovulation prediction during menstrual cycles of normal women. *Fertility and Sterility, 87*(1), 45–48.

Practice Committee of the American Society for Reproductive Medicine. (2004). Optimal evaluation of the infertile female. *Fertility and Sterility, 82*(Suppl. 1), S169–S172.

Smith, S., Pfeifer, S. M., & Collins, J. A. (2003). Diagnosis and management of female infertility. *Journal of the American Medical Association, 290*(13), 1767–1770.

Scott, R. T., & Hoffman, G. E. (1995). Prognostic assessment of ovarian reserve. *Fertility and Sterility, 63,* 1–12.

Speroff, L., Glass, R. H., & Kase, N. G. (2005). *Clinical gynecologic endocrinology and infertility* (10th ed.). Baltimore: Williams & Wilkins.

Chapter 27 The Postcoital Test

Bush, M. R., Walmer, D. K., Couchman, G. M., & Haney, A. F. (1997). Evaluation of the postcoital test in cycles involving exogenous gonadotropins. *Obstetrics and Gynecology, 89,* 45–52.

Carcio, H. A. (1998). *Management of the infertile woman.* Philadelphia: Lippincott-Raven.

Glatstein, I. Z., Harlow, B. L., & Hornstein, M. D. (1997). Practice patterns among reproductive endocrinologists: The infertility evaluation. *Fertility and Sterility, 67,* 443–450.

Speroff, L., Glass, R. H., & Kase, N. G. (2004). *Clinical gynecologic endocrinology and infertility* (5th ed.). Baltimore: Williams & Wilkins.

Chapter 28 Evaluation of the Candidate for Intrauterine Insemination

Lobo, R. A. (2007). Infertility: Etiology, diagnostic evaluation, management, prognosis. In V. L. Katz, R. A. Lobo, G. Lentz, & D. Gershenson (Eds.), *Comprehensive gynecology* (5th ed., pp. 1001–1037). Philadelphia: Mosby.

Speroff, L., & Fritz, M. A. (2005). Female infertility. In *Clinical gynecologic endocrinology and infertility* (7th ed., pp. 1013–1067). Philadelphia: Lippincott Williams and Wilkins.

Stanford, J. B., White, G. L., & Hatasaka, H. (2002). Timing intercourse to achieve pregnancy: Current evidence. *Obstetrics and Gynecology, 100*(6), 1333–1341.

Wilcox, A. J., Weinberg, C. R., & Baird, D. D. (2000). The timing of the "fertile window" in the menstrual cycle: Day-specific estimates from a prospective study. *BMJ, 321*(7271), 1259–1262.

Chapter 29 Sperm-Washing Technique
Chapter 30 Intrauterine Insemination Procedure

Carcio, H. A. (1998). *Management of the infertile woman.* Philadelphia: Lippincott-Raven.

Fanchin, R., Olivennes, F., Righini, C., Hazout, A., Schwab, B., & Frydman, R. (1995). A new system for fallopian tube sperm perfusion leads to pregnancy rates twice as high as standard intrauterine insemination. *Fertility and Sterility, 64,* 505–510.

Karabinus, D. S., & Gelety, T. J. (1997). The impact of sperm morphology evaluated by strict criteria on intrauterine insemination success. *Fertility and Sterility, 67,* 536–542.

Kerin, J., & Quin, P. (1987). Washed intrauterine insemination in the treatment of oligospermic infertility. *Seminars in Reproductive Endocrinology, 5,* 430–438.

Qasim, S. M., & Trias, A. (1996). Does the absence or presence of seminal fluid matter in patient undergoing ovulation induction with intrauterine insemination? *Human Reproduction, 11,* 1008–1010.

Ransomi, M. X., Blotner, M. B., Bohrer, M., Corsan, G., & Kemmann, E. (1994). Does increasing frequency of intrauterine insemination improve pregnancy rates significantly during superovulation cycles? *Fertility and Sterility, 62,* 303–306.

Speroff, L. L. (1990). Who benefits from intrauterine insemination with washed sperm? *Contemporary OB/GYN, 34,* 65–69.

Van Voorhis, B. J., Sparks, A. E., Allen, B. D., Stovall, D. W., Syrop, C. H., & Chapler, F. K. (1997). Cost effectiveness of infertility treatments: A cohort study. *Fertility and Sterility, 67,* 830–836.

Chapter 31 Donor Insemination

American Fertility Society. (1993). Guidelines for therapeutic donor insemination: Sperm. *Fertility and Sterility, 59,* 1S–4S.

Bordson, B. L., Ricci, E., Dickey, R. P., Dunaway, H., Taylor, S. N., & Curole, D. N. (1986). Comparison of intracervical, intrauterine, and intratubal techniques for donor insemination. *Fertility and Sterility, 59,* 339–342.

Carcio, H. A. (1998) *Management of the infertile woman.* Philadelphia: Lippincott-Raven.

Kang, B. M., & Wu, T. C. (2006). Effect of age on intrauterine insemination with frozen donor sperm. *Obstetrics and Gynecology, 88,* 93–98.

Klock, S. C. (1993). Psychological aspects of donor insemination. *Infertility and Reproductive Medicine Clinics of North America, 4,* 455–469.

Speroff, L., & Fitz, M. (2005). *Clinical gynecologic endocrinology and infertility* (7th ed., pp. 435–437). Philadelphia: Lippincott Williams & Wilkins.

Stenchever, A. (2001). *Comprehensive gynecology* (4th ed., pp. 1204–1206). St. Louis: Mosby.

Wainer, R., Bailly, M., Merlet, F., Tribalat, S., Ducat, B., & Lombroso, A. (1995). Prospective randomized comparison of intrauterine and intracervical insemination with donor spermatozoa. *Human Reproduction, 10,* 2919–2922.

Chapter 32 Vulvar Cancer and Biopsy

Cunningham, F., Kenneth, L., Leveno, S. L., Bloom, J. C., & Hauth, C. (2005). *Williams obstetrics* (22nd ed.). Norwalk, CT: Appleton & Lange.

Darney, P. D., Horbach, N. S., & Kom, A. P. (2005). *Protocols for office gyneco-logic surgery.* Cambridge, UK: Blackwell Science.

Kaufman, R. (1997). Vulvar examination and biopsy. In M. J. Evans, M. P. John-son, & K. S. Moghissi (Eds.), *Invasive outpatient procedures in reproductive medicine* (pp. 143–149). Philadelphia: Lippincott.

Pascale, A. (2007, November). *The diagnosis and treatment of vulvovaginal com-plaints.* Paper presented at Nursing Conference at Harvard Vanguard Medi-cal Associates, Boston.

Reed, B. D. (2006). Vulvodynia: Diagnosis and management. *American Family Physician, 73,* 1231–1239.

Shehnaz, K. H., Madeleine, M. M., Johnson, L. G., Du, Q., Malkki, M., Wilker-son, H.-W., et al. (1997). Risk factors for vulvar cancer. *Journal of the Na-tional Cancer Institute, 89,* 1516–1523.

Wilkinson, E. J., & Stone, I. K. (1995). *Atlas of vulvar disease.* Baltimore: Wil-liams & Wilkins.

Chapter 33 Endometrial Biopsy

Bremer, C. (1992). Endometrial biopsy. *Female Patient, 17*(10), 15–28.

Clark, T. J., Mann, C. H., Shah, N., Khan, K. S., Song, F., & Gupta, J. K. (2002). Accuracy of outpatient endometrial biopsy in the diagnosis of endometrial cancer: A systematic quantitative review. *British Journal of Obstetrics and Gynecology, 109,* 313–321.

Mihm, L. M., Quick, V. A., Brumfield, J. A., Connors, A. F., Jr., & Finnerty, J. J. (2002). The accuracy of endometrial biopsy and saline sonohysterography in the determination of the cause of abnormal uterine bleeding. *American Jour-nal of Obstetrics and Gynecology, 186,* 858–860.

Rosenburgh, D. L., Chudow, S., & Bronson, R. A. (1996). Diagnosis of luteal phase inadequacy. *Obstetrics and Gynecology, 1088,* 435.

Chapter 34 Acrochordonectomy

Strother, G. D. (1998). Acrochordonectomy made easy. *Clinician Reviews, 8*(3), 75–83.

Chapter 35 Polypectomy

Darney, P. D., Horbach, N. S., & Kom, A. P. (2005). *Protocols for office gyneco-logic surgery.* Cambridge, UK: Blackwell Science.

Chapter 37 The Simple Cystometrogram

Carcio, H. A. (2005) Urodynamic testing: A reliable indicator of urinary dysfunc-tion. *ADVANCE for Nurse Practitioners, 13*(10), 45–49.

Carcio, H. A. (2007). Mixed signals: Treating overlapping symptoms of urinary incontinence. *ADVANCE for Nurse Practitioners, 12*(10), 32–36.

Ouslander, J. G., Abelson, S., Staskin, D. R., & Blaustein, J. (1989). Simplified tests of lower urinary tract function in the evaluation of geriatric urinary in-continence. *Journal of the American Geriatrics Society, 37*(8), 706–714.

Index

559